Mosby's  of

Dermatology

Commissioning Editor: Timothy Horne
Development Editor: Barbara Simmons
Project Manager: David Fleming, Christine Johnston
Design Direction: George Ajayi

Mosby's Color Atlas and Text of

Dermatology

Robin Graham-Brown BSC MB FRCP
Consultant Dermatologist
Leicester Royal Infirmary
and
Honorary Senior Lecturer in Dermatology
University of Leicester, School of Medicine,
Leicester, UK

Johnny Bourke MD FRCP
Consultant Dermatologist
South Infirmary – Victoria Hospital, Cork
and
University College, Cork
Republic of Ireland

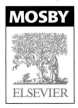

MOSBY

ELSEVIER

EDINBURGH   LONDON   NEW YORK   OXFORD   PHILADELPHIA
ST LOUIS   SYDNEY   TORONTO 2007

© 2007, Elsevier Limited. All rights reserved.

The rights of Dr Robin Graham-Brown and Dr Johnny Bourke to be identified as authors of this work has been asserted by them in accordance with the Copyright, Designs and Patents Act 1988.

No part of this publication may be reproduced, stored in a retrieval system, or transmitted in any form or by any means, electronic, mechanical, photocopying, recording or otherwise, without the prior permission of the Publishers. Permissions may be sought directly from Elsevier's Health Sciences Rights Department, 1600 John F. Kennedy Boulevard, Suite 1800, Philadelphia, PA 19103-2899, USA: phone: (+1) 215 239 3804; fax: (+1) 215 239 3805; or, e-mail: *healthpermissions@elsevier.com*. You may also complete your request on-line via the Elsevier homepage (http://www.elsevier.com), by selecting 'Support and contact' and then 'Copyright and Permission'.

First edition 2002
Second edition 2007

ISBN-10: 07234 3364X
ISBN-13: 978 07234 33644

British Library Cataloguing in Publication Data
A catalogue record for this book is available from the British Library

Library of Congress Cataloging in Publication Data
A catalog record for this book is available from the Library of Congress

Note
Knowledge and best practice in this field are constantly changing. As new research and experience broaden our knowledge, changes in practice, treatment and drug therapy may become necessary or appropriate. Readers are advised to check the most current information provided (i) on procedures featured or (ii) by the manufacturer of each product to be administered, to verify the recommended dose or formula, the method and duration of administration, and contraindications. It is the responsibility of the practitioner, relying on their own experience and knowledge of the patient, to make diagnoses, to determine dosages and the best treatment for each individual patient, and to take all appropriate safety precautions. To the fullest extent of the law, neither the Publisher nor the Authors assumes any liability for any injury and/or damage to persons or property arising out or related to any use of the material contained in this book.

The Publisher

Working together to grow
libraries in developing countries

www.elsevier.com | www.bookaid.org | www.sabre.org

ELSEVIER   BOOK AID
International   Sabre Foundation

your source for books,
journals and multimedia
in the health sciences
www.elsevierhealth.com

The
publisher's
policy is to use
**paper manufactured
from sustainable forests**

Printed in Italy

Contents

Preface and User Guide

Clinical medicine is all about patients, their problems and (sometimes) solutions. It is primarily about making diagnoses and thereby gaining access to the aetiological, pathological, prognostic and practical information that a diagnosis yields. Dermatology provides uniquely rich and diverse diagnostic challenges. It is more important, when studying dermatology than any other specialty, to start seeing patients and learning from them; from their symptoms, their signs and from the issues they raise, under the guidance of experienced clinical teachers. In preparing this book, we were both aware of our need, particularly in the early days, for a reasonably comprehensive atlas with appropriate text to complement our clinical exposure.

We therefore hope that by looking, listening, reading and asking (always with an open mind), younger doctors will find their way to becoming accomplished dermatologists, because that is what the patients need.

We further hope that, in some small way, this book will help in that process.

Robin Graham-Brown
Johnny Bourke

This book contains three different types of boxes:

Key points appear in yellow.

Clinical features appear in blue.

Definitions appear in pink.

Dedication

This book is dedicated to Margaret and Jenni, whose forbearance allowed us to put it together.

Acknowledgements

We are grateful to Timothy Horne who placed his confidence in us and to Barbara Simmons and the team at Elsevier who saw the project through with amazing patience and good humour. We could not have completed this task either without the assistance of Beverly Booker, who has for some years been a jealous guardian of clinical photographs, the Department of Medical Illustration at the Leicester Royal Infirmary, nor that of Joan McGowan whose unswerving support has kept us sane.

Robin Graham-Brown
Johnny Bourke

chapter 1

The Structure and Function of the Skin

INTRODUCTION

The skin is as complex (and, if you spend a little time reading about it, as interesting) as any other organ. It is also, by weight and by surface area, the single largest organ in the body. Without it we would be in a sorry (and highly temporary) state!

THE MICROSTRUCTURE OF THE SKIN

The skin is conventionally divided into several layers (**Fig. 1.1**).

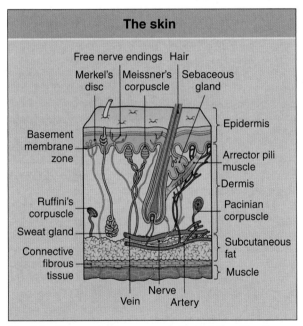

Fig. 1.1 *Diagrammatic representation of the skin:* the epidermis and its appendages, the basement membrane zone, the dermis, the subcutis.

THE EPIDERMIS

The epidermis is composed of four major cell types: keratinocytes, Langerhans' cells, melanocytes, and Merkel cells.

Box 1.1 Layers of the skin

Epidermis
The cellular external layer composed mostly of keratinocytes, but also containing melanocytes, Langerhans' cells, and Merkel cells.
Basement membrane zone
The thin layer that provides adhesion between the epidermis and the dermis.
Dermis
The area of connective tissue between the epidermis and the underlying fat; also contains blood vessels, nerves, and other specialized structures.
Subcutis
The layer beneath the dermis, whose name implies that it is not properly part of the skin — this distinction is somewhat pedantic however, since all these components function as an integrated whole.

Keratinocytes

Keratinocytes (**Fig. 1.2a**) are the major building blocks of the epidermis. They differentiate from actively dividing basal cells to become anucleate plates of keratin (horny cells or corneocytes), which are then shed.

The basal cells are anchored to the basement membrane by hemidesmosomes (*see* basement membrane zone on page 5). Each basal cell divides every 4 days or so to produce more basal cells, some of which undergo a process of maturation and differentiation.

The process of differentiation involves two transitional phases, recognized as producing the spinous (prickle cell) layer and the granular cell layer respectively. The spinous cells are interlocked and held together by a network of desmosomes, themselves stabilized within the cells by tonofilaments. It is during this period in the keratinocyte's life that keratin is formed within the cell, as keratohyaline granules, and that the cell nuclei disintegrate (**Fig. 1.2, b and c**).

Keratins are a group of fibrous proteins found in skin, hair, nails, claws, hooves, horns, feathers, and other integumental structures of birds and mammals. The word keratin derives from the Greek keras, which means horn (hence rhino-keras = rhinoceros = 'nose-horn'). Keratins are also found in all epithelial cells, forming a major part of the cytoskeleton. In human epidermal cells, keratin bundles are synthesized within the keratinocytes from basic amino acids, using a high proportion of cysteine (particularly in hair and nails). This allows for disulphide-bond cross-linking and gives added strength, with keratin bound into an insoluble proteinaceous complex with loricrin and a number of other proteins by the enzyme transglutaminase 1.

A thin film of lipid is also manufactured within these layers, in specialized organelles known as Odland bodies or membrane-coating granules. This film coats the surface of the keratinocytes in the outer layers of the epidermis, providing a degree of cohesion and waterproofing. Lipid represents approximately 10% of the stratum corneum by weight.

The epithelial keratinocyte 'transit' time, from the beginning of normal differentiation to the final shedding from the surface, is in the order of 50–70 days.

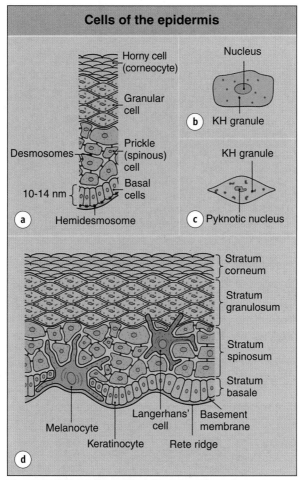

Cells of the epidermis

(a) Horny cell (corneocyte); Granular cell; Desmosomes; Prickle (spinous) cell; Basal cells; 10-14 nm; Hemidesmosome

(b) Nucleus; KH granule

(c) KH granule; Pyknotic nucleus

(d) Stratum corneum; Stratum granulosum; Stratum spinosum; Stratum basale; Melanocyte; Keratinocyte; Langerhans' cell; Basement membrane; Rete ridge

Fig. 1.2 *Cells of the epidermis: (a)* epidermal keratinocytes — differentiation involves four phases to produce the flat, protective cells of the stratum corneum; the time taken from differentiation of the basal cell to shedding of the horny cell is approximately 28 days; *(b)* epidermal keratinocytes — keratohyaline (KH) granules begin to appear in the cytoplasm of the spinous (prickle) cells; *(c)* epidermal keratinocytes — keratinohyaline (KH) granules have become larger and the cell's nucleus has begun to disintegrate; *(d)* melanocytes and Langerhans' cells interdigitate with the keratinocytes.

Langerhans' cells

Langerhans' cells (**Fig. 1.2d**) are antigen-presenting cells found in the prickle cell layer of the epidermis and represent one arm of the body's immune system.

3

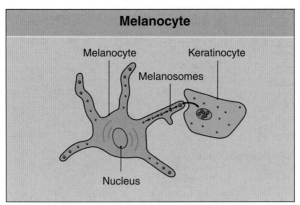

Fig. 1.3 *Melanocytes produce melanin and transport it, in melanosomes, to the neighbouring epidermal keratinocytes.*

Melanocytes

Melanocytes (**Fig. 1.3**) are large cells that are interspersed among the keratinocytes along the basement membrane at a rate of approximately one melanocyte per 10 basal cells. Melanocytes produce the pigment melanin. This is manufactured from the amino acid tyrosine, packaged into melanosomes, and then transported and delivered into the cytoplasm of surrounding keratinocytes (*see* **Fig. 1.3**). Thus, most of the cutaneous melanin is contained within keratinocytes. The reason for this is discussed on page 11. The degree to which the epidermis is

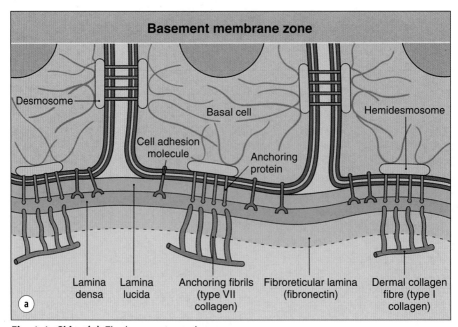

Fig. 1.4 *Skin. (a) The basement membrane zone.*

The constituent parts of the basement membrane zone

The base of the keratinocyte basal cell, containing hemidesmosomes.

A clear zone crossed by a fine network of anchoring filaments – the lamina lucida (largely composed of the structural protein laminin).

An electron dense band – the lamina densa (largely composed of type IV collagen).

The reticular lamina and its anchoring fibrils (collagen VII).

Fig. 1.4 *Skin. (b) The constituent parts of the basement membrane zone.*

melanized is under both genetic control and environmental stimulation (especially by ultraviolet radiation). Some individuals also produce a reddish pigment known as phaeomelanin.

Merkel cells

Merkel cells, although present in only very small numbers, are thought to represent specialized nerve endings within the epidermis.

THE BASEMENT MEMBRANE ZONE

The basement membrane zone (**Fig. 1.4**) is the narrow, but multilayered, structure lying between the epidermis and the dermis and supplies the cohesion between these two layers. This cohesion may be damaged by genetic defects in the proteins involved (as in some forms of epidermolysis bullosa — *see* Chapter 7) or by acquired disease processes, such as bullous pemphigoid (also covered in Chapter 7). A further degree of stability is provided by the corrugations of the basement membrane zone, in which the rete ridges of the epidermis interdigitate with dermal papillae. This occurs less often with age.

Box 1.2 Main constituents of the dermis

Fibroblasts
Spindle-shaped cells that manufacture the collagen and elastin.

Mast cells
Contain granules of vasoactive chemicals (notably histamine — *see* also urticaria in Chapter 5) and are involved in moderating immune and inflammatory responses in the skin.

Tissue macrophages
Phagocytic cells derived from blood monocytes important in immune defense.

Blood vessels
Blood supply at cellular level including small arterioles, capillaries, venules, and cutaneous lymphatics.

Nerve bundles and sensory receptors
These include nerve endings that detect pain, itch, temperature, touch and vibration.

Epidermal appendageal structures
These include hair follicles and their sebaceous glands, the eccrine and apocrine sweat glands and the nails.

THE DERMIS

The dermis is a layer, of varying thickness, between the epidermis and subcutaneous fat. The main component of the dermis is an interlacing network of connective tissue, largely made up of the protein collagen but also containing some elastin, all embedded in a matrix of mucopolysaccharides. Scattered among this are several types of cells and specialized structures.

The collagens are a family of vital structural proteins, forming a major part of the basement membrane, dermis, blood vessels, bone, cartilage, tendons, and ligaments. In the skin, collagen is manufactured by fibroblasts. The skin contains several types of collagen, the production of which is controlled by different genes: types I and III are found in the dermis; types IV and VII in the basement membrane zone; type VIII in blood vessels.

THE SUBCUTIS

The subcutis is the tissue immediately below the dermis, although in certain sites (e.g. the scrotum) the skin lies directly on muscle. It consists largely of fat traversed by nerves and blood vessels.

APPENDAGEAL STRUCTURES

It is conventional to consider three important components of the skin as 'appendages' of the epidermis: hair follicles and their sebaceous glands; the eccrine and apocrine sweat glands; and the nails. All lie within the dermis or the subcutis, but connect with the surface.

Hair follicles and sebaceous glands (or pilosebaceous units)

Almost the whole skin surface is punctuated by invaginations of the epidermis, out of which emerge the keratinized tubes we call hairs (**Fig. 1.5**). There are three types of hair seen in humans: terminal, vellus, and lanugo.

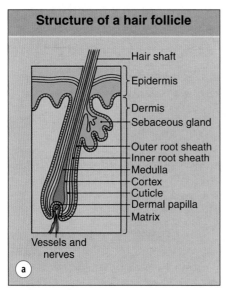

Structure of a hair follicle

Hair shaft
Epidermis
Dermis
Sebaceous gland
Outer root sheath
Inner root sheath
Medulla
Cortex
Cuticle
Dermal papilla
Matrix
Vessels and nerves

(a)

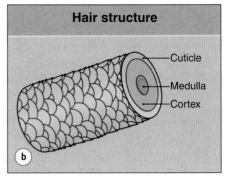

Hair structure

Cuticle
Medulla
Cortex

(b)

Fig. 1.5 *Hair: (a) the pilosebaceous unit, consisting of a hair follicle and its attached sebaceous gland; (b) a hair shaft in cross-section.*

Box 1.3 Hair classification and distribution

Terminal
Scalp, eyebrows, eyelashes, beard, axillae, pubic.
Vellus
The finer, downy hair that covers most of the rest of the body except the palms and soles.
Lanugo
The hair present *in utero*, but shed in early childhood.

Each area of the body has its own genetically determined pattern of hair, and there are variations between individuals, between families, and between ethnic groups. For example, it is obvious that some men have much more body hair than others, which may be a familial trait, and that some races (e.g. the North-European 'Norsemen') have much stronger and thicker beard growth than others (e.g. the Chinese and Afro-Caribbeans). There are well over 100 000 hairs on the average fully covered scalp. Genetic factors, combined with hormonal influences, also determine the increase in hairiness at or around puberty, throughout much of adult life, and at the menopause, as well as the apparently paradoxical loss of terminal hairs on the scalp, known as common, pattern, or androgenetic alopecia (*see* Chapter 9).

Each group of hairs has its own predetermined growth cycle: hairs grow for a set period of time. This is much longer in scalp hair (3 years plus), which can grow to the mid-back or beyond if left, than in pubic or eyebrow hair (a few months). This active growing phase is called anagen. Eventually, all hairs cease active growth and move into a resting phase known as catagen.

Finally, each resting hair is shed, during a phase known as telogen, following which a new hair normally develops. This process is not synchronized in humans, whereas in many animals it is the cause of the annual moult and coat change. Alterations to this cycle do occur from time to time and may be the cause of significant hair loss (*see* Chapter 9).

The hair follicles are set at an angle into the dermis, with the germinal portion, or bulb, sitting deep down on a modified dermal papilla, just above or in the subcutaneous fat. The bulb contains a group of cells that divide and differentiate to produce the early hair shaft. These cells gradually keratinize as the shaft matures and grows towards the mouth of the follicle. Ultimately, the hair shaft consists of tubular layers (**Fig. 1.5b**):
- The cortex, which is more or less equivalent to the prickle cell layer of the epidermis, but within which keratinization is further advanced.
- The cuticle, a layer of overlapping keratinized plates.
- The medulla, present in terminal hairs, which is a central core in which air is incorporated into the cells.

The main constituent of the hair shaft is keratin, which is especially rich in sulphur-containing amino acids.

Hair is not found everywhere on the body surface. The lips, palms and soles are hairless (glabrous). The palms and soles are interestingly characterized by remarkable whorled ridge and furrow patterns known as dermatoglyphics (**Fig. 1.6**). These are, as every schoolboy sleuth knows, unique to each human.

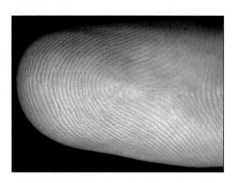

Fig. 1.6 *Dermatoglyphics* (*fingerprints*) — *unique to each individual.*

Each hair bulb also contains melanocytes, which produce pigment. Pigmentation is discussed on pages 11–12 and in Chapter 10.

Part way along the hair follicle, a duct delivers sebum — the secretion of the attached sebaceous gland — onto the surface of the hair, thus lubricating the surface.

Also attached to each follicle is a small bundle of smooth muscle, the arrector pili (*see* **Fig. 1.1**), the contraction of which causes the appearance called goosebumps. These muscles are served by adrenergic nerves of the sympathetic nervous system.

Sweat glands

Human skin possesses two kinds of sweat glands: eccrine and apocrine.

Eccrine sweat glands are coiled structures, usually lying at the junction between the dermis and the subcutis, from which emerges a duct leading through the dermis and epidermis to the surface of the skin (**Fig. 1.7a**). There are over 2 million eccrine sweat glands in the average human's skin. They are present over the whole body surface, but are more numerous in some sites: the forehead, axillae, palms, and soles. The glands are

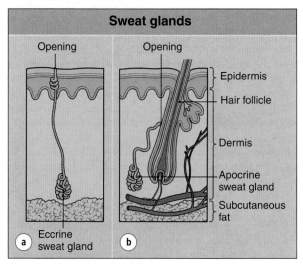

Fig. 1.7 *Sweat glands:* (**a**) *the architecture of an eccrine sweat gland;* (**b**) *the architecture of an apocrine sweat gland.*

innervated by the sympathetic nervous system, but the efferent neurones directly involved are cholinergic. Sweat glands also respond to temperature, increasing their output of salty water when the body becomes hot.

Apocrine sweat glands are also coiled structures with a duct, but they open into associated hair follicles (**Fig. 1.7b**) and are not found as widely as eccrine glands, being localized largely to the axillae, nipples, perineum, and scalp. The secretion of these glands is produced by the direct separation of parts of the apocrine cells' cytoplasm into the lumen. The gland is androgen-dependent and is also innervated by the sympathetic nervous system (with adrenergic final-pathway neurones).

Nails

A similar epidermal invagination to that seen in the hair follicle is present at the end of each digit and produces the structure we call the nail (**Fig. 1.8**). The nail plate is produced both from the lower surface of the nail fold and from the upper surface of the matrix. These elements fuse into the flat nail plate that covers the end of each digit. This is clearly a complex process, with genetically determined controls to keep the nail flat (only primates have nails, all other mammals having claws). Any disturbance to this process, either genetic or acquired (e.g. by inflammation, trauma, or a space-occupying lesion), can alter nail growth significantly. However, severe defects of the nails are surprisingly uncommon (*see* Chapter 9).

The nail plate is, like hair, largely made of keratin, rich in sulphur-containing amino acids.

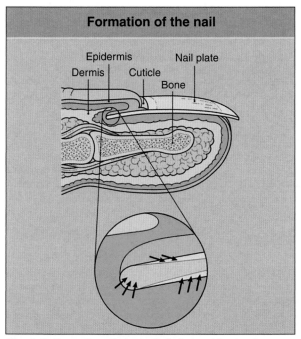

Fig. 1.8 *Formation of the nail: fusion and lamination of flat, keratinized plates arising from the nail bed and nail fold.*

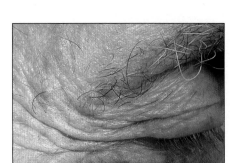

Fig. 1.9 *An area of facial skin showing the typical coarsening and wrinkling that is attributed to age but is largely due to environmental damage (particularly ultraviolet radiation).*

'NATURAL' ALTERATIONS TO THE STRUCTURE OF THE SKIN

Age and the environment alter the anatomy of the skin. Some changes are associated with normal maturation and development: for example, the development of facial, axillary and pubic hair, and the increased size and activity of the apocrine glands, all of which occur at puberty. Some are the result of a process of deterioration, part of which is age-related: for example, greying of the hair due to the cessation of pigmentary mechanisms, and the gradual loss of dermo-epidermal corrugations. Others are largely due to environmental damage, especially ultraviolet radiation: for example, wrinkling, coarsening, and yellowing of facial skin (**Fig. 1.9**). Several of these characteristics — such as thinning of hair, the age of greying, and the degree of wrinkling — are undoubtedly influenced by our genes.

Many of these changes have to be accepted as a part of life, although some people, quite naturally, try to 'hold back the waves' or sometimes try to turn back the tide of time. For example, dyeing of greying hair is very common. Many men wear hairpieces or have transplants or other augmentation techniques. Dermatologists, dermatological surgeons, and plastic/cosmetic surgeons are increasingly being asked to reduce the wrinkliness of the face by means of chemical applications (retinoids, acids), injections (collagen and other materials), botox, or surgery (blepharoplasty, full or partial face-lifts, laser resurfacing).

THE FUNCTIONS OF THE SKIN

The complex organization and structure of the skin, as described earlier, has obviously developed for many reasons, even though most people think of the skin simply as an envelope. In fact, the skin performs several important (sometimes vitally important) physiological functions.

BARRIER FUNCTION

The outer layers of the epidermis consist of several overlapping plates of keratin. These are surrounded by a thin film of lipid that is dispersed across the surface of the cells by the Odland bodies (or membrane-coating granules), which become visible under electron microscopy in the prickle cell layer. The envelope thus produced is both strong and flexible, providing a semi-permeable barrier to the outside world. Removal of the horny layer results in a marked increase in water loss, and further stripping of the epidermis leads to significant protein loss. Thus, the skin has an important role in maintaining the integrity of all that lies within. Although the horny layer repels water on first contact, it can also absorb a large amount of water and can survive a significant degree of water loss.

- Skin is the largest organ in the body by weight and surface area.
- Skin is composed of four layers: epidermis, basement membrane zone, dermis and subcutis.
- Epidermis is the outer layer composed mainly of keratinocytes but also melanocytes and Langerhans' cells.
- Dermis is a supportive connective tissue layer comprised mainly of collagen but also containing elastin embedded in a matrix of mucopolysaccharides.
- Hairs are keratinized tubes emerging from invaginations of the epidermis called follicles.
- Sebaceous glands deliver sebum into the follicle lubricating the hair surface.
- Eccrine sweat glands are found over the entire skin surface and innervated by the sympathetic nervous system, responding to temperature/psychological changes.
- Apocrine sweat glands are localized (axillae, nipples, perineum, scalp) and androgen-sensitive.
- Nails, like hair, are made largely of keratin.

Melanocyte function and pigmentation

One aspect of the skin's barrier function deserves a special mention: the role of melanocytes and melanin in the prevention of damage by ultraviolet radiation. As indicated on page 4, the melanocyte produces melanin granules at a genetically predetermined rate and transports them, via the cell's dendritic processes, into the cytoplasm of surrounding keratinocytes. Melanin absorbs ultraviolet radiation and thus protects the nuclei of the

---

Box 1.4 Functions of the skin

Barrier
The skin provides a protective barrier to: mechanical, thermal, and other physical injury, the ingress of noxious agents, the excessive loss of moisture and protein that would (and does) occur if the skin were absent or seriously compromised and the harmful effects of ionizing radiation (especially ultraviolet radiation).
Sensation
The skin is rich in nerve endings and specialized sensory receptors.
Thermoregulation
The skin is the body's principal organ of heat control.
Immunological surveillance
The skin contains immunologically competent cells.
Biochemical reactions
The best-known example is the skin's role in vitamin D synthesis, but the skin is also involved in androgen degradation and other biochemical reactions.
Social and sexual functioning
It is hard to overemphasize just how important the skin is to our whole system of interacting with others and that disorders of the skin owe much of their impact to impairing the individual's sense of well-being and self-worth.

basal and spinous cells from DNA damage. In the lower layers of the epidermis, the melanin granules are arranged as a shield or umbrella over the nuclei of the basal and spinous cells. In the outer layers, melanin granules are scattered throughout the cells.

SENSATION

We all take the skin's sensory role for granted. It is the organ of touch and of hot and cold, and we can also feel pressure and pain through our skin. The same nerve fibres that carry pain also carry the sensation of itch. This sensation, which is unique to the skin, causes considerable distress when it becomes persistent and severe. The skin is very rich in nerve endings, especially on the fingers, toes, lips, and tongue (not, perhaps, strictly 'the skin'), and this allows us to localize sensations very accurately.

TEMPERATURE REGULATION

Like all warm-blooded creatures, humans normally maintain a constant core temperature whatever the outside temperature may be. This is most important for many biological functions. The skin plays a role in this process by alterations to the blood flow through the cutaneous vascular bed (vasodilatation = more blood flow = higher direct heat loss; vasoconstriction = less blood flow = reduced heat loss). The skin also allows the body to cool itself by the evaporation of sweat from the surface.

IMMUNOLOGICAL SURVEILLANCE

The skin is an important site of immunological activity. Depending upon the 'need' for an immunological response, a variety of cells and chemical messengers (cytokines) are involved in recruiting and stimulating both cellular and humoral responses:

- Epidermal Langerhans' cells are constantly 'on the lookout' for antigens in their surroundings in order to trap them and 'present' them to lymphocytes.
- In certain circumstances, the epidermal keratinocytes themselves can express immunological markers on their surface and produce cytokines.
- Mast cells in the dermis aid the process by releasing vasoactive chemicals that help in the recruitment of cells.
- Tissue macrophages are recruited by vessel dilation and release of chemical attractants.
- So-called adhesion molecules assist by binding to surface markers on immunologically competent cells.

These functions are important in dealing with infection and tumour cells. Dysregulation leads to allergic contact dermatitis (*see* pages 184–187) and, probably to atopic dermatitis (pages 188–192), psoriasis and many other skin disorders. Defective function, in patients receiving immunosuppressive drugs for example increases the risk of infection and tumour formation.

BIOCHEMICAL REACTIONS

The skin is known to be involved in several biochemical processes, and no doubt, more have yet to be delineated. In most of these, the skin is essentially an 'end-organ', but in two — vitamin D and androgen metabolism — it is an active participant.

A vital part of vitamin D metabolism takes place in the epidermis: exposure to ultraviolet radiation, largely in the basal and prickle cell layers, converts 7-dehydrocholesterol to vitamin D3, via a precursor molecule, previtamin D3. Without this natural process, vitamin D3 deficiency leads to impaired intestinal calcium and phosphate absorption, which results in osteomalacia and rickets.

There is no doubt that androgen metabolism also takes place within the skin, with the conversion of testosterone to 5α-dihydrotestosterone by the enzyme 5α-reductase. The skin also contains receptors for other steroid hormones (oestrogens, progestogens, and glucocorticoids) and for vitamin A.

SOCIAL SIGNALLING

Even the briefest study of human history will tell you that the skin is important socially: men and women with pigmented skins have been treated as second-class citizens by many societies over the centuries; persons with albinism are often rejected because of their unusual skin colour; the presence of a major facial blemish, such as a port-wine stain, often causes even the most open-minded of us to turn our head as we pass by. The presence of 'abnormalities' that are essentially physiological — such as male balding, excessive hairiness, body odour, and the signs of ageing — also can cause major misery and anxiety.

Many people decorate their skin. Sometimes the decoration is relatively simple (e.g. the wearing of earrings and the painting of finger and toe nails); sometimes it is extremely elaborate (e.g. painting for religious and other ceremonies, tattooing — **Fig. 1.10**).

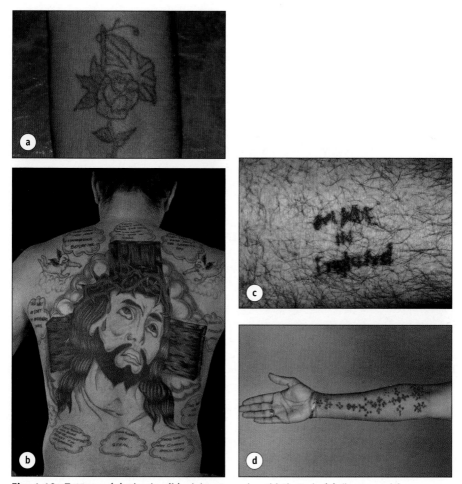

Fig. 1.10 *Tattoos: (a) simple; (b) elaborate and sophisticated; (c) 'home-made';*
(d) a reflection of ancient cultural traditions.

We all rely on our skins to present the outside world with an acceptable image. We need it to be good enough to allow us to mingle with our peers and to find our sexual partners. Different societies have encouraged different expressions of what is and what is not acceptable. The media can alter and condition these (fashions for skin change, as well as those for clothes). However, whatever the details, it is essential for anyone involved in the management of patients with skin disorders to understand that blemishes and deviations from what is considered normal in that societal framework can be enough to require aid from professionals, as real psychopathology may sometimes be caused.

- Skin provides a protective barrier to injury and prevents water and protein loss.
- Skin is rich in nerve endings and specialized sensory receptors.
- Regulation in blood flow through the skin is a principal means of thermoregulation in the body.
- Skin provides a barrier to infection and contains numerous elements of cellular immunity.
- Skin is vital to Vitamin D synthesis and androgen metabolism.
- Skin is an important element in human social interaction.

chapter 2

Diagnosing and Treating Skin Disease

INTRODUCTION

Physicians and scientists have been studying the skin and its afflictions for as long as one man has acted as medical adviser to another. As a result, many myths have emerged about the significance of this sign or that, the relationship of the skin to various internal organs, and the probable outcome of the disease process involved. To complicate matters further, the ancients provided an enormous number of diagnostic terms for changes in the skin, and these have been modified and adapted by others as the centuries have rolled by. Many non-dermatologists find the 'mumbo-jumbo' too impenetrable and simply give up. This chapter is designed to stop you doing that!

It is also designed to give a brief introduction to some of the special tests and investigations that are available to assist in dermatological diagnoses and to cover some of the basics of management; more detail on both these areas can be found in later chapters of the book.

DERMATOLOGICAL TERMINOLOGY

As indicated above, dermatologists have adopted a range of terms to describe conditions affecting the skin and its associated structures. Many of these have their roots in the classical languages of Greek and Latin, but with major influences coming in later times from clinicians working with patients and their problems. For hundreds of years, the only system of classification available to doctors was based on simple clinical observation. It is, after all, only over the last hundred years that pathology has begun to shed another perspective on disease processes, and only in the last 20 or 30 years that the advent of the technologies of immunology, molecular biology, and genetics has opened up some of the newer concepts. Certainly, new insights into aetiology and pathogenesis have altered the nosological position of some disorders in the 'old order', but many of the terms have remained and past clinical observations have been confirmed to be strikingly accurate on many occasions. The true student of dermatology will have to assimilate many unfamiliar names in his or her first brushes with the discipline, but will find that they represent situations with close parallels in other medical specialties. There is another group of terms with which you will have to become acquainted: the words that are used to describe various changes seen in the skin affected by disease. Some of these are listed in the boxes below.

Box 2.1   Characteristics of individual lesions

Macule
Flat skin discolouration.
Papule
Elevated lesion < 0.5 cm in diameter.
Nodule
Elevated lesion > 0.5 cm in diameter.
Small plaque
Elevated, flat-topped lesion < 2 cm in diameter.
Large plaque
Elevated, flat-topped lesion = 2 cm in diameter.
Wheal
Elevated area of cutaneous oedema.
Vesicle
Fluid-filled lesion < 0.5 cm in diameter.
Bulla
Fluid-filled lesion > 0.5 cm in diameter.
Pustule
Pus-filled lesion.

Box 2.2   Characteristics of the surface

Scale
Visible and palpable flakes of aggregated epidermal cells.
Crust
Dried exudates.
Horn
Projection of keratin.
Ulceration
Loss of epidermis (+/- underlying dermis and subcutis).
Excoriation
Superficial ulceration as a result of scratching.
Maceration
Softened, wettened epidermis.
Lichenification
Flat-surfaced epidermal thickening.

These terms are the 'building blocks' of dermatological diagnosis, description, and communication. They should be used accurately, but often they are not or they are qualified by phrases such as 'sort of' or 'a bit like'. The term maculopapular, for example, seems to be used by non-specialists, almost at random, to describe any rash. The essence of good communication is accuracy. We believe that learning to use words properly at the beginning is educational in itself and also leads to far fewer problems in the long term. We therefore urge you to take a little time and try to understand the differences highlighted in the boxes, and apply them to your clinical experience, as you see more and more patients with skin disease.

STARTING TO MAKE A DIAGNOSIS

Your task, in aiming to become better at dermatology, is to try to diagnose specific skin disorders as accurately as possible. You want to be able to tell Bowen's disease from psoriasis (**Fig. 2.1**), or a seborrhoeic keratosis from a melanoma (**Fig. 2.2**). You want to be able to anticipate that the eczematous dermatosis you see on a patient's skin may be due to contact with a known allergen, such as nickel in a jean-stud or footwear (**Fig. 2.3**).

As with any other specialty, in order to do this, you need to start seeing patients. You will probably want to watch a dermatologist in action initially and then have a go yourself. Although skin diseases and abnormalities present and are seen in many medical settings, such as family practice and general medical or surgical clinics, there is no doubt that the best place to begin is a specialist skin clinic. It is much harder to try and begin the process on your own, but sometimes this is thrust upon you. In both situations, a good atlas can aid immeasurably in the learning process by providing photographic examples with which to compare your own experience. However, atlases need to be augmented by good text, good teaching, guidance, and feedback, and by diligent repetition of the process of history-taking, examination, and deductive reasoning.

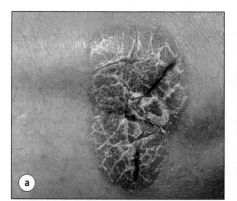
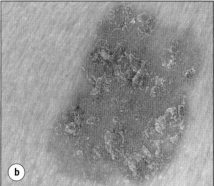

Fig. 2.1 *Diagnostic appearances of (a)* a plaque of psoriasis and *(b)* a patch of Bowen's disease.

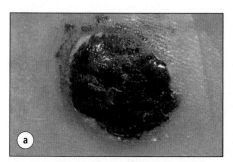
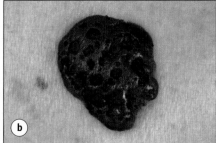

Fig. 2.2 *Diagnostic appearances of (a)* a malignant melanoma and *(b)* a darkly pigmented seborrhoeic keratosis.

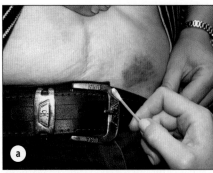 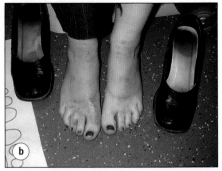

Fig. 2.3 *Dermatitis (a)* under a buckle — nickel in the buckle confirmed by dimethyl glyoxime test; *(b)* allergic contact dermatitis due to chromate in leather shoes.

DERMATOLOGICAL HISTORY-TAKING

The essentials of dermatological history-taking are listed below.

As with any other specialty, the first thing to establish is the presenting complaint: ask questions to define and qualify it, establish whether there are any other linked problems, and assess its severity. There are, however, some differences in this learning process in dermatology compared with certain other disciplines:

- It is somewhat more common in dermatology to find that several problems have been identified by the patient (and there is also a good deal of 'While I'm here, doctor, …', as the patient remembers something else they would like to show you).
- Skin signs are there for all to see and patients often put their own interpretation on the nature of their problem — this can affect the language they use to describe the problem.
- The visibility of the skin lesion(s) often also demands that it/they be examined very early on during the consultation — this can help to limit subsequent questions.
- Skin diseases present with new symptoms, most notably itch — non-dermatologists will need to take time to familiarize themselves with the phrases used by patients to describe the intensity and characteristics of itch (**Fig. 2.4**); itchy patients can be divided into two groups: those with a rash and those without; it is important to establish from the beginning whether the itch preceded or followed any skin changes.
- Skin disease has major psychological effects, especially when it affects the face — the patient will often not speak of these unless drawn out by the dermatologist.
- There are important genetic aspects to many skin diseases.
- Some skin diseases are infectious or contagious.
- There are important environmental aspects to many skin diseases — to take a good history, one may need to explore the patient's work and leisure activities.
- Patients frequently use multiple creams and ointments on their skin — these may have been: prescribed by their doctor; already present in the house for other problems or other people; bought 'over the counter' (OTC) at a pharmacy; lent by friends and family; supplied by alternative/complementary practitioners; be part of a cosmetic/toiletry regimen.
- Patients frequently forget the names of the treatments they have used on their skin — it is helpful to be able to show patients examples of the creams they might have used, as these can act as an excellent *aide memoire*.

Itch: characteristics and severity

Itch may be localized or generalized.

Some patients use very specific words to qualify itch, e.g. 'creeping' or 'like ants crawling over the skin'. These descriptions are often associated with itch due to systemic diseases, but may also apply to a psychological cause.

The distribution may be significant, e.g. in dermatitis herpetiformis, itch affects the extensor aspects of the forearms and lower legs and the lower back and scalp, scabies seldom affects the scalp and face in adults.

The time when itch is worst may be significant, e.g. itch may be a problem only when the patient is at rest, be worse at night (it characteristically is in scabies), result in loss of sleep (a frequent problem in atopic dermatitis), or be present constantly (as it is when a feature of systemic disease).

The intensity may be judged to some extent by the presence of secondary skin lesions caused by scratching (excoriations and bruising).

Fig. 2.4 *Itch:* **characteristics and severity.**

EXAMINATION OF THE SKIN

It is very common for part, if not all, of the examination to begin at the start of the consultation, and for the early findings to condition and guide the direction and nature of the history-taking and the rest of the consultation. Skin examination, like dermatological history-taking, requires some new techniques and thought-processes (**Figs 2.5 and 2.6**):

Box 2.3 Essentials of dermatological history-taking

Presenting complaint
Where?
How long?
What symptoms? — itch (*see* Fig. 2.4), bleeding?
What effect does it have on your life at work and at home?
How and with what has it been treated already? (*see below*)
Past history
Skin disease
Allergies
General disorders
Family/close contacts
Any skin disease
Any allergies or atopic diseases (e.g. hay fever, asthma)
Exposure to materials in the workplace or at home
Occupation and hobbies
Medical systemic
Therapy
Medical, systemic and topical (including other people's and old creams) this includes over the counter products and those recommended by non-medical health professionals, e.g. pharmacists, specialist nurses
Alternative/complementary
Exposure to cosmetics and toiletries

Key elements in examination of the skin

Establish the site and distribution of the lesion(s).
Describe the characteristics of the individual lesion(s). Note especially their:
type (*see* box on page 16)
size, shape, and outline, especially of tumours
colour(s)
surface characteristics (*see* box on page 16)
texture — is the lesion superficial, and therefore largely epidermal, or is it deep? probably involving dermis or subcutis?
Examine 'secondary sites' (using appropriate secondary techniques — *see* Fig. 2.6):
nails — in psoriasis, alopecia areata, fungal infections
umbilicus — in psoriasis
toe-webs — in fungal infections
mouth — in lichen planus
finger-webs — in scabies
male genitalia — in scabies

Fig. 2.5 *Key elements in examination of the skin*

Examples of secondary examination techniques that can aid diagnosis

Scratching, rubbing, or prodding the skin to elicit whealing in:
- dermographism (*see* Chapter 5)
- mastocytosis (urticaria pigmentosa and mast cell naevi) — 'Darier's sign' (*see* Chapter 6).

Application of ice, warm water, pressure, etc. to elicit whealing in the physical urticaria.
Scraping a psoriatic plaque to elicit capillary bleeding (Auspitz sign). **NB This must only be carried out using appropriate sterile instruments.**
The easy stripping of the epidermis in pemphigus and toxic epidermal necrolysis (Nikolsky's sign).
Blanching a spider angioma with a fine point.
'Diascopy' (pressure with a glass slide) in cutaneous granulomas, especially TB.
'Wood's light' examination for fluorescence in some fungal infections and for enhancing the visibility of pale patches in tuberous sclerosis.

Fig. 2.6 *Examples of secondary examination techniques that can aid diagnosis.*

- It is considered 'best practice' to examine the whole skin every time. However, in practice, this is unworkable and unreasonable — no-one wishes to be completely undressed when they come for attention to a wart on the finger or to a cyst on the scalp.
- It is critical to palpate skin lesions as well as to look at them — not only does this provide useful information but it also indicates to the patient that the doctor, at least, is not repelled or frightened by their rash.
- It is sensible to measure lesions rather than to describe them vaguely in terms related to coins or fingernails. It is a good discipline to draw tumours in their approximate location, with a note of their size (usually in millimetres).

- Take time to learn accurately key dermatological terms used to describe the characteristics of individual lesions and the skin surface.
- Essentials of dermatological history taking: presenting complaint, past history, family and close contacts, occupation and hobbies, other medical therapies (e.g. topical creams).
- Examine the entire skin surface.
- Palpate lesions to assess texture.
- Describe the site, distribution and characteristics (type, size, shape, colour, surface, texture) of individual lesion(s) using accurate descriptive terms.
- Examine 'secondary sites' (e.g. nails, hair, mucous membranes) using appropriate techniques.

- There are some 'secondary' sites that are worth examining when certain diagnoses are suspected.
- The results of the examination should be recorded using the terms outlined in the boxes on page 16.

Another early problem for the examining dermatological novice is that he or she will have to learn which lesion(s) to focus on. All rashes are dynamic and usually contain some lesions that are relatively 'young', some that are 'older', and others that are at the mid-point. Only a proportion of these lesions will bear the signs classically associated with the diagnosis that he or she is about to make. It is therefore important to receive guidance as to how and why to pick out those lesions that provide the most 'useful' diagnostic clues. This can really only come from practising the technique alongside an expert.

SPECIAL INVESTIGATIONS

As with all other specialties, dermatology has developed a number of special techniques for advancing the diagnostic information available on an individual patient. Many of these have been in use for a long time. One or two are much more recent. The box below lists the most important and gives some indication of their potential value. Examples of skin biopsies processed by different techniques are shown in **Figures 2.7 and 2.8**.

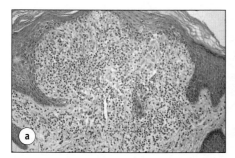 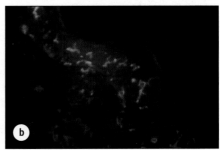

Fig. 2.7 *Skin biopsy: (a) a skin biopsy (of lichen nitidus) processed for light microscopy; (b) a skin biopsy (of lichen planus) processed for immunocytochemistry — here, the epidermal Langerhans' cells are beautifully delineated by a monoclonal antibody tagged with fluorescein.*

21

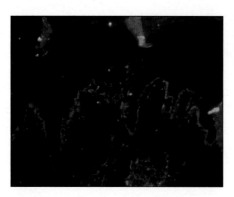

Fig. 2.8 *A skin biopsy processed for immunofluorescence:* showing a linear band of immunoglobulin (in this case, IgG in a case of bullous pemphigoid).

Box 2.4 Investigational techniques

Blood tests
For a wide range of disorders, for indirect immunofluorescence in immunobullous disease.

Swabs
Bacteriological
To ascertain nature of infecting organism, antibiotic sensitivity.
Viral
To ascertain nature of infecting organism.

Scrapes or clips
To obtain material for inspection for fungi, mites, molluscum bodies, giant cells (in herpes virus infections); to set up cultures for fungi.

Biopsy
Light microscopy
Pathological interpretation, including special stains and immunocytochemistry as necessary (*see* Fig. 2.7).
Immunofluorescence
Bullous disorders; cutaneous and systemic lupus erythematosus; vasculitis (*see* Fig. 2.8).
Electron microscopy
Especially useful in congenital and acquired blistering diseases.
Culture
The organisms causing TB, leishmaniasis, and some rarer organisms are more easily, or can only be, cultured from skin biopsies.
***In-situ* hybridization**
Subtyping human papilloma virus.

Patch tests
Investigation of allergic contact dermatitis (*see* Chapter 5).

Prick tests
Testing for IgE mediated (immediate type) hypersensitivity
Important in suspected latex allergy. Place in other disorders (e.g. urticaria, atopic eczema) less clear.

Blood tests for indirect immunofluorescence

There are circulating antibodies to skin components in pemphigus and bullous pemphigoid (*see* Chapter 7). These can be demonstrated by applying serum to animal epithelium and staining the combination with an antibody labelled with a fluorescent marker.

Skin scrapings and clippings

Skin scrapings and clippings are widely used in dermatology clinics to aid in the diagnosis of fungal infections (*see* Fig. 3.51, p. 78), mite infestations (scabies), and, occasionally, molluscum contagiosum, bullous disorders, and herpesvirus infections.
You will require:

- A good-quality microscope.
- A blunt-edged scalpel ('banana' scalpel) or a disposable scalpel blade, a pair of fine scissors, and a pair of forceps.
- Slides and cover slips.
- Potassium hydroxide (KOH) solution for epidermal scrapings, hair, and nails (usually 10% KOH, but 20–30% is better for nails).
- A bottle of Giemsa's stain for a Tzanck preparation.
- Some training and experience!

Samples should be taken from:

- The edge of cutaneous ringworm lesions.
- The blister roof of vesicular lesions (using a pair of scissors).
- Both scalp scale and hair (using forceps if necessary) in suspected scalp ringworm.
- Both infected nail plate and samples of subungual hyperkeratosis/debris, in suspected nail infections.
- A suspected herpetic blister without pus, if possible.
- The edge of a suspected pemphigus lesion.

Samples of epidermal scale, and hair and nail are placed on a microscope slide with a drop of KOH solution and a cover slip. After a few minutes (20–30 for nails), the slide can be examined for the presence of fungal elements. These are seen as mycelial strands crossing cell boundaries and, often, crossing focal planes. Scabies mites, eggs, egg cases, or immature forms are easily seen under low power.

For a Tzanck preparation, looking for *Herpes* or acanthloysis in pemphigus, the material obtained from the lesion(s) is smeared onto a microscope slide and stained with Giemsa's stain. The slide is then examined for the presence of multinucleate giant cells (herpes virus — both simplex and varicella-zoster).

Culture for fungus is very useful for both practical and epidemiological purposes in knowing the source of the infection; samples should be sent folded into paper (preferably black to make the scale easily identifiable) to a laboratory that is properly equipped to grow fungi. The standard culture medium is still that first described by Sabouraud, although some organisms require special handling (especially saprophytic moulds — *see* Chapter 3). Culture results are usually available within 6 weeks.

Skin biopsy and pathology

Two techniques are commonly used to obtain diagnostic skin samples: punch biopsy and elliptical incisional biopsy. These are illustrated in **Figure 2.9.**

Briefly, the area to be examined or removed is anaesthetized, usually using injected lidocaine. In some instances (especially in children), the skin may be deadened first by the application of a topical anaesthetic cream for 30—60 minutes. The piece of skin is then removed using the punch knife or scalpel, and the skin edges are brought together with a fine suture.

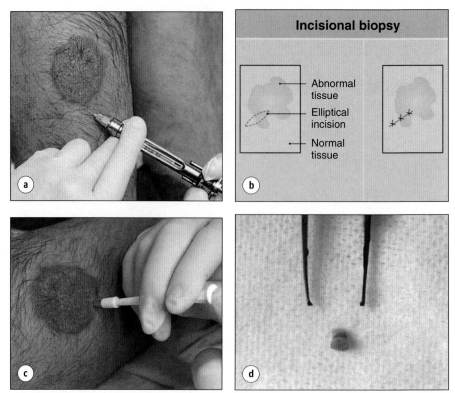

Fig. 2.9 *Skin biopsy: (a) the skin is anaesthetized; skin is removed either by cutting out an ellipse (b) of skin with a scalpel or by means of a punch biopsy (c and d).*

It is important to choose an appropriate area from which to take the sample. The skin lesion(s) should generally be fully formed. Late lesions should be avoided. In some situations (e.g. dermatitis herpetiformis and bullous pemphigoid), it is important to sample early lesions because the classic histology may be altered by the passage of time.

The specimen should then be processed by the method required by the investigative technique that is being requested. For example, 'ordinary' light microscopy specimens simply need to be transported to the laboratory, fixed in formalin. The 'standard' stain applied to skin, as with most other tissue, is haematoxylin and eosin (H&E), although there are many special stains for particular tissue components — for example: periodic-acid–Schiff (PAS) for polysaccharides in basement membrane and fungi; van Giesen for connective tissue; and Alcian Blue for mucin. Formalin-fixed and paraffin-embedded specimens can also be processed for immunopathological elements, such as the cell surface markers CD4 (T helper/inducer lymphocytes) and CD8 (cytotoxic T cell subset), using the immunoperoxidase technique.

Direct immunofluorescence, however, can only be performed on frozen tissue because fixation destroys the antibodies that are being sought. Samples will therefore need to be snap frozen, or otherwise preserved, before transportation or be taken straight to the laboratory as they are. These cryostat sections are processed and 'stained' with antibodies to the element being sought (e.g. IgG in pemphigus and pemphigoid). The antibodies are tagged with a fluorescent dye.

Similarly, specimens for culture should be sent fresh to the laboratory and those to be examined by electron microscopy held in special fixative during transfer. If there is any doubt, it is always best to consult the laboratory concerned.

Scalp and nail biopsies

It is sometimes necessary to obtain tissue from the scalp or the nail. The principles involved are essentially the same as for skin biopsy, but there are some technical differences:

- Scalp biopsies need to be deep, to include subcutaneous fat, and the specimen, whether taken by punch or by elliptical incision, must be orientated carefully so that whole hair follicles are available for analysis.
- Nail-bed tissue can be obtained either by lifting the nail plate away from the nail bed or by performing a full-thickness, longitudinal nail biopsy (**Fig. 2.10**). Both techniques require specialist training.

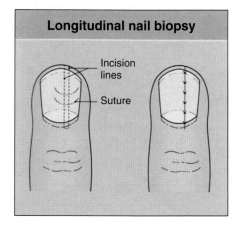

Fig. 2.10 *Longitudinal nail biopsy.*

Patch testing

The term patch test describes an investigative tool that involves the deliberate application of materials suspected of causing allergic dermatitis, to the skin under controlled conditions, and is described in Chapter 5.

Prick testing

This is a more controversial type of allergy test. It has gained a reputation for being misused by some practitioners, especially in the context of atopic dermatitis. Prick testing is unreliable at best in atopics and certainly does not identify environmental triggers for the eczema with any consistency. The technique is valuable, however, in immediate (Type I) hypersensitivity. The most important example in recent times has been the emergence of latex allergy. Latex Type I hypersensitivity peaked in the 1990s with dramatic increases in latex glove use throughout industry, but has tailed off since. Prick testing to purified latex extract is the most sensitive test for latex allergy (**Fig. 2.11**).

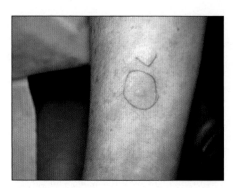

Fig. 2.11 *Positive prick test in a patient with immediate type hypersensitivity to latex.*

- Skin scrapings and clippings are used to diagnose a range of infections and infestations.
- Two techniques commonly used to obtain diagnostic skin samples are punch biopsy and elliptical incisional biopsy.
- Patch and prick testing are used to test for skin allergies.

TREATING SKIN DISEASES

Broadly speaking, skin diseases may be treated by one of the following techniques:
- Topical application of a cream, ointment, gel, tape, or spray.
- Local injection of active agents.
- Ingestion or injection of systemic agents.
- Exposure of the skin to ionizing radiation (ultraviolet, X-rays, g-rays).
- Removal of the tissue.
- Physical destruction of the tissue by heat, cold, electricity, or light.

The broad principles of each of these is discussed below, with examples being illustrated in **Figure 2.12**. Specific information is also given in the individual chapters dealing with each disorder.

Many of these treatments are 'generic' in that they are used by several specialist groups, and the reader may well have encountered them before. However, it is worth noting a few specific points about some of the treatment modalities that are not used very frequently outside dermatology.

Common examples of treatment modalities for skin diseases

Topical agents*	Emollients and moisturizers	Any condition characterized by 'Dryness' of the skin
	Salicylic acid	Scaly disorders, warts
	'Exfoliants'	Acne vulgaris
	Tar (creams/pastes/bandages)	Psoriasis, eczemas
	Dithranol (anthralin)	Psoriasis
	Steroids	Any inflammatory dermatosis (*see* Chapter 5), some infiltrates (*see* Chapter 6)
	Calcineurin inhibitors (Tacrolimus; pimecrolimus)	Eczema
	Retinoic acid derivatives	Acne vulgaris, psoriasis
	Antiseptics and antibiotics	Bacterial infections, secondary infection of eczemas
	Antivirals	Viral infections, especially herpetic infections
	Antifungals	Fungal infections, seborrhoeic dermatitis
	Vitamin D analogues	Psoriasis
	5-Fluorouracil	Actinic keratoses, Bowen's disease
	Diphencyprone	Alopecia areata
	Capsaicin	Neuralgia, intractable localized itch
	Imiquimod	Viral warts (esp genital), superficial epithelial dysplasia and BCC
	Solaraze	Superficial epithelial dysplasia
Local injection	Steroids	Inflammatory dermatoses, alopecia areata, granuloma annulare; necrobiosis lipoidica, keloid scars, cutaneous infiltrates
Systemic agents	Antihistamines (low sedation)	Urticaria
	Antihistamines (sedative)	Itch, especially in childhood eczema
	Antibiotics	Bacterial infections
	Antivirals	Viral infections, especially herpetic infections
	Steroids	Severe inflammatory skin disorders, bullous disorders, lupus erythematosus (LE)

Fig. 2.12 *Common examples of treatment modalities for skin diseases.*

	Immunosuppressives, e.g. azathioprine, ciclosporin, mycophenolate mofetil	Severe inflammatory skin disorders, bullous disorders, psoriasis, LE
	Methotrexate	Psoriasis, sarcoidosis
	Retinoids	Disorders of keratinization, psoriasis, acne
	Dapsone	Leprosy, dermatitis herpetiformis, vasculitis
	Antimalarials	LE, polymorphic light eruption
	Psoralens (+ ultraviolet A) †	Psoriasis, eczemas, vitiligo, cutaneous T-cell lymphoma, disseminated granuloma annulare
	Monoclonal antibodies (biologics)	Severe psoriasis, psoriatic arthropathy, pyoderma gangrenosum
Exposure to ionizing radiation	Ultraviolet A (+/− psoralen)†	Psoriasis, eczemas, vitiligo, cutaneous T-cell lymphoma, disseminated granuloma annulare, polymorphic light eruption and other photodermatoses
	Ultraviolet B	Psoriasis, eczemas
	X-rays	Epithelial cancers, Bowen's disease, localized areas of cutaneous lymphoma, Kaposi's sarcoma
	Gamma-rays	Disseminated cutaneous lymphoma
Removal of tissue	Curettage and diathermy/cautery	Superficial epithelial lesions, e.g. seborrhoeic keratoses, superficial basal cell carcinomas, pyogenic granulomas
	Snip and cautery/diathermy	Skin tags and other pedunculated lesions
	Excision	Cysts and tumours
Physical destruction of tissue	Cryotherapy	Warts (including anogenital), superficial epithelial tumours, basal cell carcinomas, spider angiomas
	Cautery/diathermy	Small tags, spider angiomas
	Hyfrecation/dessication	Tags, pedunculated seborrhoeic keratoses, warts, spider angiomas
	Laser (various types)	Epithelial lesions, vascular lesions, pigmented lesions, tattoos

*many of these topical agents are used in combinations
† combination of oral agent and UVA = PUVA

Fig. 2.12 (Cont'd)

THE BASES OF TOPICAL AGENTS (AND EMOLLIENTS)

All topical agents are 'held' in suspension in a base of some kind, which allows the patient to apply the material to the skin surface. Some of these bases are greases, oils, or waxes (ointments); others are emulsions of oil, grease, or wax in water (creams) or emulsions of water in oils (oily creams). There are also aqueous gel bases, alcoholic solutions (used especially on the scalp to avoid matting the hair), mousses, and liquid and powder sprays. This rather bewildering array of preparations has been produced by pharmaceutical companies as a response to the different treatment needs of different disorders and patient requirements.

In general terms, the greasier a base is, the more occlusive it is. This also generally implies a greater degree of emolliency or moisturizer effect, as it prevents water loss to a greater degree. On the other hand, a lighter cream is much easier to use and is much more cosmetically acceptable to most patients. Some of the more modern oily creams aim to achieve a balance between these two extremes, by providing a higher degree of occlusion and emolliency with a lower and more acceptable degree of 'greasiness'. Some agents designed purely to be emollients contain additional ingredients (such as urea, allantoin, or aloe vera) which are claimed to increase the moisturizing effects.

The needs of each patient must be judged individually, although the old 'rule of thumb' still has an element of truth to it: if the skin is 'dry', use an ointment; if it is wet and weepy, use a cream.

SALICYLIC ACID

Salicylic acid 'softens' keratin and helps to remove scale from psoriasis and from other very scaly disorders, especially in the scalp. It is therefore often added to mixtures of tar and steroids. Salicylic acid in higher concentrations is also used to treat viral warts.

TAR AND DITHRANOL

Tar is soothing when applied to itchy, inflamed skin. It is also a valuable adjunct in the management of psoriasis, where it seems to augment the effects of ultraviolet radiation. Dithranol is a strange material, originally isolated from Goa powder, which can return psoriatic skin to normal. It can cause quite nasty burns, however, and it also oxidizes to a brownish-purple dye. It is used in creams and ointments and in a complicated, stiff paste known as Lassar's paste.

TOPICAL CORTICOSTEROIDS

Topical corticosteroids are undoubtedly the mainstay of the treatment of all the eczema/dermatitis group of conditions and of many other inflammatory dermatoses (e.g. lichen planus and lupus erythematosus). They also have a valuable role in psoriasis, especially on certain sites. However, topical corticosteroids need to be handled with care. They have the potential to cause significant skin atrophy if they are applied to the same area of skin repeatedly over many weeks or months. They reduce the skin's resistance to superficial infections. They can inhibit the pituitary–adrenal axis if sufficient quantities are applied to lead to significant systemic absorption.

It is important to appreciate that topical corticosteroids are by no means 'all the same': some are much stronger than others (**Fig. 2.13**). Furthermore, several factors increase the potential for atrophogenicity and absorption:
- The base — ointments>creams>gels>lotions.
- The site of application — the face and flexures are much more vulnerable.
- The size of the patient — children have a higher surface-area-to-body-mass ratio and are more susceptible to absorption of steroids.
- The use of occlusive dressings over the steroid (especially polythene).

Potency of some topical steroids (UK classification and nomenclature)

Group	Approved name	Proprietary name
I (very potent)	Clobetasol propionate	Dermovate®
	Diflucortolone valerate 0.3%	Nerisone forte®
II (potent)	Triamcinolone acetonide	Adcortyl®
	Betamethasone valerate 0.1%	Betnovate®
	Betamethasone dipropionate	Diprosone®
	Beclomethasone dipropionate	Propaderm®
	Fluocinolone acetonide 0.025%	Synalar®
	Fluocinonide	Metosyn®
	Hydrocortisone 17-butyrate	Locoid®
	Mometasone furoate	Elocon®
	Fluticasone propionate	Cutivate®
III (moderately potent)	Flurandrenolone	Haelan®
	Desoxymethasone	Stiedex®
	Fluocinolone acetonide 0.00625%	Synalar 1:4®
	Clobetasone butyrate	Eumovate®
	Alclometasone dipropionate	Modrasone®
	Betamethasone valerate 0.025%	Betnovate R.D.®
IV (mild)	Hydrocortisone 1%	various
	Hydrocortisone 2.5%	various
	Fluocinolone acetonide 0.0025%	Synalar 1:10®

Fig. 2.13 *Potency of some common topical steroids (UK classification and nomenclature).*

Thus, topical corticosteroids need to be treated with respect. For acute episodes, it is safe to use high-potency agents for a short period of time. For longer-term treatment, however, care must be taken to minimize the amount and the strength of the agent(s) applied as far as possible — always bearing in mind that it is of no use whatsoever if no improvement follows.

TOPICAL IMMUNOMODULATORS

Two agents that modulate immune function after topical application have been introduced are primarily for the treatment of atopic dermatitis: tacrolimus and pimecrolimus. Both exert their effect predominantly by calcineurin inhibition, which alters T cell reactivity. They have both been shown to be effective in atopic dermatitis, and successful use in other disorders is being reported. They have the obvious advantage of not being corticosteroids and therefore avoiding steroid side-effects, notably cutaneous atrophy. Some rather crude animal data suggests that there might be an increased risk of UV-induced carcinogenesis, but there is no evidence of this in humans to date.

RETINOIC ACID

Retinoic acid, a topical derivative of vitamin A, has been used for many years in the treatment of acne. More recently it has been shown that regular use can reduce facial wrinkles. They have also been used with some success in psoriasis.

VITAMIN D ANALOGUES

Vitamin D analogues are relatively new, but have quickly found an important place in the management of plaque psoriasis. Reports of improvement have also been recorded in other hyperkeratotic disorders such as pityriasis rubra pilaris, ichthyosis, porokeratosis and epidermal naevi.

DIPHENCYPRONE

There are good studies that have shown that the application of agents that induce an allergic contact dermatitis can encourage regrowth in alopecia areata, although the percentage who derive persisting benefit is small. Diphencyprone appears to have replaced some of the earlier alternatives because it is safer (not oncogenic) and is not found in normal everyday life.

ULTRAVIOLET RADIATION (PHOTOTHERAPY AND PHOTOCHEMOTHERAPY)

Dermatologists have been using various forms of light treatment for years in the management of psoriasis, eczema and vitiligo. The range of conditions for which various regimens are used has increased significantly over the last few years and now includes, paradoxically, some of the photodermatoses. The addition of a psoralen, a chemical that interacts with DNA in the presence of long-wave ultraviolet (UVA) radiation, has resulted in greater efficacy for some patients. However, there are risks: ultraviolet radiation is carcinogenic.

X IRRADIATION

Although once used for chronic inflammatory dermatoses, X irradiation is now reserved for neoplastic disorders.

METHOTREXATE

Methotrexate is a folic acid antagonist and was first developed as an anticancer drug. Its use in severe psoriasis is well-established, where it is one of the most reliable agents available. The drug is associated with some side effects, notably marrow suppression and liver fibrosis, but these can generally be avoided if patients are monitored properly. Avoidance of alcohol and awareness of drug reactions is important.

DAPSONE

Dapsone is used extensively as a first-line agent in leprosy. It also has important effects on several other diseases with no apparent common features (apart, perhaps, from the pathological involvement of polymorphs): dermatitis herpetiformis, vasculitis, acne, and relapsing polychondritis.

ORAL RETINOIDS

There are two vitamin A derivatives that are useful when taken orally. Acitretin (which is replacing, or has replaced, etretinate) is used in the ichthyoses, Darier's disease, and other disorders where keratinization is abnormal. Psoriasis often responds well and a combination of oral retinoids and ultraviolet B phototherapy is widely used for severe disease. Isotretinoin is very commonly prescribed for severe acne. Both drugs cause the skin to become rather 'dry' and give rise to a characteristic cheilitis. They both also raise lipid levels and can cause hepatitis, although this is rare. There has been much debate about the risks of depression with isotretinoin use. The consensus is that, although this may be a rare complication, much of the reported psychological disturbance is not drug-related.

IMMUNOMODULATORS

A number of systemic immunomodulators have been used for treating skin disease: azathioprine, hydroxycarbamide (hydroxyurea), ciclosporin, cyclophosphamide, mycophenylate mofetil. Azathioprine and ciclosporin have certainly stood the test of time. Their side-effect profile restricts their use to severe skin disorders. Agents such as mycophenolate mofetil and fumaric acid esters are still being assessed.

MONOCLONAL ANTIBODIES (BIOLOGICS)

The latest breed of immune modulator is a range of agents genetically engineered to target specific molecule or receptors involved in inflammation. At the time of going to press, two have become fairly widely used: infliximab and etanercept — both used in psoriasis with or without arthropathy. Many others are in the pipeline.

CURETTAGE AND CAUTERY/DIATHERMY

In curettage and cautery/diathermy, the skin is anaesthetized and a curette used to scrape the lesion away. The bleeding from the raw, oozy base is then stopped by gentle diathermy or hyfrecation.

EXCISION

The technique for excision is essentially the same as for an incisional biopsy except, of course, that the ellipse passes around the whole lesion (**Fig. 2.14**). It is important to give any tumour a wide enough margin to be sure of complete excision.

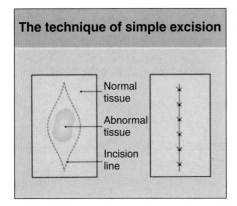

The technique of simple excision

Normal tissue

Abnormal tissue

Incision line

Fig. 2.14 *The technique of simple excision.*

- In the use of topical agents for skin treatment apply the old 'rule of thumb': if the skin is 'dry', use an ointment; if it is 'wet and weepy', use a cream.
- Treat topical steroids with respect.
- Use high-potency agents for a short period of time in acute episodes.
- Use with care in longer-term treatment and minimize the amount and the strength of the agent(s) applied as far as possible.
- UV is a well-proven treatment for psoriasis, vitiligo and an increasing range of conditions but there are risks.

PSYCHOLOGICAL ASPECTS OF THE DERMATOLOGICAL CONSULTATION

The dermatologist should also be aware that skin disease has a major impact on the well-being of the patient, both physically and psychologically. Patients cannot easily work with severe hand or foot dermatitis. Severe itch can disrupt sleeping and, therefore, the rest of life completely. Patients with skin disease find it equally difficult to cope in society as those with visible skin blemishes or deviations from the 'norm'. This is true for acne, facial eczema, psoriasis and other inflammatory dermatoses on the hands, vitiligo (especially in pigmented skins), hair loss, port-wine stains, hand warts, nail dystrophies, and many other disorders. It is not easy to form close personal relationships when your skin is covered in scaly, red patches or you scratch so much at times that you bleed. Quality of life surveys indicate that chronic skin disease may be as socially and physically disabling as diabetes and heart disease.

The dermatologist must therefore show, by his or her actions, that this is understood and that there is no need to apologize for seeking help because of issues of this kind. Touching the skin is a critical part of the consultation. Offering opportunities for the patient to discuss the affected areas is also important. Not everyone will accept the chance the first time, and there need to be other occasions when the opening is made. It may be necessary to point out to accompanying friends and family the misery that skin disease can cause.

In short, patients with skin disease invariably feel better when they know that you know a little of how they feel.

chapter 3

Cutaneous Infections

INTRODUCTION

The skin is prone to many infections, and may reflect the presence of infectious agents elsewhere. Many factors influence the ease and frequency with which infection may penetrate the skin:
- The prevalence of the infecting organism in the environment.
- The virulence of the infecting organism.
- The presence of appropriate environmental conditions.
- The state of the skin — skin that is already damaged is more prone to infection.
- The immunocompetence of the individual.

Worldwide, skin infection probably causes more discomfort and disability than any other disease process. It can also be life-threatening.

BACTERIAL INFECTIONS

STAPHYLOCOCCI

The ubiquitous staphylococcus is ever-present on the skin surface: *Staphylococcus epidermidis* is a normal commensal. True infection generally only occurs when the pathogenic *Staphylococcus aureus* invades the skin, although this organism, too, may be carried as a harmless passenger by many healthy people. However, such a carriage state usually only involves certain sites, such as the nasal passages. An exception to this is the skin of patients with atopic eczema (*see* Chapter 5) and some other scaly disorders, where *S. aureus* multiplies and survives on the skin surface.

The treatment of such *S. aureus* infections varies according to the severity and extent. If systemic antibiotics are required, they must be active against *S. aureus*, which is notorious for its ability to develop resistance. Methicillin resistant *Staph. Aureus* (MRSA) is the most serious example. It is therefore good practice to send appropriate samples for culture and sensitivity-testing to a range of antibiotics. Topical agents such as mupiricin and fusidic acid, or even simple antiseptics, may be sufficient for localized or minor infections.

Staphylococci are responsible for several different clinical infections, including folliculitis, furuncles, carbuncles, impetigo, and the 'staphylococcal scalded-skin syndrome'.

Folliculitis

In folliculitis, small aggregations of organism develop in the superficial part of the hair follicle (**Fig. 3.1**). This is very common on the buttocks and thighs. Treatment is not always required, but antibiotics and topical antiseptic washes are sometimes needed.

> ## Box 3.1 Common staphylococci skin infections
>
> **Folliculitis**
> Infection of superficial part of hair follicle.
> **Furuncles**
> Deeper and more substantial infection of a hair follicle with red, tender lesions.
> **Carbuncles**
> Deeper infection in follicle forming an indurated, red mass in which the centre may
> break down, leaving a sizeable hole.
> **Impetigo**
> Superficial skin infection of outer epidermis due to staphylococci and/or streptococci.

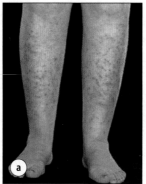 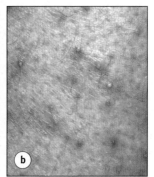

Fig. 3.1 Folliculitis — (a) *Follicular pustules on the legs of a woman.* **(b)** *Close-up of the same patient.*

Furuncles (boils)

Furuncles comprise a deeper and more substantial involvement of a hair follicle (**Fig. 3.2**). Lesions are usually red and tender and begin to 'point' after a day or so. The content of the pustule discharges and the area heals over, sometimes leaving a small scar. Treatment depends on the frequency and severity, but most lesions will settle with simple oral antibiotics and local antisepsis. Older-fashioned remedies include magnesium sulphate paste to encourage drainage. Large boils may need lancing to reduce the acute discomfort they can cause. Some people develop crops of boils that recur over months and years. Occasionally, this may be a presenting feature of diabetes, but patients are usually entirely well. Investigations of immune status are generally unrewarding, although very occasionally some specific bacterial killing defect may be identified (as, for example, in chronic granulomatous disease — *see* Chapter 11). In most patients, however, it would appear that the skin simply seems receptive to a strain of *S. aureus* that is pathogenic to the individual concerned. Empirically, these patients are probably best managed by a long-term course of antibiotics together with an antiseptic skin scrub. The tendency often disappears in time.

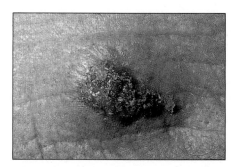

Fig. 3.2 *Furuncle, or boil, on the forehead.*

Carbuncles

Carbuncles represent an even deeper and more extensive infection of hair follicles. Several adjacent pilosebaceous units are involved and a large, indurated, red mass develops. After a few days, several 'heads' appear, discharging pus. The centre may break down, leaving a sizeable hole. Carbuncles generally occur in the elderly, the ill, in patients with diabetes, and in patients on systemic steroids. Systemic antibiotics are needed and a search for underlying systemic problems should be undertaken.

Impetigo

Impetigo is a much more superficial infection, the organism remaining within the outer layers of the epidermis. Impetigo is more common in children than in adults, particularly in temperate climates. It is, however, extremely common in countries where people live in crowded and unhygienic conditions.

- Infection occurs frequently on the head and neck, although any area of the body may be affected.
- Often complicates other skin disorders, notably eczema and ectoparasite infections.
- Lesions are classically round or oval, beginning as small pustular areas which rapidly extend.
- Superficial bulla may remain intact or may rupture, leaving an oozy surface covered in honey-coloured crusts (**Fig. 3.3**).

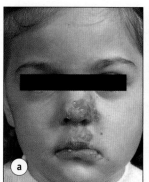
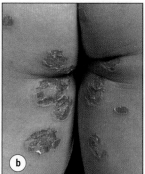
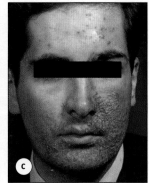

Fig. 3.3 *Impetigo — (a) bullae and crusts on the face of a child; (b) annular lesions on the buttocks and thighs; (c) extensive 'golden' crusts on the face.*

Impetigo is highly contagious and is spread easily from site to site, and from person to person. Very rarely, an outbreak may occur in neonates in intensive care facilities. This situation (pemphigus neonatorum) can be devastating, with a high mortality rate. Topical treatment may be adequate for very limited disease, but systemic antistaphylococcal antibiotics are indicated in most cases. Usually, a degree of isolation is also a good idea, to avoid the infection spreading. Impetigo heals without scars, but may leave temporary discolouration.

Secondary staphylococcal infection (impetiginization) is also very common, particularly in association with the eczemas, when superimposed on viral infections (e.g. herpes simplex), and in cutaneous ectoparasite infections such as scabies and head lice.

The 'staphylococcal scalded-skin syndrome'

The 'staphylococcal scalded-skin syndrome' is extremely rare. A specific group of staphylococci appear capable of producing a toxin that causes the epidermis to cleave through the granular cell layer. Sheets of skin peel away, producing an appearance resembling that seen with a severe burn from boiling water (hence the name — **Fig. 3.4**). Adequate treatment with antibiotics, probably parenterally, is required. As important is good general nursing and metabolic support, without which the outcome is not nearly as successful.

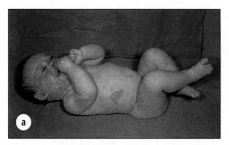 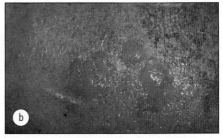

Fig. 3.4 *Epidermolysis due to staphylococcal infection (staphylococcal scalded-skin syndrome) — **(a)** an affected child; **(b)** close-up.*

- Staphylococcus is present on the skin surface as a normal commensal (*Staphylococcus epidermis*).
- Skin infection generally occurs with the pathogenic *Staphylococcus aureus*.
- Treatment of such *S. aureus* infections varies according to the severity and extent and systemic antibiotics must be active against *S. aureus* which can develop resistance.
- Send appropriate samples for culture and sensitivity-testing to a range of antibiotics.
- Topical agents such as mupirocin and fusidic acid, or even simple antiseptics, may be sufficient for localized or minor infections.
- Staphylococci are responsible for several different clinical infections, including folliculitis, furuncles, carbuncles, impetigo, and the 'staphylococcal scalded-skin syndrome'.

STREPTOCOCCI

Unlike staphylococci, the Gram-positive organisms streptococci are not normally carried on the skin surface. Most infections are due to the species known as the b-haemolytic streptococcus (or *Streptococcus pyogenes*). The bacteria can spread easily through the dermis and subcutis because the organism produces enzymes that destroy the continuity of connective tissue. Fortunately, streptococci remain sensitive to penicillin, but it is often necessary to administer the drug parenterally to obtain adequate tissue levels, especially in the first day or two of treatment.

Streptococci are involved in several important infections of the skin and subcutaneous tissues, including impetigo, scarlet fever and scarlatina, erysipelas and cellulitis, necrotizing fasciitis, perianal 'cellulitis', and secondary immunological reactions.

Box 3.2 Common streptococci infections

Impetigo
Superficial skin infection of outer epidermis due to staphylococci and/or streptococci.
Erysipelas
Acute infection of dermis by *Strep. Pyogenes*.
Cellulitis
Acute *Strep. pyogenes* infection of dermis extending into subcutaneous fat.
Necrotizing fasciitis
Dangerous streptococcal infection extending beyond the subcutis and into the fascia and underlying muscle.

Impetigo

In many parts of the world, streptococci can be cultured from impetigo lesions (*see* page 37), although this is rare in the United Kingdom. The condition behaves in the same manner irrespective of which organism is the primary infecting agent, and treatment principles are the same.

Scarlet fever and scarlatina

Some strains of streptococci produce toxins that induce a widespread erythema. The illness caused by these organisms is generally less severe nowadays than it was in the past, perhaps because a different toxin is now responsible. The disease usually begins with a high fever, vomiting, and an acute pharyngitis. Sometimes the portal of entry of the organism is an infected wound. The tonsils are classically bright red and swollen, and whitish stippling is seen on the palate. The tongue is coated with white fur initially, but this peels off to leave a colour and appearance, classically described as 'strawberry tongue'. A day or so later, a punctate, lobster-red rash develops on the neck and evolves downwards to involve the whole body. There is a degree of follicular prominence throughout the active phase. Subsequently, the skin peels and desquamates.

Erysipelas and cellulitis

Erysipelas and cellulitis are most commonly seen on the head and neck (**Fig. 3.5a**) or on the leg (**Fig. 3.5b**). Some authorities differentiate these two states, but the difference lies only in the depth of the infection: in erysipelas only the dermis is involved, while in cellulitis the

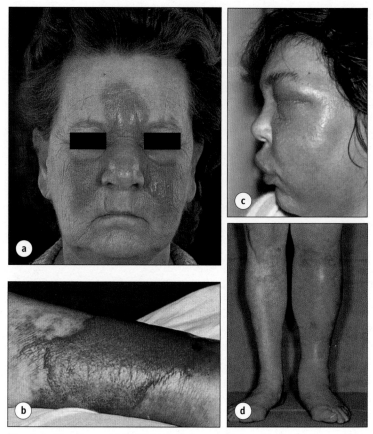

Fig. 3.5 *Streptococcal infections:* **(a)** *erysipelas on the face;* **(b)** *erysipelas on the leg;* **(c)** *cellulitis of the face;* **(d)** *cellulitis of the leg.*

infection spreads deeper into subcutaneous fat (**Fig. 3.5c and d**). In practice, the fat is involved in most instances when infection occurs in a fatty area. On the head and neck, where subcutaneous fat is less prominent, 'pure' erysipelas is more common. The streptococcal organisms require a portal of entry. These may be breaches in the skin (e.g. leg ulcers, eczema, tinea pedis) or deeper infections of sinuses or the middle ear. Besides having the local symptoms and signs of pain, redness, and heat, patients are often pyrexial and unwell. Septicaemia may occur. Swabs are of no value, but blood cultures may yield the organism. However, treatment should not wait until the results are known but be instituted as soon as the diagnosis is suspected. Ideally this should be with high doses of parenteral penicillin, flucloxacillin, or a suitable alternative in the penicillin-allergic patient. After a few days, the patient can be transferred on to oral medication.

Necrotizing fasciitis

Necrotizing fasciitis is a highly dangerous state which most commonly occurs when streptococcal infection extends beyond the subcutis and into the fascia and underlying muscle. Other aerobes and anaerobes may be involved. Massive necrosis results in rapid and widespread tissue destruction, septicaemia, and, often, death. Urgent surgical debridement of all infected tissue, together with high doses of intravenous antibiotics and general support, is the only hope of cure.

Perianal streptococcal dermatitis (Fig. 3.6)
Previously called *perianal cellulitis*, bright red, shiny skin around the anal area is accompanied by pain or itching. This is most commonly seen in children and responds well to penicillin, erythromycin, or a cephalosporin. There are several reports of this entity being a precursor to guttate psoriasis.

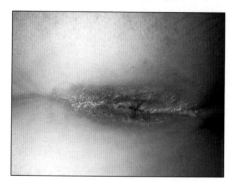

Fig. 3.6 *Perianal streptococcal cellulitis.*

Secondary phenomena
Streptococci are associated with a number of immunological reactions that may follow an initial infection. These may result in important skin changes such as erythema nodosum, leucocytoclastic vasculitis, and the erythema marginatum of rheumatic fever.

- Streptococci are not normally carried on the skin surface.
- Streptococci are sensitive to penicillin; often administered parenterally in the first day or two of treatment.
- Streptococci are involved in several important skin infections including impetigo, scarlet fever and scarlatina, erysipelas and cellulitis, necrotizing fasciitis, perianal 'cellulitis', and secondary immunological reactions.
- Necrotizing fasciitis is a highly dangerous state which most commonly occurs when streptococcal infection extends beyond the subcutis and into the fascia and underlying muscle.

'MINOR' BACTERIAL INFECTIONS
- Erythrasma — an infection of flexures and toe-webs caused by the organism *Corynebacterium minutissimum* (**Fig. 3.7a**). The areas are usually brownish and slightly scaly, and are frequently asymptomatic. Examination under Wood's light reveals a highly characteristic coral-pink fluorescence (**Fig. 3.7b**). Treatment with topical azole creams or systemic erythromycin is usually effective.

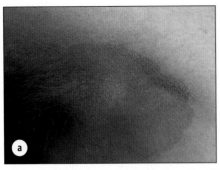 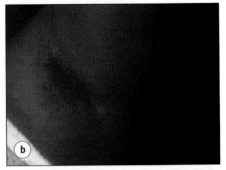

Fig. 3.7 *Erythrasma — (a) of the axilla; (b) showing coral-pink fluorescence under Wood's light.*

- Trichomycosis axillaris — the name given to the beaded appearance of axillary hair caused by infection with various species of *Corynebacterium* (including *C. tenuis*).
- Erysipeloides — caught from direct inoculation, usually involving food and animal carcasses, especially pigs. The infecting organism is *Erysipelothrix insidiosa*. This generally causes a mild, erysipelas-like infection, beginning around the inoculation site. Occasionally, more widespread lesions develop, and systemic involvement has been reported. Treatment with penicillin, erythromycin, or a cephalosporin is usually curative within a few days.
- Keratolysis plantare sulcatum (pitted keratolysis) — a common condition that is frequently overlooked, dismissed, or misdiagnosed as mosaic viral warts (*see* page 58). The characteristic clinical features include an unpleasant and pungent foot odour, hyperhidrosis of the sole or soles involved, and a thickened plantar horny layer. Multiple pits or depressions are visible within the thickened areas (**Fig. 3.8**) — these are more easily seen after the feet have been immersed in water for a few minutes. It is these that both give the condition its name and lead to the diagnostic confusion with verrucas.

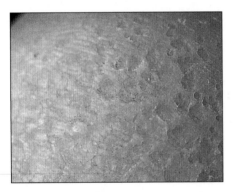

Fig. 3.8 *The characteristic plantar pits seen in pitted keratolysis.*

GRAM-NEGATIVE BACTERIAL INFECTIONS

Occasionally the skin and subcutaneous tissues are invaded by Gram-negative organisms such as *Escherichia coli*, *Proteus* spp., and *Pseudomonas* spp. The resulting cellulitis can be very destructive. For correct treatment, a diagnosis must be made, usually from tissue or blood cultures, so that antibiotics to which the organism is sensitive can be deployed.

CLOSTRIDIAL INFECTIONS

Dirty wounds may become infected with many bacteria, but the impact of the anaerobic Gram-positive bacilli *Clostridia* can be particularly devastating. One, *Clostridia tetani*, is, of course, responsible for tetanus. Others, including *Clostridia perfringens*, are implicated in gas gangrene, in which severe subcutaneous necrosis spreads out from the initial wound site. There is an accompanying systemic toxic state, and crepitus due to gas formation is apparent on palpation. As with necrotizing fasciitis, the immediate need is for wide debridement and high-dose parenteral antibiotic therapy, usually including penicillin in a cocktail to cover other potential complicating organisms.

MIXED BACTERIAL INFECTIONS

More often than is sometimes suspected, two or more organisms are involved in an infective process. Secondary bacterial colonization of viral and ectoparasite infections has already been mentioned, but there are two important situations where two or more different bacteria appear to be involved in skin infections: ecthyma and synergistic gangrene.

Ecthyma

Ecthyma is generally seen only in the malnourished. Deep necrotic ulcers develop, often on the lower limbs (**Fig. 3.9**), and yield a mixed bacterial flora on culture. Such lesions need to be differentiated from other causes of lower-leg ulceration and from some forms of nodular vasculitis/panniculitis such as erythema induratum (Bazin's disease — *see* cutaneous tuberculosis on page 48). A biopsy may, therefore, be required. Treatment involves adequate, broad-spectrum antibiotics and better nutrition. Lesions often heal to leave scars.

Synergistic gangrene

In synergistic gangrene, two micro-organisms (aerophilic micrococci and *S. aureus*), acting synergistically, produce a rapidly spreading necrotic area, frequently around a wound. The major differential diagnosis is severe pyoderma gangrenosum. Cultures should be taken in

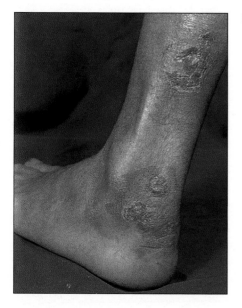

Fig. 3.9 *Ecthyma (gangrenosum).*

all cases and therapy commenced with intravenous antibiotics. Surgical debridement may also be indicated.

THE SKIN IN SYSTEMIC BACTERIAL INFECTION

Meningococcal infection
The meningococcus is a highly virulent organism that causes a severe and progressive meningitis, and septicaemia. One of the consequences of the latter is disseminated intravascular coagulation, which leads to a highly characteristic eruption consisting of rapidly spreading purpura. This clinical sign should alert any clinician to the impending disaster that may befall the patient if adequate investigation and urgent treatment are not instituted.

Gonococcal infection
Gonococcal infection occasionally results in systemic features, including an arthritis and an eruption of papulopustules.

LYME DISEASE (AND ERYTHEMA CHRONICUM MIGRANS)

Box 3.3

Lyme disease
Multisystem disorder caused by the spirochaete *Borrelia burgdorferi* which is transmitted to humans by bites of the tick *Ixodes*.

Lyme disease is important to the dermatologist in that most patients develop an eruption known as erythema chronicum migrans. A pink or red ring begins to spread out from the initial tick bite, usually some days later. The involved skin may be macular or, more commonly, elevated at the active edge. There may be some scaling. The lesion eventually becomes static and fades, but may last for up to a year. Patients also develop a variety of systemic manifestations, including arthritis, neurological disorders, and myocarditis.

Much later in the course of the disease, the skin may also be affected by a change known as acrodermatitis chronica atrophicans, in which atrophic plaques appear over the hands, feet, knees, and elbows. This is rarely seen outside Europe.

If Lyme disease is suspected, blood should be taken for serological screening. The treatment of choice is one of a range of antibiotics, of which amoxicillin (amoxycillin) and the tetracyclines are probably the best. The treatment should be given as early as possible, before dissemination of the organisms has proceeded too far.

There has been some debate about a possible aetiological role of *B. burgdorferi* in morphoea (*see* Chapter 8).

MYCOBACTERIAL INFECTIONS
Mycobacteria are an important cause of death and disability worldwide. Invasion of the skin occurs in:
• Cutaneous tuberculosis.
• Leprosy (Hansen's disease).
• Atypical mycobacterial infections.

Cutaneous tuberculosis

The cutaneous signs associated with active tuberculous infection are many and varied. They were also well known to ancient physicians, because of the high prevalence of tuberculosis in general during those times. Consequently, there is a fine array of dermatological terms that can be applied to the different clinical presentations. A complementary approach is to consider the route by which the changes have arisen. To some extent, the two 'systems' can usefully be used together (Fig. 3.10) to give a greater understanding of the nature and implications of the disease.

Lupus vulgaris — Lupus vulgaris is probably the most common clinical pattern of active tuberculous skin infection seen in clinical practice. As indicated in Figure 3.10, lesions may arise as a consequence of direct inoculation, in which case the site is determined by the point of contact with the bacilli, by haematogenous or lymphatic spread. Most of the cases of lupus vulgaris seen in Europe probably arise by the latter route.

- Area of predilection is the head and neck, especially around the nose and ears.
- Initial lesion often a small, rather nondescript papule or plaque (Fig. 3.11a) but as time passes the area gradually spreads to produce more definitive clinical changes: most commonly, a plaque of reddish-brown, infiltrated skin (Fig. 3.11b).
- Surface is frequently slightly scaly, and there may be textural irregularity due to areas of fibrosis within the plaque.
- Diascopy (pressure over the area with a glass slide) reveals the classical 'apple-jelly' nodules, especially at the edge.
- May be considerable tissue distortion due to fibrosis and scarring, particularly if the process affects the nose or ears (Fig. 3.11c).
- Lesions of lupus vulgaris occasionally ulcerate, particularly with mucosal involvement commonly occurring by direct extension.
- Lupus vulgaris slowly extends if left untreated, leaving a variable degree of scarring in its wake.
- Fibrosis may lead to considerable distortion and deformity, and this probably accounts for the appellation 'lupus' being given to this disease in ancient times.
- Squamous cell carcinomas may develop in old areas of lupus vulgaris.

Warty tuberculosis (tuberculosis verrucosa cutis) — Warty tuberculosis arises from direct inoculation of the micro-organisms into the skin of a patient who has previously been exposed to the organism, usually by another route. In the past, this was a problem for anatomy students, doctors, and autopsy technicians (hence another alternative name: 'prosector's wart'). A warty papule develops at the site of entry and, if left, extends to produce a verrucous plaque (Fig. 3.12). Common sites include the hands, feet, and buttocks (from sitting on infected material). The disease is also said to result from auto-inoculation in patients already suffering from pulmonary disease.

Orificial tuberculosis (tuberculosis cutis orificialis) — Orificial tuberculosis is rare. It occurs in patients with severe systemic disease of the upper or lower respiratory tract, or with gut or genitourinary involvement. Nodules and ulcers develop around the mouth, anus, or external genitalia.

Cutaneous disorders recognized as being due to tuberculosis

Lesions due to the active presence of tubercle bacilli

Clinical presentation	Route of inoculation/spread/pathogenesis
Lupus vulgaris	Inoculation from exogenous source haematogenous spread, lymphatic spread, direct extension from endogenous source.
Warty tuberculosis	Inoculation from exogenous source †auto-inoculation.
Tuberculous chancre	Inoculation from exogenous source.
Scrofuloderma	Direct extension from endogenous source.
Orificial tuberculosis	Spread from endogenous source, with auto-inoculation.
Miliary tuberculosis	Haematogenous spread.
Tuberculous gumma	Haematogenous spread.

Lesions due to tuberculosis but where tubercle bacilli are not directly involved

Clinical presentation	Pathogenesis
The tuberculides: Papulonecrotic tuberculide Lichen scrofulosorum Erythema induratum (Bazin's disease) Erythema nodosum † this is uncertain	Hypersensitivity phenomen.

Fig. 3.10 *Cutaneous disorders recognized as being due to tuberculosis.*

Scrofuloderma — In scrofuloderma — a rather more common form of involvement — an area of skin overlying a tuberculous lymph node or an infected bone or joint usually becomes red and infiltrated (**Fig. 3.13**) before breaking down to produce ulceration and sinuses. There is often surprisingly little discomfort despite quite extensive tissue breakdown. The areas heal with considerable fibrosis and scarring.

Tuberculous chancre — Tuberculous chancre is rare and only occurs when tubercle bacilli are inoculated into the skin of someone who has not been exposed before. In other words, this is the cutaneous equivalent of the pulmonary 'Gohn focus'. Clinically, lesions consist of ulcers with undermined, ragged edges. The draining lymph nodes may be enlarged. Most tuberculous chancres heal in time, but some progress to become a patch of lupus vulgaris.

Miliary tuberculosis — In miliary tuberculosis, which is extremely rare, a widespread papular or vesiculopustular rash develops. The patient is nearly always a child and is unwell.

Tuberculous gumma — In tuberculous gumma, another very rare form of cutaneous tuberculosis, the lesion (it is usually solitary) consists of a nodule or fluctuant mass that can arise anywhere, although the limbs are the most common site. Eventually, the skin breaks down to leave an indolent, ulcerated area.

Investigation and treatment of lesions directly due to tubercle bacilli — There are three main routes of investigation in these circumstances:
• Samples should be obtained for histology.
• Samples should be obtained for culture.
• A search should be undertaken to locate systemic infection.

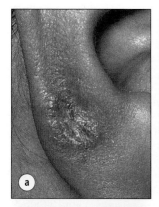

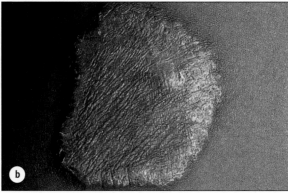

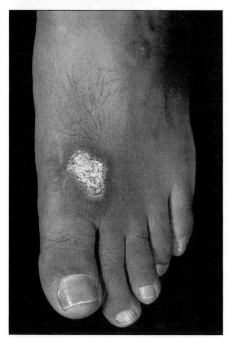

Fig. 3.11 *Lupus vulgaris* — *(a)* a small, early area; *(b)* a larger, later area; *(c)* scarring and loss of tissue in lupus vulgaris of the ear.

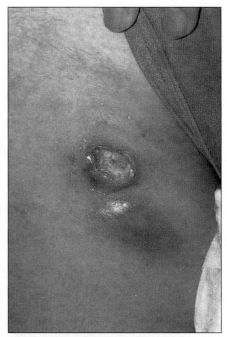

Fig. 3.13 *Scrofuloderma.* Cutaneous extension from underlying tuberculous lymph nodes.

Fig. 3.12 *An area of warty tuberculosis.*

In lupus vulgaris the histology is that of a tuberculous granuloma, without caseation in most instances. Other forms of cutaneous tuberculosis may show more caseation and necrosis, especially when the patient's level of immunity is lowered. Acid-alcohol-fast bacilli are almost invariably present. These may be numerous in some form of cutaneous tuberculosis, but are surprisingly infrequent in lupus vulgaris. They are usually present, nevertheless, and can be found if specimens are examined with care. DNA can also be identified in histological samples by polymerase chain reaction (PCR).

Deeper-seated infection may be found in many sites: lungs, gut, urinary tract, bone, and lymph nodes. Often, however, there is no obvious systemic involvement.

Treatment of all forms of tuberculosis consists in giving appropriate antituberculous chemotherapy. Nowadays, this generally involves a combination of agents: rifampicin, isoniazid, ethambutol, and pyrazinamide are the most commonly used. It is wise to discuss the patient's treatment with a physician experienced in treating systemic tuberculosis.

The 'tuberculides' — The 'tuberculides' comprise rather curious eruptions that are believed to be the result of tuberculosis of internal organs. The skin lesions do not contain bacilli — and none can be grown on culture — but invariably clear with antituberculous treatment.

Papulonecrotic tuberculide — In papulonecrotic tuberculide, recurrent, firm, dull-red papules develop, particularly over the lower legs, elbows and knees. These may break down to leave small punched-out ulcers which may linger for weeks. Occasionally, lesions involving digits have resulted in gangrene and significant loss of tissue. Lesions may occasionally be seen with erythema induratum.

Lichen scrofulosorum — Lichen scrofulosorum manifests when a patient with bony or glandular tuberculosis, and a high degree of immunity, develops a flat-topped papular eruption. Histology reveals neat tuberculous granulomas. The eruption disappears with appropriate treatment.

Erythema induratum (of Bazin) — In erythema induratum, deep-seated nodules develop, especially on the calves. These tend to wax and wane, but, frequently, gradually become more fixed and break down to leave ulcers (**Fig. 3.14**). The histology of these areas tends to

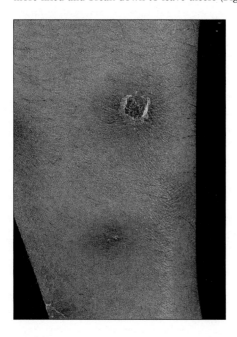

Fig. 3.14 *Erythema induratum (of Bazin).*

be that of a nodular vasculitis (*see also* Chapter 8), but often with typical tuberculoid granulomas in some parts of the specimen. As with the other 'tuberculides', the lesions clear relatively rapidly with antituberculous chemotherapy.

Erythema nodosum — This is dealt with in Chapter 8. Tuberculosis is rarely the cause in western countries.

Leprosy (Hansen's disease)

Leprosy is endemic in many parts of the developing world, especially Africa, India, South-East Asia, and Central and South America. Cases are also seen in southern Europe, the Middle East, and the southern USA. Infection was at one time prevalent in northern Europe, but is now only seen here in immigrants from endemic areas.

Box 3.4

Leprosy
Extremely destructive infection caused by direct skin contact with the bacterium *Mycobacterium leprae*.

Clinical features — The clinical expression of the disease is largely due to the interplay between the organism and the immunity of the host. This concept has led to the subclassification of the condition into five broad categories: lepromatous (LL), borderline lepromatous (BL), borderline (BB), borderline tuberculoid (BT), and tuberculoid (TT). At the extreme ends (or 'poles') of the spectrum, cell-mediated immunity to *M. leprae* is either virtually absent (LL) or good (TT). BL, BB, and BT reflect levels of immunity between these points. There is a corresponding inverse relationship between the level of immunity and the presence of bacilli in the lesions. In TT and BT leprosy, there are few bacilli ('paucibacillary'), whereas the lepromatous end (LL, BL) of the spectrum is also sometimes referred to as 'multibacillary'.

M. leprae has a predilection for nervous tissue and the skin. The organism can also disseminate by haematogenous spread and, particularly in lepromatous disease, may involve the eyes, ears, facial skin, hands, feet, testes, bones and superficial muscles. Such extensive invasion results in a disorder that can produce severe disability. Also recognized are 'reaction' states which may complicate the clinical picture.

Generally, the infection begins with direct contact of *M. leprae* on the skin surface — the combination of poor hygiene, crowded housing conditions, and the prevalence of patients with LL (who excrete organisms from their nasal passages) provides the conditions for infection in most instances. This contact may result in a rather nondescript patch of slightly pale or numb skin ('indeterminate' leprosy), or pass unnoticed. As indicated previously, the next phase of the condition depends on the host's level of immunity to the infecting organism. This may, to some extent, have a hereditary component, but it is likely that other factors, such as nutrition and the presence or absence of other diseases, are more important determinants.

In TT leprosy, the patient presents with a few patches of cutaneous infiltration and evidence of nerve damage. Typically, there is a plaque of slightly scaly, thickened skin (**Fig. 3.15**) in which sensory impairment is almost always demonstrable. Indeed, the area may be entirely without sensation, but partial loss is more common, and temperature appreciation is often the first modality to be lost. It is also often possible to feel thickening of adjacent nerves. These may be palpable branches of cutaneous nerves close to individual lesions, or complete nerve trunks. The lesions are often significantly hypopigmented.

In LL, the picture is entirely different. Quite often the patient suffers with symptoms related to the involvement of other organs before cutaneous lesions are evident. In particular, many patients complain of nasal stuffiness and discharge at an early stage in their disease. When skin lesions appear, they are generally multiple, poorly defined, and may be macular or palpable, occasionally exhibiting a mild degree of hypopigmentation and occasionally mild erythema (**Fig. 3.16**). The lesions can appear anywhere, but favour 'cooler' sites such as the arms, legs, face, and buttocks. They are rarely seen in the scalp. The surface may be normal to the touch or rather shiny, but there is no scaling as seen in tuberculoid lesions. Sensation is usually normal in the first instance. Occasionally, large areas of the dermis become diffusely infiltrated.

As the disease progresses, lesions become more diffuse and thickened. This is particularly striking on the face, where the skin often takes on a so-called leonine appearance. The nasal mucosa may perforate.

In essence, the borderline forms of leprosy (BT, BB, and BL) represent stages on a spectrum of clinical features between the two polar extremes. Lesions are more numerous in BL (**Fig. 3.17a**) than in BB or BT (**Fig. 3.17b**) disease, and nerve damage is correspondingly variable. The importance of recognizing these subcategories is increased by the fact that they are potentially unstable — lesions may 'upgrade' towards the tuberculoid end of the spectrum, or 'downgrade' towards the lepromatous end. Such alterations in the pattern of the disease may be associated with immunological alteration and with treatment.

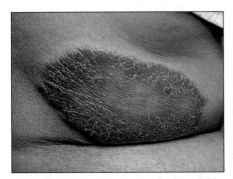

Fig. 3.15 *Leprosy.* *A plaque of tuberculoid leprosy (TT) (courtesy of Dr P E Hutchinson).*

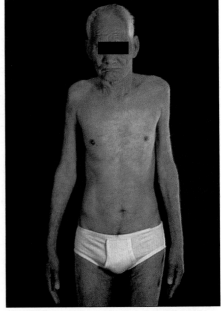

Fig. 3.16 *Leprosy.* *Leonine facies in lepromatous leprosy (LL) (courtesy of Dr P E Hutchinson).*

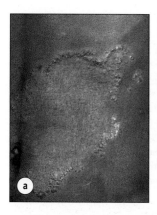
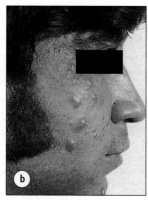

Fig. 3.17 *Leprosy —* *(a)* *borderline lepromatous (BL) (courtesy of Dr P E Hutchinson);* *(b)* *borderline tuberculoid (BT).*

The clinical picture may also be obscured by the so-called leprosy (or lepra) reactions. In type-1 lepra reactions, a patient with borderline disease suddenly develops new lesions and, often, older lesions also become more inflamed and uncomfortable. This may happen entirely unexpectedly, but quite commonly follows the commencement of therapy. The inflammation can cause increased nerve damage.

Type-2 lepra reactions are only seen in patients with LL or BL disease, and appear to be due to a vasculitic response to dead *M. leprae.* The most common manifestation is erythema nodosum leprosum (ENL) (which, despite its name, should never be confused with erythema nodosum) (*see* **Fig. 3.18**). Multiple red nodules develop in the skin, especially on the face and limbs. The individual lesions are smaller than those seen in

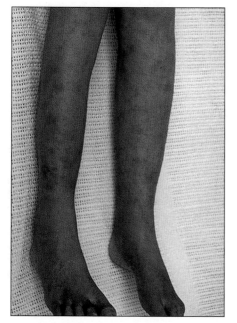

Fig. 3.18 *Leprosy.* *Erythema nodosum leprosum (ENL) (Courtesy of Dr P E Hutchinson).*

'ordinary' erythema nodosum, and the lesions do not fade through the colours of a bruise in the same way. Type-2 reactions may also affect the eye and nerves, and the patient is often febrile and unwell.

Nerve involvement is clearly one of the most important aspects of this disease. In general, nerve damage becomes more and more prominent in all forms of leprosy if they are left untreated, although the ravages are worse towards the lepromatous end of the spectrum. Peripheral nerves are severely damaged, resulting in gross loss of sensation to affected areas, including the eyes. As the disease progresses, autonomic and motor functions are also impaired, resulting in loss of sweating, hand deformities, and wrist and foot drop.

In addition to repetitive trauma due to sensory deficits, bony changes are seen in the phalanges. As a consequence, the hands and feet may become severely deformed (**Fig. 3.19**). Patients are frequently very disabled by leprosy.

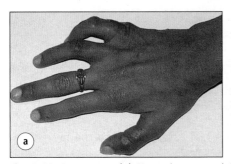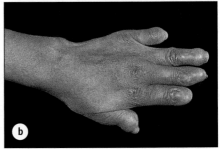

Fig. 3.19 *Leprosy* — *(a) Nerve damage and **(b)** auto-amputation of digits (courtesy of Dr P E Hutchinson).*

Investigations and treatment — The most important single investigation in the diagnosis and assessment of leprosy is of its histology, which varies considerably between the various categories. In essence, TT disease has a granulomatous pathology with inflammation particularly centred on the neurovascular bundles, while in LL the dermis and subcutis is replaced by an infiltrate of foamy macrophages with lymphocytes and plasma cells. In LL, BL, and BB leprosy, it is possible to find organisms on slit-skin smears. In this technique, a superficial wound is made in the lobe of the ear. Scrapes from the surface are placed on a microscope slide and stained with modified Ziehl–Neelsen. Similarly, nasal scrapes may reveal organisms in patients with LL.

Leprosy can now be treated effectively. In patients with paucibacillary disease, the usual regimen is a combination of daily dapsone and once-monthly rifampicin for 6–12 months. In multibacillary disease, clofazimine is added and treatment is continued for at least 2 years. Lepra reactions may also need therapy. Type-1 reactions usually respond to oral prednisolone, but courses occasionally need to be given over remarkably long periods. Type-2 reactions may respond to thalidomide or oral steroids.

As important as chemotherapy is, there is also a need for this to be combined with good physiotherapy and measures to prevent ongoing traumatic damage to the hands, feet and eyes.

Atypical mycobacterial infections

Occasionally, the skin may be invaded by other mycobacteria. The most common of these is *M. marinum*, which is acquired from swimming pools or fish tanks. Cutaneous infections have also rarely been described with a number of other organisms, including *M. ulcerans*, *M. kansasii*, *M. avium*, *M. fortuitum*, and *M. chelonae*.

Fish-tank (or swimming-pool) granuloma

Box 3.5

Fish-tank granuloma
Infection of the skin with *M. marinum*, usually presenting as a nodule over the site of inoculation.

Although obviously varying from case to case, possibly the most frequent site is the dorsum of the hand, or the finger. Subsequently, further lesions appear along the line of the lymphatic drainage of the area involved (**Fig. 3.20**), in what is sometimes described as 'sporotrichoid' spread (owing to the similarity to the expansion of lesions in sporotrichosis — *see* page 85). Individual lesions are typically erythematous nodules, but they may break down and ulcerate. Usually, lesions resolve spontaneously after a few months, but new lesions can continue to appear for up to 3 years. Most, if not all, patients with lesions on the hands and arms keep fish and may have been noticeably unwell. Others will often give a history of minor abrasions while swimming.

The diagnosis can usually be confirmed by biopsy for histology and culture. Histologically, there may be tuberculoid granulomas, but, more typically, there is a rather non-specific inflammatory infiltrate. Organisms can sometimes be seen on direct microscopy. It is essential that the personnel in the microbiology laboratory are warned about the suspected organism because its growth is poor under standard culture conditions at 37°C. The organism needs to be incubated at 30–33°C. Treatment should not, however, rely on unequivocal laboratory confirmation but be initiated on clinical grounds. In truth, it is not always necessary to treat the infection actively, because spontaneous resolution is the rule, but patients usually want to see something active being done. There are reports of reasonable responses to rifampicin, co-trimoxazole and minocycline. The drug should be given for about 6 weeks.

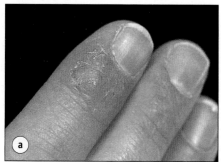

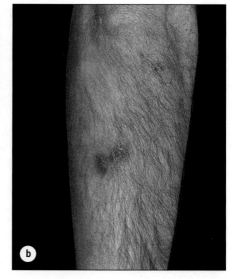

Fig. 3.20 *Fish tank granuloma.* *Lesions on the finger (**a**), and others (**b**), following the line of lymph nodes up the arm ('sporotrichoid spread').*

SYPHILIS AND OTHER TREPONEMAL INFECTIONS

Box 3.6

Syphilis
Infection of skin by *Treponema pallidum* presenting to the dermatologist in a variety of ways:
- primary chancre
- eruption during the 'secondary' phase
- one of a number of late manifestations
- in congenital infection.

Primary syphilis

In primary syphilis, chancres typically present as indurated painless ulcers. The most common sites are the male and female genitalia, the cervix, the anus and rectum, and the lips and mouth. This phase of the infection often passes unnoticed in women.

Secondary syphilis

Most patients develop the secondary stage of the disease about 2–3 months after initial exposure. There may be an early macular eruption, but this is often either absent or missed. Patients may feel unwell, spike a mild fever, and often develop widespread lymphadenopathy. The dermatologist may be consulted because of the eruption that accompanies these systemic symptoms and signs. This is notoriously variable in its overall appearance, but is said always to be symmetrical and non-itchy. The rash most commonly consists of a shower of reddish-brown, scaly papules. Lesions classically appear across the forehead (**Fig. 3.21a**), where they are known as the corona veneris. Lesions also occur on the palms and soles (**Fig. 3.21b**). Lesions are also frequently found in the anogenital area, where the soft, moist papules known as condylomata lata appear (**Fig. 3.21c**), and in the

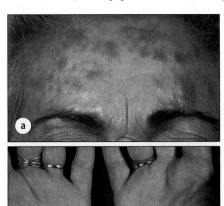

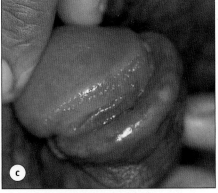

Fig. 3.21 *Secondary syphilis —*
(a) 'corona verneris'; (b) a typical lesion on the palm; (c) condylomata lata.

mouth, causing snail-track ulcers. However, as mentioned previously, the appearance of the cutaneous eruption may be quite variable, resembling pityriasis rosea, psoriasis, or lichen planus. Hypopigmentation may occur in dark skins. It is important to keep a high degree of suspicion in order to diagnose syphilis.

Late syphilis

If the early phases of the disease pass untreated, and if the patient manages to survive for a long time without courses of penicillin or other antibiotics, late syphilis may develop. Skin lesions are usually of two kinds: infiltrated granulomatous nodules (**Fig. 3.22**) and ulcerative gummas.

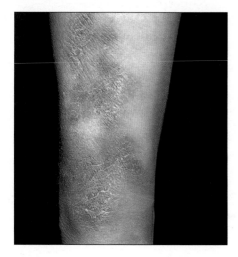

Fig. 3.22 *Tertiary syphilis. Infiltrated granulomatous areas on the lower leg.*

Congenital syphilis

Cutaneous infiltration is reported to be a common feature in congenital syphilis, and the child often also has significant systemic involvement, including hepatosplenomegaly, and eye and neurological damage.

Investigation and treatment

Syphilis serology should be requested for any patient in whom the disorder is suspected. Treatment consists in giving antibiotics, preferably penicillin by injection. If the patient is allergic to penicillin, tetracyclines or erythromycin are generally satisfactory alternatives. Patients should also be screened for other sexually transmitted diseases, and there is a case for HIV testing, especially in those with high-risk sexual behaviour. In the USA, the UK, and those countries where dermatology and genitourinary medicine are practised separately, the patient should be referred to the appropriate department for his or her management.

Other treponemal infections

Yaws and pinta are infections seen only in tropical regions of the world. Yaws is found along a band straddling the equator through South America, Africa, and Asia, whereas pinta is exclusively a disorder of Central and South America.

Yaws is predominantly a disease of childhood and, like syphilis, has several stages. Initially, there is a localized, infiltrative, and often ulcerative, lesion at the site of entry of the organism. Later, multiple papules develop and enlarge to become oozing masses that are said to resemble raspberries ('framboeisiform'). These are known as daughter yaws. Later still, ulcers, nodules, and hyperkeratotic skin lesions accompany bone and joint involvement.

Pinta derives its name from the pigmentary anomalies that are commonly seen in the later stages of the disease. Early lesions are erythematous; however, as the disease progresses, pigmentary changes become increasingly prominent, particularly a loss of pigment, which may closely resemble vitiligo. There is a predilection for the knees and elbows.

- Disseminated intravascular coagulation leading to rapidly spreading purpura is an important clinical sign of meningococcal infection (bacterial meningitis).
- Lyme disease consists of multi-system disorders caused by the spirochaete *Borrelia burgdorferi* transmitted by tick bite and characterized by the skin eruption erythema chronicum migrans.
- Mycobacterial infection of the skin occurs in cutaneous tuberculosis, leprosy (Hansen's disease) and other atypical conditions such as fish-tank granuloma.
- Lupus vulgaris is probably the most common clinical pattern of active tuberculous skin infection seen in clinical practice.
- Syphilis is a relatively rare treponemal infection which presents with a range of dermatological manifestations depending on stage but typically with a primary chancre.

VIRAL INFECTIONS

WARTS (HUMAN PAPILLOMAVIRUS INFECTIONS)

DNA hybridization has revealed that there are over 50 different 'types' within the human papillomavirus (HPV) family, not all of which are associated with simple skin infections (**Fig. 3.23**). Some appear to be relatively site-specific; others are associated with different clinical patterns. Importantly, too, some HPV types can induce dysplastic and neoplastic change in the skin, cervix, and other epithelia.

Box 3.7

Viral warts
Among the most common skin lesions seen in clinical practice and are due to infection of the skin with one of a number of DNA viruses known as human papilloma viruses (HPV).

Clinical disease patterns and most commonly associated types of human papilloma virus (HPV)	
Disease pattern	**HPV type(s)**
Common warts	1, 2, 4, 7*, 26–29
Plantar warts	1, 4
Mosaic plantar warts	2
Plane warts	2, 3, 10, 41
Genital warts	6, 11, 16, 18, 31, 32, 42–44, 51–55
Cervical dysplasia/neoplasia	16, 18, 31–33, 35, 39, 42, 51–54
Penile dysplasia (including bowenoid papulosis)	16, 18, 31, 32, 34, 39, 42, 48, 51–54
Dysplasia/neoplasia of vulva	16
Dysplasia/neoplasia of anus	6, 11, 16
Dysplasia/neoplasia of mouth	16
Laryngeal papillomas/neoplasia	6, 11, 30, 43, 44, 55
Epidermodysplasia verruciformis and/or keratoacanthomas	5, 8, 9, 12, 14, 15, 17, 19–25, 36–38, 46, 47, 49, 50
	*in meat handlers

Fig. 3.23 *Clinical disease patterns and most-commonly associated types of human papillomavirus (HPV).*

Common warts, plantar warts

Warts may occur at any age, although they are most prevalent in childhood and adolescence. As many as 10% of children may be infected at any one time. This high prevalence means that their clinical appearances are well known to parents, schoolteachers, family doctors, and dermatologists alike (**Fig. 3.24**). There may be one or many. The hands and feet are the most customary sites, with those on the plantar surface often being called verrucas. Common viral warts can, however, occur virtually anywhere. They may be especially troublesome around the nails and on the soles, where they may be painful or interfere with normal function.

Warts may arise, or be spread, as a consequence of trauma (the Koebner phenomenon — *see* **Fig. 3.24d**). Indeed, it is thought that most are acquired as a result of minor cuts and abrasions while exposed to viral particles, especially in communal areas. One notorious site where this is thought to happen is the swimming pool, but sports changing-room floors and similar surfaces are probably also implicated. Trauma to the warts themselves (e.g. by picking or nibbling hand warts, or by shaving facial warts) may also help to spread them.

Very rarely, plantar warts may progress to the very slow-growing, but invasive, carcinoma cuniculatum (*see* Chapter 4). If there is any diagnostic doubt about a warty lesion on the foot, a biopsy should be taken, although even this may be hard to interpret.

Warts are not always as easily treated as patients may expect. Although there are a number of techniques that appear to increase the clearance rate, the results are often disappointing and are certainly not as rapid as many would wish. For example, wart paints — containing salicylic acid, formalin, glutaraldehyde, and other agents — require close attention to a daily regimen for several weeks, and patience with this soon wanes unless immediate visible gains are achieved. Cryotherapy (freezing, usually with liquid nitrogen) works well for smaller, elevated warts, but is not as effective at dealing with deep plantar warts and can be excruciatingly painful. Since common warts resolve spontaneously over

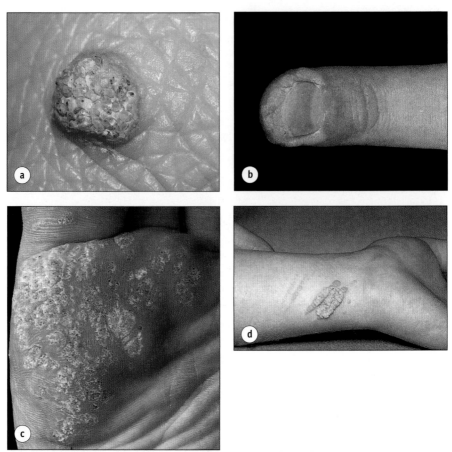

Fig. 3.24 Warts — **(a)** close up of a wart; **(b)** viral warts affecting the nails; **(c)** mosaic warts on the sole; **(d)** viral warts arising in scratches (the Koebner phenomenon).

time, it may be reasonable to leave them completely alone unless they are causing significant symptoms or functional impairment. This is especially true in smaller children. If more aggressive therapy is necessary, however, there is a wide range from which to choose: curettage, CO_2 laser, contact sensitization, intralesional bleomycin, interferons, oral retinoids, and radiotherapy. All of these have been used with apparent success. Certain doctors still use the age-old technique of 'wart-charming' as well. Some control over very widespread wart infections can be achieved by the use of the oral retinoid acitretin.

Plane warts

Plane warts sometimes give rise to diagnostic difficulty. They are also a therapeutic problem, particularly when they occur on the face (**Fig. 3.25**), because they respond poorly to cryotherapy and most of the simple painting techniques are inappropriate on facial skin. Although they do resolve eventually, usually after a few days of sudden redness and inflammation around the warts, they sometimes last for years.

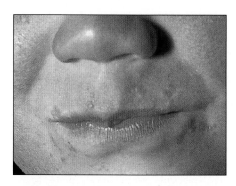

Fig. 3.25 *Plane warts on the face of a child.*

Anogenital warts (condylomata acuminata) and their complications

Warts of the anogenital area are extremely common (Fig. 3.26). Many, but not all, are sexually transmitted, apparently at a very high rate. Indeed, some authors suggest that all sexual contacts of a patient with a genital wart infection should be assumed to be infected too, even if this is not clinically apparent.

The clinical appearances are quite variable, but commonly lesions are flat, rather moist-looking papules or plaques or filiform projections. Occasionally, lesions become so large and numerous as to create cauliflower-like masses which interfere with normal functions (*see* Fig. 3.26b). This may occur on the vulva during pregnancy.

Some lesions are very difficult to see with the naked eye, and the use of dilute acetic acid solution will highlight many previously invisible infected areas. In women, the problem is

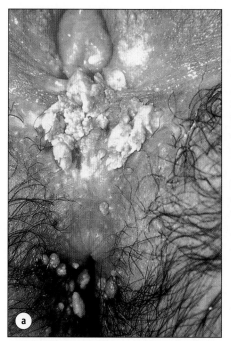

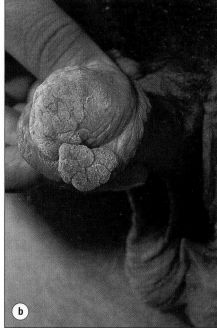

Fig. 3.26 *Viral warts* — *(a)* *around the anus (condyloma acuminata); (b)* *a large mass on the penis.*

compounded by the fact that infection may be intravaginal or present only on the cervix, hence a proper examination should include colposcopy wherever possible. Furthermore, some patients with genital warts also have other sexually transmitted infections. It is therefore our view that anogenital wart infection should generally be managed by experts in genitourinary medicine or by gynaecologists. Treatment will normally involve some form of destructive technique such as cryotherapy, diathermy, or snipping under local or general anaesthesia, but painting with podophyllin also works well for lesions of relatively limited extent. More recently imiquimod has been found highly effective. The agent appears to work by stimulating interferon gamma production. It is less useful for common warts, although variants undergoing trial at present may be more effective.

As indicated in Figure 3.23, some of the HPV types associated with genital warts are also capable of inducing dysplastic and neoplastic changes in cervical, vulval, and penile epithelia. There are several clinical forms of this, some of which may present to the dermatologist:

- Vulval intraepithelial neoplasia — biopsies of lesions reveal marked dysplasia. This group of conditions needs treatment and gynaecological follow-up.
- Cervical dysplasia/neoplasia — women with genital HPV infections should have regular smears and gynaecological follow-up.
- Bowenoid papulosis (**Fig. 3.27**; *see also* Fig. 4.20, p. 120) — flat-topped lesions (often with a degree of hyperpigmentation) appear on genital and perigenital areas and may be confused with melanocytic naevi or seborrhoeic keratoses. The histology shows relatively mild dysplasia. Lesions rarely progress to invasive malignancy.
- Penile Bowen's disease and squamous cell carcinoma (*see* Chapter 4).
- Bushke–Lowenstein carcinoma — a rare form of wart-virus-induced carcinoma seen on the penis. It is slow-growing and rarely, if ever, metastasizes.

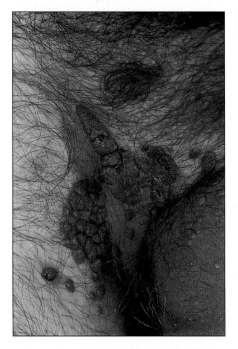

Fig. 3.27 *Bowenoid papulosis (see also* **Fig. 4.20***).*

Anogenital warts are also seen in children. Apart from the implications that this may have if the HPV type is one of those associated with dysplastic or neoplastic changes, it is important to bear in mind the possible source of such infections. In very small babies, it seems likely that this is usually due to direct transmission from the mother during birth. In others, it may occur as a result of transfer of non-genital HPV strains from hand warts. However, wart viruses can be transmitted sexually in children too, and childhood sexual abuse should always be considered as a possibility. Referral to an appropriately qualified paediatrician may be necessary.

Epidermodysplasia verruciformis

Epidermodysplasia verruciformis is a condition in which HPV infection becomes increasingly widespread and in which dysplastic and truly malignant changes occur. The disorder is hereditary and there seem to be both autosomal recessive and X-linked forms. The reason for the apparent lack of control of the proliferation of wart virus in affected individuals is unclear. Defects in cell-mediated immune function have been described in many patients, but these are not consistent. Clinically, warty lesions usually first appear in childhood. They are often rather flat-topped, but may be more verrucous. Lesions persist indefinitely and new ones appear, resulting in a remarkable clinical appearance. Dysplastic changes and squamous carcinomas may develop, especially on light-exposed skin. Patients should therefore be advised about sun exposure. The oral retinoid acitretin may be useful in controlling the extent of the lesions.

MOLLUSCUM CONTAGIOSUM

Molluscum contagiosum is another extremely common superficial skin infection, and, like warts, is most commonly seen in children. The infection is thought to be passed predominantly by direct contact, although the occurrence of outbreaks associated with

- Lesions are highly characteristic: small (5–10 mm), dome-shaped, semi-translucent, pearly papules with a central plug or 'dell' (**Fig. 3.28**); lesions occasionally may be much larger ('giant' mollusca).
- Tendency to form clusters, especially on the upper trunk, around the axillae, in the pubic region, or on the face.
- Background eczematous change may also occur, especially in children with a tendency to atopic disease, in whom the infection seems to be more common and may also be more widespread than usual.

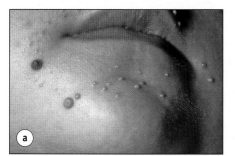
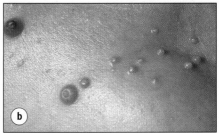

Fig. 3.28 *Molluscum contagiosum — (a) typical cluster of lesions; (b) close-up.*

swimming pools and other communal activities suggests that indirect transmission may also occur.

Infection may last from a few months to several years, but spontaneous resolution invariably occurs. However, lesions may become sore and infected, and parents often urge for some form of treatment. Gentle cryotherapy is probably the most tolerable effective modality, although some dermatologists favour curettage (which may certainly be useful if there is diagnostic doubt) and others opt for the time-honoured remedy of a phenol-impregnated pointed stick. Other options include topical salicylic acid, weak solutions of potassium hydroxide, cantharidin and imiquimod.

- Viral warts result from skin infection by human papilloma viruses (HPV).
- Common warts resolve spontaneously over time.
- Cryotherapy works well for smaller, elevated warts but is less effective with deep plantar warts.
- Anogenital wart infections are generally managed by cryotherapy or other destructive techniques although imiquimod cream is proving useful.
- Molluscum contagiosum is a superficial skin infection seen commonly in children; cryotherapy is the common therapy although lesions will usually remit spontaneously over a period of months.

HERPES INFECTIONS

Herpes simplex virus

There are two antigenic strains of the ubiquitous herpes simplex virus (HSV): HSV1 and HSV2. To some extent, these segregate by site of infection, with HSV2 being particularly common in genital infections, but both strains may occur anywhere. In common with the herpes varicella-zoster virus (*see* pages 64–65), HSV, once acquired, persists in nerve tissue throughout life, and most attacks are not new infection but recrudescences of existing disease. However, active lesions are infectious both to others and to the patient, by direct inoculation of virus-containing material into the skin.

Box 3.8

Herpes simplex
Common acute self-limiting vesicular eruption due to infection with *Herpesvirus hominis* (HSV).

Many patients have no memory of their first contact with the virus, and primary infections may presumably be subclinical. However, some patients develop acute symptomatic infections that can be quite dramatic. One of these is herpetic gingivostomatitis, which is most often encountered in children. The mouth becomes studded with small vesicles that rapidly break to leave ulcers. The child may be constitutionally unwell for a day or two beforehand, and lymphadenopathy is the rule.

The lesions continue to crop for a few days before subsiding. A similar process may affect the genital area when the virus is encountered — by sexual contact — for the first time. Primary infection may also occur by inoculation into other parts of the body, such as the finger ('herpetic whitlow'), or around the eye.

Once infection has been established, the virus shelters in sensory nerve ganglia and only reappears intermittently. HSV2 is more prone to produce recurrent disease, hence genital herpes is more susceptible to this problem. However, wherever the recurrence occurs, the same symptoms and signs are seen. The same area or areas are involved over and over again. The skin often tingles for a few hours before visible changes appear. Initially, the area becomes red and slightly swollen, before vesicles emerge on the surface. After a day or so, these become pustular and then crust over. The lesion eventually settles after about 7–10 days, leaving mild erythema. Sites of predilection are well known — lips and face (**Fig. 3.29a** and **b**), male and female genitalia, and fingers and hands (**Fig. 3.29c**) — but lesions may occur virtually anywhere. Patients also often report that recurrences are easily triggered by minor infections (hence the name 'cold sore'), trauma, or sunlight.

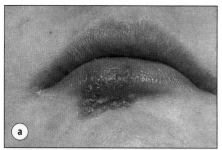

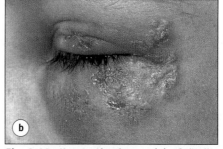

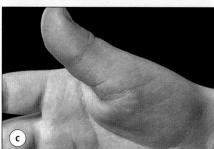

Fig. 3.29 Herpes simplex — **(a)** of the lips (cold sore); **(b)** a nasty infection around the eye — the patient should also be referred for an ophthalmic examination; **(c)** on the right thumb.

Kaposi's varicelliform eruption — Kaposi's varicelliform eruption is a potentially severe form of herpetic infection which occurs in patients with atopic eczema and in some other dermatoses, notably Darier's disease (*see* Chapter 11) and pemphigus foliaceus (*see* Chapter 7). When it occurs in atopic dermatitis, the disorder is often called eczema herpeticum (*see* Chapter 5 and Fig. 5.26, page 192). A patient with one of the susceptible skin conditions develops a shower of vesiculopustular lesions that superficially resemble those seen in chicken-pox. The patient may be systemically unwell, especially when the attack is their first exposure to the virus. There may be a viraemia and a meningoencephalitis.

Investigation and treatment of HSV infections — The diagnosis of recurrent disease is usually evident from the history. However, if there is any doubt, or in dealing with a primary attack, samples may be sent for electron microscopy and culture. It is important to try and obtain fluid from the lesions if possible.

The use of antiviral agents, such as aciclovir (acyclovir), can reduce viral replication and may shorten attacks if applied topically early enough in the course of an attack. In eye infections, idoxuridine is an alternative. Systemic treatment is seldom required unless there are complications, but is essential in Kaposi's varicelliform eruption. However, long-term prophylactic treatment may be indicated for recurrent disease which is occurring frequently or in which the symptoms are very severe.

Herpes varicella-zoster virus

The herpes varicella-zoster virus is the one that causes both chicken-pox and herpes zoster, or shingles. As with HSV, there is an initial infection (in this case chicken-pox), following which the virus rests in a nerve ganglion and re-emerges when conditions result in its reactivation.
Chicken-pox — Chicken-pox is a common infectious disease, with an incubation period of about 14 days. It usually presents with mild prodromal symptoms such as malaise, fever, and headache. Occasionally, the systemic illness is more severe, with a high swinging fever and marked constitutional symptoms (one of the authors suffered this during an attack of chicken-pox at the age of 21 years). A few days into the illness, the eruption appears. Initial lesions are pink papules, but these rapidly become vesicular and then pustular (**Fig. 3.30**),

---

Box 3.9

Chickenpox
Acute self-limiting initial infection by herpes varicella-zoster virus presenting with vesiculopustular eruptions, most commonly in children.

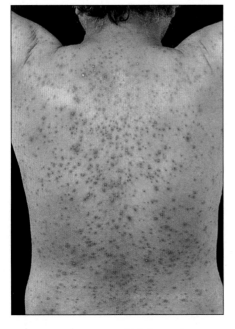

Fig. 3.30 *Chicken-pox — only rarely presents to the dermatology department.*

before a crust forms on the surface. Resolution and healing occur within 3 to 4 days, leaving a pink macule or depression, but further crops of new lesions continue to appear and this may last for several days. Itching may be trivial or very unpleasant. Usually there is no significant scarring, but some lesions may become secondarily infected, which may result in small, permanent 'pock-marks'. The virus can also cause an encephalitis, pneumonia, and thrombocytopenia.

Herpes zoster (shingles) — Herpes zoster represents the re-emergence of the varicella-zoster virus from its resting place in a nerve ganglion. The clinical picture therefore depends on which nerve root is involved. Initially, the patient may only complain of pain or discomfort in the 'to-be-affected' area. However, particularly in younger patients, there may be no pain at all. A few days later (rather more in spinal-nerve zoster than in cranial-nerve disease), an eruption of papules develops. As with chicken-pox, these rapidly become vesiculopustular and crusted. Crops of lesions can continue to appear over a number of days, and follow the line and extent of a single nerve or dermatome (**Fig. 3.31**), or, occasionally, two adjacent dermatomes. Scattered lesions may occur elsewhere as well, but large numbers of disseminated lesions should suggest the possibility of underlying immunosuppression. Healing takes a further week or so, if there are no complications, but can sometimes be significantly slowed by secondary infection and general ill-health in the patient.

Box 3.10

Herpes zoster
Acute self-limiting infection caused by recrudescence of the varicella-zoster virus causing vesiculopustular eruption.

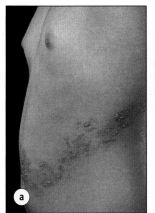 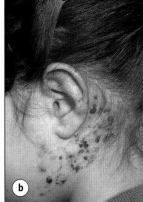

Fig. 3.31 *Shingles* — *(a) affecting a spinal nerve; (b) affecting the mandibular branch of the trigeminal nerve.*

Complications of shingles

Ocular damage may follow lesions in the ophthalmic division of the trigeminal nerve.

Lesions may appear in the mouth in maxillary or mandibular zoster, and facial pain may be confused with other causes, such as sinusitis or toothache.

If the virus originates in the geniculate ganglion, the facial nerve may be involved, leading to a temporary facial palsy (the Ramsay Hunt syndrome). Lesions may also occur in the external auditory meatus, giving rise to earache.

Motor involvement can also occur, leading to ocular palsies. Sacral-root disease can lead to retention of urine and difficulty with defaecation.

There may also be a significant degree of scarring after the resolution of zoster lesions.

Permanent nerve damage is an important complication which can lead to nagging post-herpetic pain and dysaesthesia. Patients may find this extremely distressing, especially with trigeminal nerve involvement.

Occasionally there is such significant alteration of sensation that repetitive trauma may lead to trophic changes in the previously affected area.

Fig. 3.32 *Complications of shingles.*

There are a number of complications that may accompany an acute attack of shingles (**Fig. 3.32**).

Investigation and treatment of varicella-zoster virus infections — Chicken-pox seldom requires active antiviral therapy as the condition is self-limiting, and simple supportive measures are all that should be necessary. Occasionally, however, an attack causes such severe systemic symptoms that aciclovir (acyclovir) may be considered. Furthermore, intravenous therapy is indicated if an encephalitis or pneumonia develops. There is some controversy over whether shingles should routinely be treated with antiviral medication. There is some evidence that a course of aciclovir (acyclovir), or one of the newer agents, may reduce the incidence and severity of postherpetic neuralgia. However, doses need to be high (at least 800 mg five times daily for 7 days) to have any effect at all. If neuralgia occurs, this will need separate attention and often requires careful management by a specialist in pain control.

Other herpes viruses

HHV 8 is the cause of Kaposi's sarcoma (*see* pages 169–170).

HHV 6 and 7 may be associated with pityriasis rosea (*see* pages 224–5).

Epstein–Barr virus (EBV), which is also a herpes virus, is the causative organism of infectious mononucleosis (glandular fever). An exanthematic, morbilliform rash is commonly seen in patients with this infection and almost always develops if the patient is given ampicillin.

EBV is also found in the lesions of oral hairy leucoplakia, which occur in patients with AIDS (*see* page 70).

ORF

Orf is a disorder encountered in those who handle sheep and lambs. The typical lesion is a solitary pustular mass on the hand, at the site of inoculation (**Fig. 3.33**). Lesions may occasionally be multiple. Spontaneous resolution occurs over 4–6 weeks. Orf may trigger an attack of erythema multiforme (*see* Chapter 8).

- Herpes simplex virus (HSV) persists in nerve tissue and most attacks are recrudescences of existing disease.
- HSV lesions may occur anywhere but sites of predilection are well known (lips and face, genitalia, fingers, hands).
- Kaposi's varicelliform eruption is a potentially severe form of HSV infection occurring in patients with atopic eczema and in some other dermatoses.
- Antiviral agents, such as aciclovir, can reduce HSV replication and may shorten attacks.
- Herpes varicella-zoster virus causes both chicken-pox and herpes zoster, or shingles.
- Herpes zoster is due to recrudescence of virus from nerve ganglion.
- Distribution of herpes zoster follows line or extent course of single nerve or dermatome(s); disseminated lesions suggest possible underlying immunosuppression.
- Neuralgia requires careful management by a specialist in pain control.

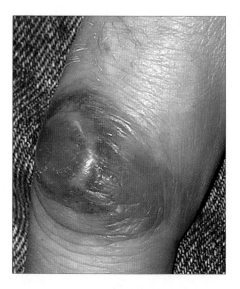

Fig. 3.33 *A lesion of ORF.*

ERYTHEMA INFECTIOSUM ('FIFTH' DISEASE; SLAPPED-CHEEK DISEASE)

Erythema infectiosum is a mild infectious disease caused by parvovirus B19. It occurs in mini-epidemics, usually in the early spring. The typical patient is a child, who suddenly develops hot, swollen, red cheeks (which look as though they have been slapped). A more widespread eruption follows over the succeeding 3–4 days, but this is quite variable in its extent. Older individuals sometimes develop arthralgia as well.

CUTANEOUS MANIFESTATIONS OF SYSTEMIC VIRAL INFECTIONS

There are a number of well-known systemic viral diseases in which cutaneous involvement is a conspicuous component:

- Measles — the rash follows a short prodromal illness in which upper respiratory symptoms, conjunctivitis, and fever predominate. Classically, the rash starts behind the ears on day 4, and spreads to involve the whole body surface. Small punctate lesions appear in the mouth (Koplick's spots). Most patients recover completely, but pneumonia, otitis, and encephalitis may affect some.
- Rubella — a very short illness, there often being little or no prodromal element and the rash often having cleared within 3 or 4 days. Tender lymphadenopathy is common. The major complication is that the virus wreaks havoc in pregnant women, causing severe handicaps in the unborn child.
- Viral hepatitis — rashes are quite common during the early phases of infection with the hepatitis viruses A, B, and C. They may be non-specific, maculopapular eruptions, but urticarial lesions due to an immune-complex-mediated vasculitis also occur. Patients may also, of course, become jaundiced. The Gianotti–Crosti syndrome (see next page) may be triggered by hepatitis B virus.

Coxsackieviruses

Coxsackieviruses can cause a wide range of cutaneous changes, including exanthematic eruptions, the Gianotti–Crosti syndrome (see next page), and hand-foot-and-mouth disease. The exanthems associated with coxsackieviruses are generally mild and non-specific, but some are more florid. One variant causes a striking vesicular eruption, for example.

Hand-foot-and-mouth disease is a common, mild infection, characterized by vesiculopustular lesions in the mouth and along the sides of the fingers and toes (**Fig. 3.34**). The lesions generally clear within a week of the onset.

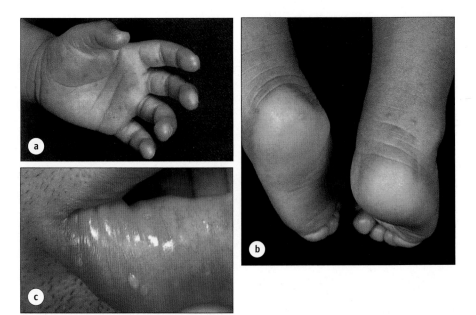

Fig. 3.34 Hand-foot and mouth disease — (a) hand; (b) feet; (c) mouth.

Papular acrodermatitis of Gianotti and Crosti (papular acrodermatitis of childhood)

The classical eruption of Gianotti–Crosti syndrome, an uncommon condition, consists of clusters of red papules on the buttocks, knees (**Fig. 3.35**), and elbows. There may be mild-to-moderate systemic symptoms, and the lymph nodes are often enlarged. The lesions are more persistent than in many virus-induced disorders, often not clearing completely for 2 months. The virus most commonly associated with these changes is the hepatitis B virus, but several other agents also appear to be capable of inducing identical changes.

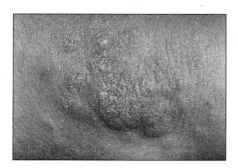

Fig. 3.35 *Papular lesions on the elbows in acrodermatitis.*

Kawasaki disease (mucocutaneous lymph node syndrome)

The cause of Kawasaki disease is still not known, but a virus is suspected. Children develop a fever and cervical lymphadenopathy. The cutaneous changes are striking (**Fig. 3.36**), with an acute erythema of the hands and feet, which peel after a few days. There is also prominent involvement of the mouth and lips, which may become extremely sore and fiery-red. The appearance of the tongue is indistinguishable from that seen in scarlet fever. Later, a more generalized rash may occur. The importance of the disease lies in its ability to damage the heart. Patients may also develop joint problems.

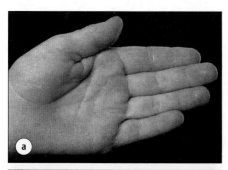

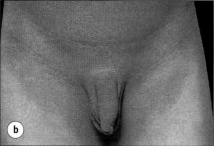

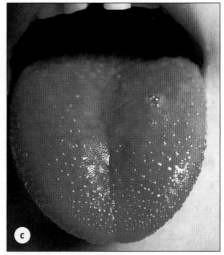

Fig. 3.36 *Kawasaki disease — (a) hand; (b) trunk; (c) tongue in a child.*

CUTANEOUS MANIFESTATIONS OF RETROVIRUS INFECTIONS

Since the first descriptions of AIDS, and the establishment of its cause as infection by the retrovirus HIV, much has been written about the effects of this startling agent. The reader is referred to Penneys NS (1995) Skin Manifestations of Aids, 2nd edition, published by Martin Dunitz Ltd., for a full account. The skin may be involved in many different ways (Fig. 3.37).

Cutaneous manifestations of HIV infection

Xerosis
Drug eruptions
Infections
• Candidiasis, dermatophyte infections, warts, molluscum contagiosum, herpes zoster, recurrent and severe herpes simplex, infections, folliculitis, oral hairy leukoplakia.
Seborrhoeic dermatitis
Psoriasis
• which may appear for the first time or deteriorate.
Kaposi's sarcoma
(*see also* Chapter 4)

Fig. 3.37 *Cutaneous manifestations of HIV infection.*

• Orf is endemic in those who handle sheep and resolves spontaneously but may trigger erythema multiforme.
• Erythema infectiosum (slapped-cheek disease) is a mild viral infection affecting mainly children and presents with hot, swollen and red cheeks.
• Rashes occur in systemic viral infections including measles, rubella and viral hepatitis.
• Kawasaki disease with its characteristic cutaneous manifestations is an important diagnosis due to potential heart damage in children.

FUNGAL INFECTIONS

INTRODUCTION

Fungi are ubiquitous. They are members of the plant kingdom, but are unable to photosynthesize. They generally live a saprophytic existence but are occasionally parasitic on other living organisms.

A number of fungal organisms are capable of inducing disease in humans. Most are only superficially invasive, involving skin alone, but some may cause deeper infections of subcutaneous tissue, bones, and muscle. Occasionally, fungi become much more widespread and infect deeper structures still, especially in the immunocompromised host.

DERMATOPHYTE (RINGWORM) INFECTIONS

The nomenclature associated with these infecting organisms is somewhat circular in that the term 'dermatophyte' is used to describe a group of fungi that cause the infections that are considered together as being 'ringworm'. However, the system works well. In practice, there are three groups (or genera) involved in human ringworm infections: *Microsporum*, *Trichophyton*, and *Epidermophyton*. Although these organisms can induce marked inflammatory responses, they are restricted to the keratin layer of the epidermis, nail plate, or hair shaft.

There are two epidemiological points that are worth noting about ringworm fungi:

- Different organisms within these groups predominate in different parts of the world — for example, scalp ringworm is mostly caused by *Microsporum* spp. in the United Kingdom and Europe, but is more often due to *Trichophyton* spp. in the USA, the Middle East, and Asia. These patterns can change over time: *T. Tonsurans* is now the commonest cause of scalp ringworm in London.
- Some dermatophytes are adapted to living as 'full-time' parasites in humans and are known as anthropophilic; others, more usually found in animals but capable of infecting humans from time to time, are zoophilic; a third group are acquired from soil and are called geophilic. This has obvious implications in the investigation and treatment of an outbreak of ringworm within a family or other social group.

The most widely used subclassification of the dermatophyte infections, however, is based on the region of the body that is affected. The Latin for the appropriate anatomical site has the prefix 'tinea' added, to produce a classically derived term designed largely (or so it seems) to keep the unsuspecting patient in the dark and to maintain dermatological mystique!

Box 3.11 Dermatophyte infections

Tinea capitis
Scalp ringworm.

Tinea barbae
Ringworm of the beard area.

Tinea faciei
Facial infection outside the beard area.

Tinea corporis
Ringworm of the body with annular (circinate) lesions.

Tinea cruris
Ringworm of the leg but generally applied to infection in the groin and on the upper, inner thighs.

Tinea manuum
Ringworm infection of the hand(s).

Tinea pedis
Fungal infections of the feet.

Tinea unguium
Fungal invasion in nails.

'Tinea incongnito'
Ringworm infections with clinical features masked by treatment with topical or systemic steroids.

Tinea capitis

Scalp ringworm is primarily a disorder of children, although the very severe form known as favus may be seen in adults. The clinical picture is essentially one of hair loss with a variable degree of inflammation and scaling, but the features vary greatly. This is partly because of the immune response generated by the organism involved. In general, the zoophilic species tend to cause more inflammation than the anthropophilic ones. However, this is also partly due to the way different infecting organisms invade the hair shafts. For example, *Microsporum canis*, the most common cause of scalp ringworm in white UK residents, is one of a group of fungi in which there is a mixture of invasion and growth over the surface of the hair. This situation (known as ectothrix) results in the hairs breaking part-way along the shaft (**Fig. 3.38**). This organism fluoresces under Wood's light (**Fig. 3.39**). In so-called endothrix infections (largely caused by *Trichophyton* spp.), the organism remains entirely within the hair, which becomes very fragile and tends to break close to its emergence from the scalp. Sometimes there is marked swelling of the hair follicles, resulting in the appearance of black dots across the surface.

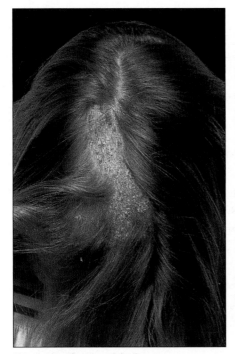

Fig. 3.38 *Tinea capitis due to* **Microsporum canis.**

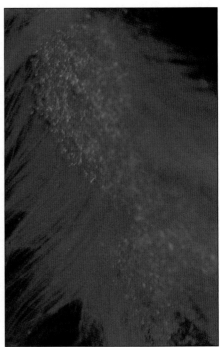

Fig. 3.39 *Fluorescence of* **Microsporum canis.**

Another characteristic change that can occur in scalp ringworm is the development of kerion. In essence, this state is the most severe end of the inflammatory response and therefore occurs mostly with animal ringworm fungi such as *Trichophyton verrucosum* (cattle) or *Trichophyton mentagrophytes* (rodents). The scalp becomes covered with a boggy mass of sinuses (**Fig. 3.40**). The importance of this clinical appearance is two-fold: firstly, it is often misdiagnosed and treated inappropriately; secondly, although the affected

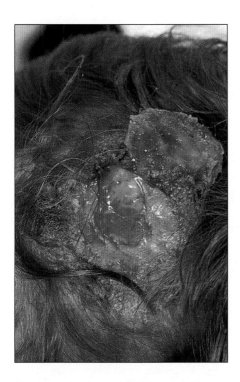

Fig. 3.40 *Kerion in a child.*

areas will respond well to antifungal drugs, hair loss is occasionally permanent, especially if treatment is delayed. This form of scalp ringworm does not fluoresce.

The most severe form of scalp ringworm is favus, in which the scalp becomes covered in matted crusts known as scutula and a scarring alopecia develops. The organism involved is *Trichophyton schoenleinii*, which is found in the Middle East, Pakistan, and some parts of North Africa. Cases have also been reported from South Africa and Australia.

Tinea barbae and tinea faciei

Hair invasion is also seen in ringworm of the beard area (tinea barbae), where a patch or patches of inflammation, sometimes studded with follicular pustules, classically develop (**Fig. 3.41**). This is most often caused by infection with animal-associated species of *Trichophyton* and should therefore be suspected in anyone who has had contact with cattle or other animals. Occasionally, *Trichophyton tonsurans* is responsible, and outbreaks of tinea barbae have been associated with communal shaving arrangements in long-stay hospital patients.

When facial infection is outside the beard area, it is known as tinea faciei. This is frequently misdiagnosed — and therefore mistreated — as some form of eczema (**Fig. 3.42**). Infection may occur by direct inoculation or by extension from ringworm of the scalp, body, or beard.

Tinea corporis

Ringworm of the body may be caused by any dermatophyte. In some instances the infection is an extension of a more localized form covering larger parts of the body, while in others the infection is due to the direct invasion of the skin from an external source such as a cat or other animal (**Fig. 3.43**). Lesions are often annular, or at least have a circinate border (an

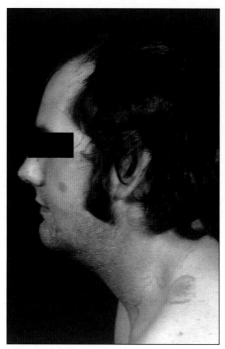

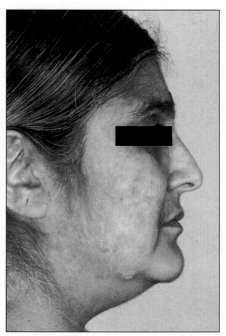

Fig. 3.41 Tinea barbae.

Fig. 3.42 *Tinea faciei.* *This woman's fungal infection had been treated with topical steroids and had spread gradually across her face.*

Fig. 3.43 *Tinea corporis.* *These annular lesions were caused by* Trichophyton mentagrophytes, *caught from laboratory animals.*

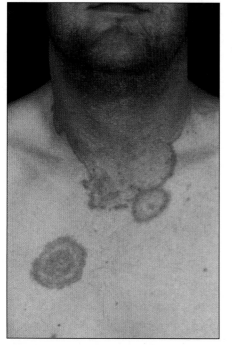

alternative name is tinea circinata). The use of topical steroids may confuse the picture considerably (*see* tinea incognito on page 78).

Tinea cruris

Taken literally, tinea cruris means ringworm of the leg, but the term is generally applied to infection in the groin and on the upper, inner thighs. Typically, the infection causes a scaly red, marginated eruption, which spreads outwards from the groin crease (**Fig. 3.44**) and may extend onto the buttocks and hips. Itching is a common feature. Tinea cruris is much more common in men than in women. The overwhelming majority of cases are due to anthropophilic organisms, particularly *Trichophyton rubrum* and *Epidermophyton floccosum*, which are also frequently implicated in tinea corporis and tinea pedis. Tinea cruris tends to be recurrent, with autoinfection from accompanying disease elsewhere being a factor in this.

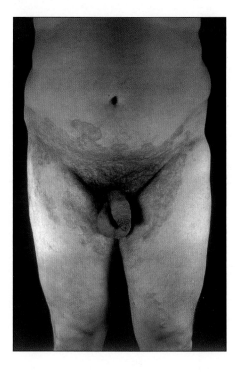

Fig. 3.44 *Extensive tinea cruris spreading onto the thighs and abdominal skin.*

Tinea manuum

There are several clinical patterns associated with ringworm infection of the hand(s), including blisters similar to those seen on the feet (*see* next page), sheeted, red scaly areas on the dorsa of the hand (**Fig. 3.45a**), and more annular or inflammatory lesions involving animal fungi. Perhaps the most striking, and certainly the most common, however, is the dry, scaly, sweatless hand associated with *Trichophyton rubrum* infection (**Fig. 3.45b**). This can be mistaken for eczema. However, it is often unilateral, which would be unusual for an eczema. Furthermore, inspection of the nails will often show changes of fungal invasion.

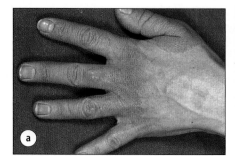
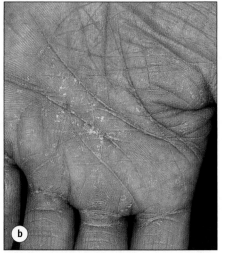

Fig. 3.45 *Tinea manuum* — *(a) there is clearly a demarcated erythematous eruption; (b) the dry, scaly palm caused by infection with* Trichophyton rubrum.

Tinea pedis

Fungal infections of the feet are extremely common. There are three quite distinct forms encountered in clinical practice:

- Toe-web space infection (athlete's foot), in which the interdigital toe clefts become fissured, macerated, and itchy (**Fig. 3.46a**). The fourth or fifth interspace is the most commonly affected, and may be involved alone. The changes frequently recur endlessly, following treatment. It is important to note that infections other than with dermatophytes may be responsible for such changes, including candidiasis and erythrasma. Soft corns (**Fig. 3.46b**) are also commonly misdiagnosed as fungal infections.

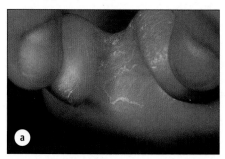
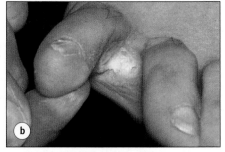

Fig. 3.46 *(a) Tinea pedis. Toe-web disease. (b) Soft corn. Easily confused with tinea pedis.*

- Vesicular patches, particularly on the soles and the sides of the feet (**Fig. 3.47**). These may become widespread and confluent, leading to quite big blisters. The areas are generally extremely itchy. This form of tinea pedis may be associated with a 'dermatophytide' (*see* pages 77, 78–9).

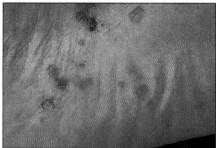
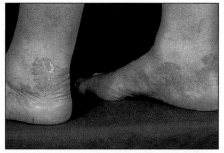

Fig. 3.47 *Vesicular form of tinea pedis.*   Fig. 3.48 *'Moccasin' type of tinea pedis.*

• Dry, scaly changes, which may extend to cover the whole of the sole, and extend up around the sides of the feet to produce a demarcated line (the so-called moccasin pattern — **Fig. 3.48**). The infection may also extend on to the dorsa of the feet and up the back of the leg, and is frequently treated as eczema or psoriasis, leading to 'tinea incognito' (see below). Accompanying nail disease is very common. This pattern is particularly associated with *Trichophyton rubrum* infection.

Tinea unguium

The nails are frequently involved in fungal invasion, but this is most commonly seen in the toenails and in association with chronic or recurrent tinea pedis. Indeed, a reservoir of infection in the nails is an important cause of continued skin infection. One or just a few nail plates may be affected initially, but as time goes on there is a tendency for more to become involved. The nails become thickened and discoloured (**Fig. 3.49**), classically producing a yellowish-brown appearance. There may be a significant degree of subungual hyperkeratosis.

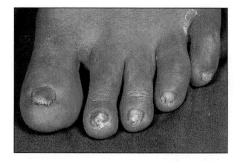

Fig. 3.49 *Tinea unguium.*

'Dermatophytides'

Very occasionally, a fungal infection, particularly of the acute vesicular variety on one or both feet, is associated with a more widespread eczematous eruption or with pompholyx of the hands.

'Tinea incognito'

'Tinea incognito' is the name given to ringworm infections whose clinical features have been modified by treatment with topical or systemic steroids (**Fig. 3.50**). This may occur at any site, but is most commonly seen on the feet and lower legs, or in the groin. Occasionally scalp ringworm is affected in this way. There are some features that should alert one to this possibility:

- A history of initial improvement of a rash with topical steroids, but with subsequent relapse and extension.
- The appearance of persistent follicular nodules and pustules — these are sometimes glorified with the name 'Majocchi's granuloma'.
- The presence of signs of fungal infection in adjacent areas (e.g. tinea cruris or tinea unguium).

Investigation of dermatophyte infections

The easiest way to confirm whether a rash is due to a fungal infection is to take specimens for microscopy and culture. Microscopic examination is simple enough to be performed in an outpatient clinic (**Fig. 3.51**; *see also* Chapter 2).

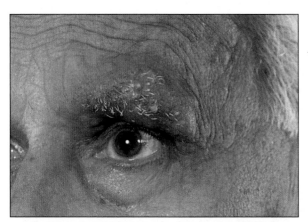

Fig. 3.50 *Tinea incognito.* *This lesion was due to a fungal infection but was treated with a topical steroid.*

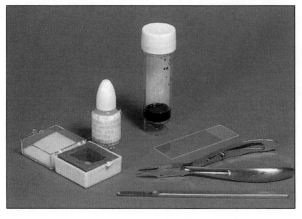

Fig. 3.51 *The equipment required for taking scrapings and clippings for microscopy (the ink is used when looking for Pityrosporum — see page 80).*

Samples should always be taken from:
- The edge of cutaneous ringworm lesions.
- The blister roof of vesicular lesions (using a pair of scissors).
- Both scalp-scale and hair (using forceps if necessary) in suspected scalp ringworm.

If culture is also required (and it may be useful for both practical and epidemiological purposes to know the source of the infection), samples should be sent to a laboratory equipped to grow fungi.

As mentioned on page 72, if scalp ringworm is suspected of being due to *Microsporum canis*, examination under Wood's light may also be helpful.

Treatment of dermatophyte infections

Once a diagnosis of fungal infection has been made, the most important decision is whether it should be treated systemically or with topical treatment alone. As a rule of thumb, systemic therapy is nearly always indicated if:
- Disease involves hair or nails.
- More than one site is involved.
- Lesions are extensive.
- Topical treatment has already failed.
- The diagnosis is 'tinea incognito'.

Therefore, topical treatment is satisfactory only for disease in one site and of limited extent. A number of topical agents are available:
- Benzoic acid compound (Whitfield's ointment) is cheap and old-fashioned, but it works.
- Undecenoate creams.
- Tolnaftate cream.
- Imidazole creams (e.g. clotrimazole, miconazole, econazole, ketoconazole) have for some years been the agents of first choice for most infections; some are available in combination with hydrocortisone, which can help reduce inflammatory symptoms.
- Terbinafine cream is highly effective and possesses some anti-inflammatory properties.
- Tioconazole and amorolfine are available in paints for the treatment of nail disease, if systemic therapy is not tolerated or is otherwise contraindicated.

The systemic therapies currently in use are:
- Griseofulvin, which has been in use for nearly 40 years. It is safe and remains the first choice for children with scalp ringworm, where the dose required is 20 mg/kg/d for 6–8 weeks. The cure rate for nail infections is, however, poor, and treatment must be continued for over a year.
- Imidazoles (ketoconazole, itraconazole, fluconazole) are effective. Ketoconazole induces hepatitis in a small proportion of patients.
- Terbinafine is also effective against virtually all dermatophyte infections, although it is relatively less effective against *M. canis*, where griseofulvin remains the treatment of choice at present.

Terbinafine or one of the imidazoles are now the systemic agents of choice for most situations in adults, unless there are cost problems. Recommended regimens for nail infections vary around the world, but 3 months' treatment at adequate dosage (terbinafine, 250 mg daily; itraconazole, 200 mg daily) is usually satisfactory with either group of agents. Some advocate higher doses over shorter periods or pulsed therapy.

The addition of appropriate antibiotics may also speed up the response when treating a child with kerion. There may be a role for a short course of systemic steroids in the very rare instances of a true dermatophytide and, occasionally, in extremely severe scalp ringworm.

YEAST INFECTIONS

Yeasts are another group of fungi capable of inducing human disease. However, many are also true commensals and only become invasive under certain conditions: for example, *Candida albicans* may only cause 'thrush' when the patient receives a course of broad-spectrum antibiotics. The superficial infection known as pityriasis versicolor and the disease states caused by *Candida* are considered below.

Pityriasis (or tinea) versicolor

Box 3.12

Pityriasis (tinea) versicolor
Very common, superficial fungal infection caused by a species of *Pityrosporum* (reclassified into 7 species), of which *Malassezia furfur* is the responsible type.

Pityriasis (sometimes 'tinea') versicolor is a very common, superficial fungal infection caused by a species of *Pityrosporum*, which has now been reclassified into 7 species, of which the more attractively named *Malassezia furfur* is the responsible type.

The most typical clinical picture is of slightly scaly patches on the upper trunk, upper arms, and neck, although treatment with topical steroids can result in the lesions becoming much more widespread and confluent. In pale skin, the patches appear to be a slightly dirty brown colour (**Fig. 3.52a**), while in skin that is either genetically darker or has been exposed to ultraviolet radiation, the areas are hypopigmented (**Fig. 3.52b**). This has been attributed to the inhibition, by the organism, of normal melanogenesis.

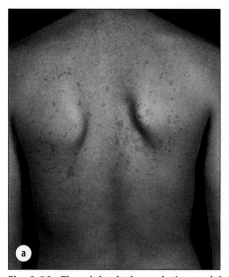
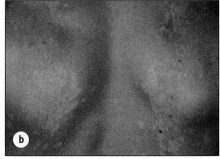

Fig. 3.52 *Tinea/pityriasis versicolor* — *(a)* hyperpigmented areas in pale skin; *(b)* hypopigmented areas in dark skin.

Scrapes from affected skin can be directly examined under the microscope — the addition of a drop of ink to the usual 10% KOH solution reveals a characteristic mixture of yeast-forms and mycelia, graphically compared to 'spaghetti and meatballs'. Initial treatment and clearance is relatively straightforward, but recurrence is common. The organism is sensitive to Whitfield's ointment, selenium sulphide, and the imidazoles. One approach that we have found successful is to combine a topical imidazole cream twice daily, with a daily wash with half-strength selenium sulphide shampoo. If the infection is very widespread, a week's course of oral itraconazole, 200 mg daily, is highly effective. Recurrence may be prevented by using selenium sulphide in the shower from time to time. Patients should also be warned that the hypopigmentation will require longer to resolve and, in fact, may not improve until the skin is exposed once again to sunshine and that it is likely to recur and need periodic treatment.

Malassezia yeasts are also involved in dandruff and seborrhoeic dermatitis, and a form of folliculitis (see Chapter 5).

Candidiasis (candidosis)

Box 3.13

Candidiasis
Disease states resulting from invasion of tissues by one of the yeasts of the *Candida* family — by far the most important of which is *C. albicans*.

Defining the diseased state in candidiasis is sometimes difficult, since *Candida* is found naturally in the mouth or lower intestinal tract in 50–60% of people, and is occasionally a commensal in the normal vagina as well. However, true invasion, with symptoms and signs, may occur in a number of sites:

- Oral — candidal infection in the mouth may be seen at any age, but is most common in children, older adults with dentures, the immunocompromised, and in patients receiving antibiotics or steroids, either orally, by inhalation, or locally to the mouth itself. In the classic form, known as thrush, lesions consist of whitish, creamy patches, which peel off to leave a red, oozy, and bleeding base. This may affect any part of the oropharynx and may extend to involve the upper airways and the oesophagus. Occasionally, candidal infection may leave painful atrophic areas when the more superficial component has apparently cleared. A variant of oral candidal infection produces hypertrophic, keratinized plaques, which may closely resemble malignant or premalignant changes. The diamond-shaped patch — commonly called median rhomboid glossitis — that is sometimes seen on the dorsal surface of the tongue is undoubtedly a variant of this in most instances (**Fig. 3.53a**). *Candida* is also involved in angular stomatitis, although gum resorption and ill-fitting dentures are also important factors in many patients. *Candida* may occasionally produce a hypertrophic, persistent plaque at the corner of the mouth (**Fig. 3.53b**).
- Vulvovaginal — thrush is characterized by a creamy-yellow discharge, erythema, oedema, and itching (**Fig. 3.54**). Lesions may spread onto the surrounding skin, and the perianal area may also be involved. Infection is often recurrent, with some women seeming to be much more prone to infection. The problem is also commoner in

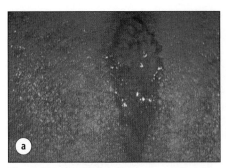
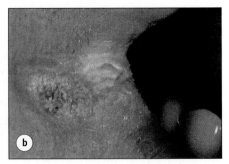

Fig. 3.53 _Candidal infection_ — _**(a)** close up of tongue showing median rhomboid glossitis;_ _**(b)** hypertrophic plaque at the angle of the mouth._

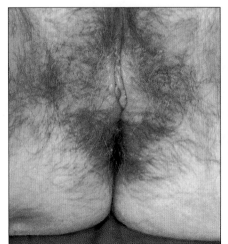

Fig. 3.54 _Vulval candidiasis._

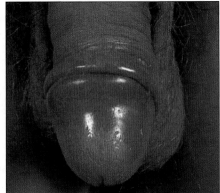

Fig. 3.55 _Candidal balanitis._

pregnancy and in those receiving courses of broad-spectrum antibiotics. Very occasionally, diabetes presents with vulvovaginal candidiasis.

- Penile — candidal balanitis (**Fig. 3.55**) usually occurs in the partner of an infected individual, although oral and anal carriage may be the source in some patients. The glans becomes red and inflamed, with white, cheesy plaques developing on the surface. Some men seem to harbour _Candida_ asymptomatically and may be the source of recurrent infection in their partner.
- Perianal — infection of the perianal skin may occur alone or in association with genital infection, or infection of the groin and scrotum.
- Paronychial (_see_ Chapter 9) — _Candida_ is probably involved, at least as a co-pathogen, in many instances of chronic paronychia.
- Ungal — it is rare for _Candida_ to be the sole cause of primary nail infection, but this can happen. A nail dystrophy is common in chronic paronychia, and, very occasionally, the nail plate may be invaded distally. Involvement of the nails is an important feature of chronic mucocutaneous candidiasis (see below).

- Skin and flexures — *Candida* is an important cause of skin inflammation in intertriginous areas. As indicated on page 76 some 'athlete's foot' is caused by intertriginous candidal infection in toe-web spaces. *Candida* is also frequently isolated from intertrigo in the infra-mammary folds, axillae, and groin, where the presence of small 'satellite' pustules around the edge of the characteristic glazed erythema of intertrigo should raise suspicion. One highly characteristic form of flexural *Candida* infection occurs in the finger-webs (**Fig. 3.56**). It has been given the typically dermatological, but erroneous, name erosio interdigitale blastomycetica!

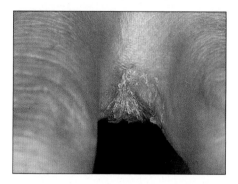

Fig. 3.56 *'Erosio interdigitale blastomycetica'*. Finger-web candidiasis.

- Napkin (diaper) infection — infants and young children are prone to rashes in the napkin area (*see* Chapter 5) and *Candida* is a common secondary invader.

Chronic mucocutaneous candidiasis — Chronic mucocutaneous candidiasis is rare. However, it is important that the diagnosis is made early because there may be significant underlying disease and because treatment is now reasonably effective in controlling the problem. A number of clinical features are seen (**Fig. 3.57**):
- Persistent oral infection.
- Nail invasion and destruction, with or without paronychia.
- Skin involvement by candidal infection. This may occur anywhere on the body surface and may not, at first, be easily recognized as candidal infection unless it is in a typical site.

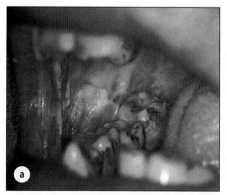
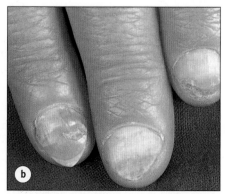

Fig. 3.57 *Chronic mucocutaneous candidiasis* — oral *(a)* and nail *(b)* involvement.

Some patients, especially those with significant immune deficiencies, may present with other infections as well.

Most patients with this disorder present in childhood, although it may also appear for the first time later in life. Many immunological defects have been described and any patient suspected of having chronic mucocutaneous candidiasis will need a thorough immunological review. However, there are also some other important features which should be noted:

- Some childhood-onset disease is genetically determined.
- Some patients have associated endocrinopathies. Two main variants are described: one with failure of the parathyroids and adrenals; one characterized by hypothyroidism. Other endocrine functions may also be affected.
- In adult-onset disease, there may be an associated thymoma, and immune deficiency must be excluded. HIV infection may present as chronic mucocutaneous candidiasis.

Treatment of candidal infections — Topical imidazole creams, combined with pessaries, are effective in genital disease. It is often sensible to treat the partner at the same time. Nystatin is an alternative topical agent and is probably the easiest to use in oral disease, as it is available in a suspension, although some patients may find it easier to suck amphotericin lozenges. Systemically, the imidazoles itraconazole and fluconazole are the drugs of choice, although flucytosine is also effective.

SKIN INFECTIONS CAUSED BY OTHER FUNGI AND MOULDS

There are several other fungi that are occasionally responsible for skin infections and, in some instances, cause changes similar to those seen in dermatophyte infections:

- *Hendersonula toruloidea* is found in the soil of tropical and sub-tropical areas and can infect the nail plate, classically causing dystrophic changes which begin laterally and spread towards the middle of the nail from the edge (**Fig. 3.58**). If this organism is suspected, the laboratory should be warned, because culture must be undertaken using plates without cycloheximide. There are currently no truly effective treatments available.

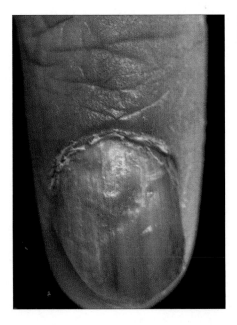

Fig. 3.58 *Nail dystrophy due to infection with Hendersonula.*

- *Scopulariopsis brevicaulis* is a saprophytic mould that is occasionally cultured from dystrophic nail plates.
- *Aspergillus alternaria* and *A. fusarium* may occasionally be isolated from skin scrapings and from nail clippings. These are considered usually to be non-pathogenic, but they may be involved in infections of damaged tissue and may become pathogenic in immunodeficiency states.
- Blastomycosis, coccidioidomycosis, paracoccidioidomycosis, and histoplasmosis are diseases seen in North, Central, and South America. These are primarily systemic infections, especially of the lungs. Skin involvement may occur, however, particularly later in the disease, when the infecting organism becomes widely disseminated. This is more common in immunodeficiency states such as AIDS. Occasionally, erythema nodosum is due to systemic infection with one of the fungi responsible (*see* Chapter 8).
- *Cryptococcus neoformans* is an organism found in bird droppings and can cause a severe meningitis, most typically in immunocompromised states. Skin involvement is rare, but is another infection encountered in AIDS patients.
- *Sporothrix schenckii*, a soil fungus, causes sporotrichosis when inoculated into the skin. This is seen in the Americas, Australia, and parts of Africa. The most common presentation is of ulcerating nodules, which appear to progress steadily upwards along the line of draining lymphatics in a manner simulated by atypical mycobacterial infections (*see* page 52).
- A variety of fungi or higher, branching bacteria cause deep infections, collectively termed mycetoma. These infections may affect any part of the body, although the feet are much the most common site (**Fig. 3.59**). The organisms gain entry by inoculation, but spread deep into subcutaneous tissues, where they invade bone and other structures. The area gradually becomes more and more swollen, indurated, and distorted, and sinuses often develop. Treatment with chemotherapy is relatively disappointing, although some organisms are sensitive to antibiotics and others, at least in theory, are sensitive to ketoconazole. Surgical excision of relatively localized disease may be appropriate.

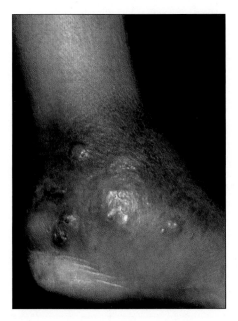

Fig. 3.59 *Mycetoma of the foot* (courtesy of Dr D A Burns).

- Most pathogenic fungal organisms are only superficially invasive, involving skin alone.
- Fungal infections can be especially serious in the immunocompromised.
- Dermatophyte (ringworm) infections can present in the scalp, body, groin, hands, feet and nails.
- Use systemic agents in the treatment of dermatophyte infections if the lesions are extensive or involving more than one site; use topical treatments for disease at a single site or of limited extent.
- Candidiasis is an opportunistic infection of the body folds, mouth, genitals and nails and is more common in immunocompromised patients and others with various predispositions including diabetes.
- Topical imidazole creams or nystatin are effective for most cases of candidiasis

PARASITIC INFECTIONS

Humans, for the most part, live in peace with the arthropods, protozoa, and worms in their environment. However, arthropods may cause disease in a variety of ways, including carrying other organisms (e.g. plague, malaria, leishmaniasis) or by causing allergic reactions (e.g. house-dust mite). Similarly, protozoa and worms may cause a variety of skin problems. This section is predominantly concerned with those situations in which diseases are caused directly by parasites, and which may present to the dermatologist.

FLEAS, LICE, AND OTHER BLOOD-FEEDERS

Many arthropods are adapted to feeding on the blood of homoiothermic creatures: for example, fleas, various mites, lice, bugs, and flying insects such as mosquitoes. The puncture and penetration of the host by the creature often causes little or no significant injury and many people are completely unaware that they have been bitten. However, reactions may occur to chemicals or to insect parts (or to both), either as an irritant or an allergic response. The clinical picture varies with the arthropod concerned and with the site affected.

Fleas

Fleas are small insects that inhabit the dwelling-place of a particular species to which they are adapted. Infestation by the human flea (*Pulex irritans*) is rare in the Western world and is only seen in individuals living in highly congested conditions. Outbreaks do occur from time to time in refugee camps and other such situations. The human flea, together with the rat flea, are the vectors of plague. Most flea problems arise from the bite of animal fleas, most commonly those associated with domestic pets (**Fig. 3.60a**), or, occasionally, birds in adjacent nests.

The characteristic clinical picture is of recurrent crops of irritable papules (**Fig. 3.60b**). These are most common on the lower legs, but may occur elsewhere and may appear under clothing. This clinical picture is called papular urticaria. Occasionally, the reaction is so marked that blisters may form. The lesions are itchy and often continue to be symptomatic for some days, or even up to 4 weeks, with irritation coming in spasms. Secondary infection is quite common and lesions may heal to leave small depressions and pigmentary anomalies.

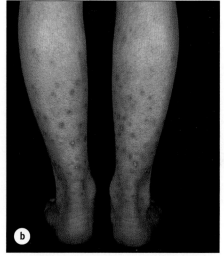

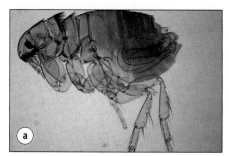

Fig. 3.60 *(a) Cat flea; (b) Papular urticaria of the legs (both courtesy of Dr D A Burns).*

Examination of any domestic pet will usually reveal the presence of 'flea dirt' (small specks of brownish material) in the coat or fur. However, the fleas themselves are easier to find in the animal's bedding, as a flea colony contains many thousands of individuals at various stages of development, while the animal itself may carry only a few at any one time. Occasionally, the source of infestation is not immediately apparent, and a search of the local environment may be necessary. As an illustration, the authors offer this brief case-history: a male patient presented one spring with typical flea bites on the upper trunk, neck, and forearms; he kept no pets and had lived in the same house for 20 years; a search revealed a bird's nest, which had not been occupied as usual that year, in the roof of his garage; the fleas were activated by the starting of his car each morning and dropped down to bite him on the way to work!

Fleas need to be eradicated from the environment and not just from the animal source itself. There are a variety of agents and delivery systems available, but it is often useful to involve the local veterinary surgeon or the environmental health department.

Lice

Humans are unique in having more than one type of louse infestation. Lice are wingless insects and there are several different species. Some feed on the skin and hair of their hosts, but those that cause problems in humans are blood-feeders. There are three important clinical infections in humans:

- Head-louse infestation (pediculosis capitis) — this remains an extremely common infection, occurring endemically in the developing world and epidemically in 'the West', where outbreaks typically appear in schools and in other communities where children predominate. The infection is generally passed by direct head-to-head contact, although some authorities believe that hats and brushes may be vehicles of transmission. The most important symptom is pruritus, and any child with any itchy scalp should be examined very carefully for evidence of head lice. Sometimes there is a papular, excoriated eruption in the occipital area and on the nape of the neck. Secondary infection with *Staphylococcus aureus* is common and may be severe. The most

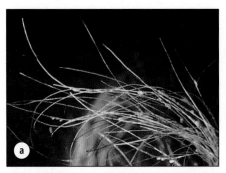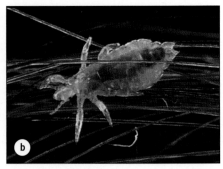

Fig. 3.61 *(a) 'Nits'. (b) Head louse (both courtesy of Dr D A Burns).*

important physical sign is the presence of 'nits', the egg-cases of the insect which are stuck on to hair shafts (**Fig. 3.61a**) and are visible with a hand lens. They are often best seen at the back of the head. Occasionally, an adult louse may be seen scuttling away from the peering eyes of the examiner (**Fig. 3.61b**).

- Body-louse (clothing-louse) infestation (pediculosis corporis) — in developed countries, this infection is only seen in vagrants; however, like fleas, body lice will appear in overcrowded conditions such as refugee or prisoner-of-war camps, and infestation is still prevalent in poorer communities with bad housing conditions. The louse lives in the seams of clothing, but feeds on the blood of the wearer. Most patients complain of itching and are covered in scratch marks. Secondary bacterial infection is, again, very common. Once the clothes have been removed, the problem subsides, unless the patient returns to the same living conditions. Body lice are important vectors of disease, especially typhus.
- Pubic-louse infestation ('crab lice', phthiriasis pubis) — this infection is caused by an entirely separate louse (the head louse and body louse are essentially identical) known as *Phthirus pubis* (**Fig. 3.62**). It is seen almost exclusively among sexually active young adults. The lice are generally found in the pubic hair, on the lower abdomen or inner thighs, clinging to hair shafts along with their egg-cases. Occasionally, lice are also found on the chest, in the axillae, on the scalp margins, and in the eyelashes and beard hair. There may be little or no other sign of the infection, although most patients complain of some itching and there may be blood spots on underwear and other clothing.

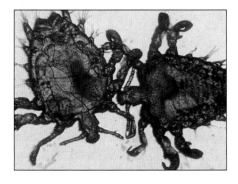

Fig. 3.62 *Crab lice.*

Lice are all susceptible to simple insecticides such as malathion, but do develop resistance. More recently, permethrin has been added to the range of available treatments. Scalp treatments should be carried out with lotions rather than shampoos. Body-louse infection requires little more than a change of clothes.

Bed bugs

Bed bugs live in the furniture, floors, and walls. At night they move out in search of food and may be attracted towards the warmth of the (usually) sleeping victim. They feed by sucking blood from exposed sites and may leave little or no trace. However, in a patient sensitized to the bite, large urticarial wheals develop. Occasionally, the reaction is severe enough to cause blisters. The bugs need to be eradicated from the dwelling, but can survive without food for over a year, as one of the authors can personally confirm!

Mosquitoes, gnats, and midges

Almost everyone will be familiar with the flying blood-suckers mosquitoes, gnats, and midges. Apart from producing insect-bite reactions in sensitized individuals, many are vectors of diseases such as malaria, yellow fever, filarial infections, and leishmaniasis. The insect-bite reactions are similar in nature to those seen with fleas and bed bugs: urticarial wheals, which may persist for some days or even 1–2 weeks. More extreme reactions may result in the swelling of parts of limbs or in blister formation. Lesions are most common on exposed sites, although the insects can penetrate hosiery and light clothing. The legs are frequently affected, especially in women. Sandflies may transmit leishmaniasis.

Ticks

Ticks are arachnids, belonging to the same group of arthropods as spiders and mites. They feed on their host by implanting their mouthparts into the skin and remaining attached for some considerable time. As they feed, they swell with blood, and they are often identified as small blobs on the skin surface, and urticarial reactions may occur around the site. They are generally acquired by humans passing through infested vegetation. Ticks should be removed with care, to avoid leaving mouth-parts behind.

The importance of these creatures for humans lies in their ability to transmit other diseases, particularly the rickettsial infections, (e.g. Rocky Mountain spotted fever), some forms of viral encephalitis, relapsing fever, some forms of typhus, and Lyme disease (*see* page 44).

FLY LARVAE (MAGGOTS)

Some flies complete their life-cycle in the skin of living animals. They have various ways of achieving this, and the infection is not always an essential part of their development. However, when the development of fly larvae (maggots) occurs in the skin, this leads to a condition called myiasis. Most parts of the world have flies that infect animals, particularly cattle, but human infections are generally acquired in the tropics. Typically, the patient develops a boil-like lesion, which breaks down and suppurates (**Fig. 3.63a**). Careful inspection may reveal the moving maggots within the lesion (**Fig. 3.63b**). The larvae can be removed surgically, but the condition will resolve itself naturally in due course as the maggots die or mature.

SCABIES AND OTHER MITE INFECTIONS

Humans can be affected by a large number of mites. One of the more common human–mite interactions is with *Dermatophagoides pteronyssinus*, the ubiquitous house-dust mite. Its role in some allergic processes (asthma, rhinitis) seems clear, and there is increasing

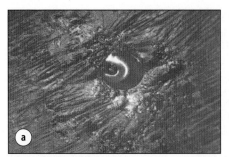
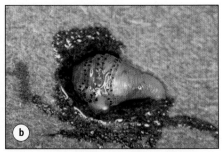

Fig. 3.63 *Myiasis: (a) an indolent, suppurating lesion on the upper arm due to (b) the larva of the fly Dermatobia hominis.*

evidence of a role for it in atopic dermatitis (*see* Chapter 5). Other problems are due to more direct involvement by the mite, but are also often associated with a significant hypersensitivity component.

Human scabies

Scabies is very common. The infection is due to the invasion of the host by the mite *Sarcoptes scabei var. hominis* (**Fig. 3.64**), which passes from person to person almost exclusively by direct contact. The typical clinical picture begins with the onset of pruritus, usually about 6 weeks after exposure in a first attack. The itching is most severe at night. Characteristically, other members of the family are also affected by itch, but this is not always the case. There have been several reports of outbreaks in institutions, especially those caring for the elderly.

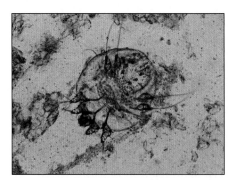

Fig. 3.64 *The scabies mite* — *microscopic view.*

The onset of symptoms is accompanied by the appearance of a widespread, papular or eczematous rash which spares the head and neck in all except very small babies. The rash is often more pronounced around the anterior axillary folds. It may also become secondarily infected. Careful inspection will also reveal the presence of the cardinal lesion: the burrow. These may be very numerous (especially if the patient has been treated with topical corticosteroids) or quite sparse (especially if the patient has received some, but not adequate, scabicidal therapy).The clinical features are sometimes obscured by inflammation (**Fig. 3.65a**). The sites of predilection are the sides and webs of the fingers, the palms, the soles and sides of the feet, and the male genitalia (**Fig. 3.65b**). Indeed, papules on the penis

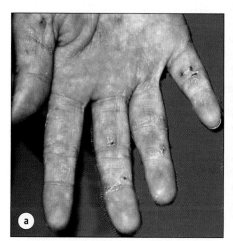
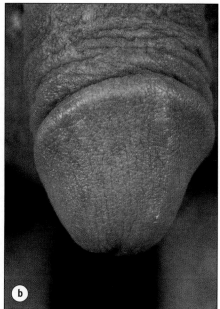

Fig. 3.65 *Scabies burrows* — *(a) on the palms, hard to see here because of intense inflammation and secondary infection; (b) on the glans penis.*

and scrotum in a male with itch will prove to be scabies in 99% of cases. In small children, the burrow may become vesicular and is more common on the palms and soles. Lesions may also appear on the cheeks and even the scalp in infants.

Very rarely, mites proliferate hugely without apparently giving rise to much itching or other symptomatology. This situation, known as crusted or Norwegian scabies, is usually seen in those with neurological, immunological, or mental deficits. The clinical picture is variable, often simulating an eczema, psoriasis, or another inflammatory skin disease.

The condition is best diagnosed by the examination of scrapings of a burrow in 10% KOH under low power microscopy. Mites, nymphs, eggs, and egg cases (**Fig. 3.66**; *see also* Fig. 3.64) are all confirmatory evidence of infection. Treatment should be undertaken with one of the proven acaricides:

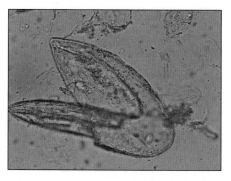

Fig. 3.66 *Egg cases of scabies mites* — *microscopic view.*

- Benzyl benzoate, which has to be applied from chin to toes three times in 24 hours; it is an irritant and is unsuitable for small babies and patients with pre-existing eczema; treatment should not be repeated without further advice because irritation and sensitization become more troublesome with multiple applications.
- Gamma-benzene hexachloride, which should be applied to the same areas as for benzyl benzoate and left in place for 6–24 hours; there have been worries over its neurotoxicity in infants and in pregnant or lactating mothers.
- Malathion, which should be used twice over the course of a week, being left on for 24 hours on each occasion.
- Permethrin, which has recently become the treatment of first choice in many centres; the cream is applied once to the trunk, limbs, and genital areas; some authorities recommend a second application a few days later.
- Crotamiton (present in Eurax®) a weak acaricide but a useful general antipruritic which can be used to help relieve the symptoms both before and after treatment with a more active agent.
- Resistant cases, particularly where there is an institutional outbreak, may be managed by the use of ivermectin orally in a single dose (200 µg/kg).

All those living and sleeping in the same house, all sexual contacts, and, where appropriate, all close friends should be treated simultaneously. Patients should be warned that itching may persist for several days even after the live mites have been successfully eradicated. Occasionally, patients develop small irritable lumps which persist for weeks or months following scabies. These lumps, which are known as postscabitic nodules, can be treated by intralesional steroid injection, but sometimes have to be excised.

Other mites

Animal scabies and mange mites occasionally cause an eruption of irritable papules that may defy diagnosis unless the source is suspected and examined. A mite known as *Cheyletiella* infests short-haired dogs and can cause itchy papules in their owners. Various grain and bird mites have been reported to cause similar problems. The harvest mite (or chigger) causes widespread dermatitic rashes in endemic areas (especially the USA, parts of Europe, and Asia).

Animal *Demodex* mites can cause an awful mange, but there has been much controversy over whether the human form, the follicle mite *Demodex folliculorum*, is associated with skin disease, particularly rosacea.

SPIDERS, WASPS, BEES, AND OTHER ARTHROPODS

Many other arthropods may cause skin problems by directly biting or stinging. The effects are variable and depend on the extent of the injury, the virulence and nature of any chemical or venom implanted, and the sensitivity or otherwise of the individual so bitten or stung. Some arthropods have highly poisonous bites or stings, and urgent action may be required. Others are no more than a temporary, if extremely unpleasant, nuisance. Some patients develop anaphylaxis after bites and stings (*see* Chapter 5).

PROTOZOAL INFECTIONS

Many protozoal infections, such as amoebiasis and trypanosomiasis, occasionally affect the skin. However, one protozoal infection primarily involves the skin: leishmaniasis, caused by the group of organisms known as *Leishmania*. Leishmaniasis can conveniently be divided into Old World and New World forms. In the Mediterranean basin, North Africa, the

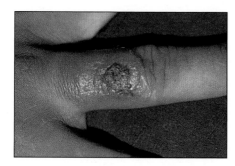

Fig. 3.67 *Leishmaniaisis of the finger.*

Middle East, and Asia, the causative organisms are *L. donovani*, *L. major*, *L. tropica*, and *L. aethiopica*. In the Americas, the prevalent strains are different and include *L. mexicana mexicana*, *L. brasiliensis brasiliensis*, and *L. peruviana*. Similarly, the clinical features are different. All forms, however, are transmitted by insect vectors of the sandfly family.

The systemic form of leishmaniasis, known as kala-azar, is a severe disorder causing hepatosplenomegaly, lymphadenopathy, fever, and malaise, and is associated with a significant mortality. A few patients develop widespread hypopigmentation after recovering from the systemic illness.

The forms of cutaneous leishmaniasis seen in the Old World depend on the causative organism. One of the most commonly encountered infections in travellers, and endemic in rural areas around the Mediterranean and in the Middle East, is with *L. major*. This usually produces a firm, red papule or nodule at the site of the original insect-bite. Frequently, this progresses to form an indolent ulcer with a granulomatous-looking edge (**Fig. 3.67**) which can enlarge to several centimetres in diameter before regressing and healing to leave a scar. A similar, but less aggressive, process occurs with *L. tropica*, which is prevalent in urbanized environments. Other clinical patterns of Old World leishmaniasis may also produce a diffuse cutaneous infiltration and facial involvement, with tissue destruction, closely resembling lupus vulgaris.

In New World disease, lesions are more frequently multiple, exuberant, and nodular, and more destructive. Lymphatic extension is relatively common, particularly in infections due to *L. mexicana mexicana*. Another distinguishing feature is the prominent tendency for mucocutaneous lesions to develop, especially with South American strains. Here, nasal passages, the mouth, and the oropharynx may become involved. The disease is chronic and slowly progressive, and can lead to severe disfigurement.

The investigation and treatment of leishmaniasis begins with samples being taken by scrape or biopsy and examined by light microscopy and submitted to culture (on specialized media such as NNN, Novy-McNeal-Nicolle medium). Some forms heal spontaneously, and it may be best to wait, treating secondary infection as and when necessary. Some authorities advocate cryotherapy. Other patients, particularly those with more severe forms, will require active intervention. The drugs of choice are antimonials, such as sodium stibogluconate, which have to be administered parenterally.

WORMS

Several worm infections have cutaneous manifestations:

- As part of the primary invasion of the skin and subcutis by the worm.
- As a consequence of active migration of worms within the skin (= larva migrans — seen with various hookworms).
- Secondary to the effects of the worm infection in underlying tissues (e.g. the lymphatics in filariasis).

- Flea or other insect bites may trigger reactions to chemicals or insect parts (or both), either as an irritant or an allergic response, forming itchy and often blistering papules.
- Head lice infestation is extremely common in school children (spread by head contact); secondary infection is common.
- Body lice in the developed world occur mainly in vagrants.
- Pubic lice are spread almost exclusively by sexual activity and often present with itching.
- Scabies is spread by direct contact and presents with intense itching commonly around the fingers, the palms, soles and sides of the feet, and the male genitalia; treatment of all contacts should be undertaken with one of the proven acaricides.
- Leishmaniasis is a protozoal infection transmitted by insect vectors of the sand fly family and is associated with a variety of cutaneous manifestation depending on the specific causative organis.

chapter 4

Tumours and Naevi

INTRODUCTION

The skin, as we have seen in Chapter 1, is composed of a large number of different tissue elements. Each of these has the potential to form new growths, or tumours, both benign and malignant. **Figure 4.1** gives a working classification of the most common and the most important lesions encountered in clinical practice, but it must be stressed that this is by no means exhaustive.

Some of the many tumours seen in the skin are the cutaneous equivalent of hamartomas: collections of essentially normal tissue elements present in abnormal amounts or distributions. These are known as naevi and will be covered here alongside acquired tumours.

A classification of naevi and acquired skin tumours

Tissue of origin			
Keratinocytes and epidermal appendages	Naevi	Epidermal	Linear, systematized, and inflammatory, Becker's naevus, linear porokeratosis.
		Appendageal	Naevus sebaceus, (also contains epidermal elements), Fordyce spots, steatocystoma, hair follicle naevi (including naevus comedonicus), sweat gland naevi.
	Benign acquired	Epidermal	Seborrhoeic keratosis (basal cell papilloma), clear cell acanthoma.
		Epidermal cysts	Epidermoid, milia, trichilemmal (pilar).
		Hair follicle malformations/ tumours	Trichofolliculoma, trichoepithelioma (including desmoplastic variant),

Fig. 4.1 *A classification of naevi and acquired skin tumours.*

Tissue of origin			tricholemmoma, trichodiscoma, pilomatricoma, fibrofolliculoma, inverted follicular keratosis.
		Sebaceous gland tumours	Sebaceous adenoma/hyperplasia.
		Sweat gland tumours	Syringoma, eccrine and apocrine hidrocystomas, eccrine spiradenoma, eccrine poroma and eccrine duct tumours, hidradenomas, syringocystadenoma papilliferum, cylindroma.
	Dysplastic/ malignant acquired	Epidermal	Keratoacanthoma, actinic (solar) keratosis (-es), squamous cell carcinoma, *in situ* (Bowen's disease, bowenoid papulosis, vulval *in-situ* carcinoma/ intra-epithelial neoplasia or VIN, and erythroplasia of Queyrat/penile intraepithelial neoplasia or PIN), invasive, carcinoma cuniculatum, basal cell carcinoma, Paget's disease (mammary; extra-mammary).
		Appendageal	Sweat gland carcinomas, porokeratosis, sebaceous carcinoma. Merkel cell tumour.

Fig. 4.1 *(cont.)*

Type of origin

Melanocytes	Naevi	Congenital	Giant; medium/small.
		'Acquired'	Junctional, compound, intradermal, atypical, Sutton's halo naevus, 'en cockarde' naevus, Spitz naevus, spindle cell naevus of Reed, blue naevus, speckled lentiginous naevus.
		Dermal melanocytosis	Mongolian blue spot naevus of Ota, naevus of Ito.
	Benign acquired		Freckle (ephelid), lentigo, labial melanotic macule.
	Dysplastic/ malignant acquired		Lentigo maligna, malignant melanoma.
Dermal components	Naevi		Connective tissue naevi, vascular naevi and angiokeratomas, mast cell naevi.
	Benign acquired		Dermatofibroma (histiocytoma), fibrous papule of the nose, acrochordons (skin tags), acquired digital fibrokeratoma, fibrous tissue, angiomas (including Campbell de Morgan spots), pyogenic granuloma, neurofibroma, leiomyoma.
	Dysplastic/ malignant acquired		Dermatofibro-sarcoma protruberans, atypical fibroxanthoma, malignant fibrous histiocytoma, neurofibrosarcoma, angiosarcoma, Kaposi's sarcoma.

Fig. 4.1 *(cont.)*

Lymphomas	Cutaneous T-cell lymphoma (mycosis fungoides), B-cell lymphomas.
Pseudo-tumours	Chondrodermatitis nodularis helicis chronicus, keloids and hypertrophic scars.
Subcutaneous tissue	Lipoma.

Fig. 4.1 *(cont.)*

NAEVI AND TUMOURS OF THE EPIDERMAL KERATINOCYTES AND EPIDERMAL APPENDAGES

NAEVI

BOX 4.1

Naevi
Benign proliferation of one or more of the constituent cell types found in normal skin.

Epidermal naevi

Epidemiology and aetiology

Epidermal naevi are thought to result from a single, aberrant, epidermal keratinocyte line. Some seem to be inherited. Very rarely, systematized epidermal naevi and sebaceous naevi may be associated with other defects — the so-called epidermal naevus (Feuerstein–Mims) syndrome.

Clinical features

- Most adopt a linear or a whorled appearance following the lines of Blaschko (*see* Chapter 11), resulting in anything from a single, small area of hyperkeratotic skin (**Fig. 4.2**) to a long streak of abnormal tissue affecting the length of a limb or the whole of one side of the body (naevus unius lateris; **Fig. 4.3**).
- Surface is usually rough and may be markedly so.
- Individual lesions are porokeratoses (*see* page 130) in some cases.
- Some lesions are also itchy and inflammatory, so-called inflammatory verrucous epidermal naevus (ILVEN — **Fig. 4.4**).
- Lesions may be present at birth but often appear in early childhood and extend for a variable period before stabilizing.
- Main differential diagnosis in a child is lichen striatus (*see* Chapter 5), and sometimes only time will differentiate between the two; parents should therefore be given a guarded prognosis in any linear lesion appearing in childhood.

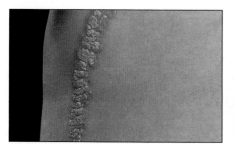

Fig. 4.2 *A typical epidermal naevus on the thigh.*

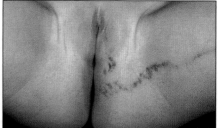

Fig. 4.3 *Naevus unius lateris. This lesion extended the whole length of this little girl's leg.*

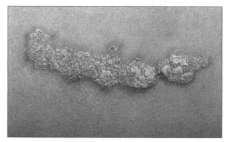

Fig. 4.4 *Inflammatory verrucous epidermal naevus. Although very similar to the lesion in Figure 4.2, this patient's main complaint was not the appearance, but the intense itching she experienced.*

Pathology

Most epidermal naevi show acanthosis with hyperkeratosis. Some have a more psoriasiform pathology, while others may be quite eczematous. A few have more distinctive changes, including epidermolytic hyperkeratosis identical to that seen in bullous ichthyosiform erythroderma (*see* Chapter 11), and dyskeratosis and acantholysis.

Investigation and treatment

Investigation of epidermal naevi is generally not necessary, although a biopsy may sometimes be helpful. Systemic investigation may be indicated in a child with multiple or with very widespread lesions, if there are accompanying symptoms and signs.

Treatment is difficult. Local destruction with cryotherapy will flatten smaller lesions, but the effect is temporary. Once the extent has become clear, excision may be an option.

Becker's naevus

Epidemiology and aetiology

Becker's pigmented, hairy, epidermal naevus usually appears for the first time at or around puberty, suggesting that hormonal influences are important. It is much more common in men than in women.

Clinical features

- Flat, brown patch with an irregular, edge (typically) (**Fig. 4.5**).
- Area enlarges over the course of 2–3 years, the skin becomes thicker, and the hairs within it become longer, darker, and more numerous.

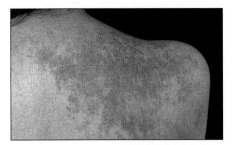

Fig. 4.5 *A typical Becker's naevus on the shoulder of a teenager.*

Site(s) of predilection

Most of these naevi occur on the shoulder or on the upper back, although they are occasionally seen elsewhere on the trunk.

Pathology

There may be some epidermal thickening, and there is a relative increase in epidermal melanization.

Investigation and treatment

There is no satisfactory treatment, although depigmenting agents such as hydroquinone and azaleic acid have their advocates.

Sebaceous naevi

Epidemiology and aetiology

Naevus sebaceus is one of the most prominent of the 'organoid' naevi, in which several tissue elements are involved in the congenital malformation.

Clinical features

- Most begin as flat, often yellowish, patches, visible from early childhood (**Fig. 4.6**a).
- Alopecia is the rule with lesions in hair-bearing areas and may be the presenting problem.
- Area becomes thicker and the surface becomes rougher over time (**Fig. 4.6b**); extensive sebaceous naevi are very rarely associated with multiple defects in the epidermal naevus syndrome.
- Other tumours can develop within these naevi, notably low-grade basal cell carcinomas (**Fig. 4.6c**) and the benign, apocrine-derived tumour syringocystadenoma papilliferum (*see* page 115); sebaceous carcinomas are much less common.

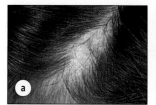
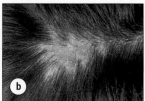
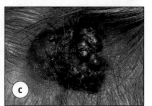

Fig. 4.6 *Naevus sebaceous* — *(a)* this little girl presented with a patch of alopecia; *(b)* this is another sebaceous naevus in an older child; the area has thickened; *(c)* a pigmented basal cell carcinoma arising in a naevus sebaceus in a 50-year old man.

Site(s) of predilection

Most sebaceous naevi occur on the head and neck.

Pathology

The histology is characteristic, but does not fully develop until later in life, when the epidermal hyperplasia is clinically apparent. There are masses of isolated sebaceous glands high in the dermis, beneath a thickened, papillomatous epidermis. There are also, almost always, collections of apocrine glands at the junction of the dermis and subcutis, and there may be eccrine elements as well. The appearance of basaloid change is fairly common in later lesions and does not always signify a truly malignant basal cell carcinoma. However, the histological features of the tumours described above may, of course, also develop.

Investigation and treatment

If there is any clinical doubt, a biopsy will confirm the diagnosis and is essential if there is any change within a pre-existing sebaceus naevus. Many can be excised satisfactorily and this should generally be undertaken in adolescence unless there are compelling disadvantages, in order to prevent trouble at a later date.

Fordyce spots

Epidemiology and aetiology

Fordyce spots represent ectopic, aberrant collections of sebaceous glands.

Clinical features and site(s) of predilection

Clusters of small, yellowish papules are seen along the vermilion border of the lips or further inside the buccal cavity. Lesions tend to increase in numbers over time.

Pathology

There are lobules of otherwise normal sebaceous glands.

Investigation and treatment

- Epidermal naevi usually adopt a linear or a whorled appearance, with a rough surface, and can be itchy and inflammatory; treatment is difficult but cryotherapy or excision may be options.
- Becker's epidermal naevi are pigmented and hairy and commonly appear in the shoulder or upper back region of young men.
- Sebaceous naevi are congenital, occurring in early childhood as flat yellowish patches commonly on the head and neck; excision in adolescence is recommended to avoid potential malignant change.

None is required, although some is often requested, and patients may become obsessed with what they see as a major abnormality.

Steatocystoma (multiplex)

Epidemiology and aetiology

These are the true sebaceous cysts, those usually accorded the name being epidermoid or trichilemmal cysts (*see* pages 106, 107. Many patients give a clear history of autosomal dominant inheritance.

Clinical features

Patients usually present in adolescence with multiple, smooth, dermal, cystic swellings (**Fig. 4.7**). There may also be many comedones.

Site(s) of predilection

Lesions occur on the trunk, particularly the upper chest.

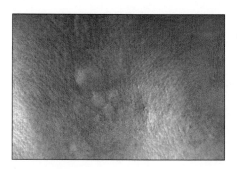

Fig. 4.7 *Small cysts on the chest in steatocystoma multiplex.*

Pathology

The individual lesions consist of an epithelial-lined cyst with sebaceous gland lobules in the wall.

Investigation and treatment

There are usually too many lesions for excision to be a practical solution.

Hair follicle naevi

Epidemiology and aetiology

These are cutaneous hamartomas derived from hair follicle epithelium.

Clinical features

A number of lesions are considered to be hair follicle naevi (*see also* trichofolliculoma on page 108). The most commonly encountered in clinical practice is the comedo naevus (or naevus comedonicus): usually a localized area of blackheads (**Fig. 4.8**). Although typically present from birth, these lesions may become much more prominent at puberty.

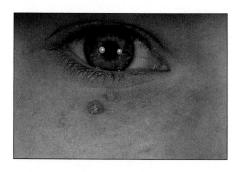

Fig. 4.8 *Naevus comedonicus. There is a patch under the right eye in which there are a number of blackheads and other follicle-derived abnormalities.*

Site(s) of predilection

Most hair follicle naevi are seen on the head and neck.

Investigation and treatment

Treatment is purely cosmetic except that some lesions become inflammatory and may require antibiotics (*see* treatment of acne in Chapter 5).

Sweat gland naevi

Epidemiology and aetiology

There are two main forms of sweat glands, eccrine and apocrine (*see* Chapter 1), and each may give rise to naevoid malformations. Apocrine glands are the origin of the benign tumour syringocystadenoma papilliferum (*see* page 101) and this may arise early enough in life to be considered a naevus. Eccrine elements may be found histologically in a variety of lesions, all of which are rare.

BENIGN EPIDERMAL TUMOURS

BENIGN TUMOURS OF THE EPIDERMAL KERATINOCYTES AND EPIDERMAL APPENDAGES

Seborrhoeic keratosis (seborrhoeic wart; basal cell papilloma)

BOX 4.2

Seborrhoeic keratosis
Common, usually pigmented, benign proliferation of basal kerinocytes.

Epidemiology and aetiology

Seborrhoeic keratosis is one of the most common benign skin tumours encountered in clinical practice. These tumours are much more common in the elderly, although in some families a genetic predisposition may result in lesions appearing at an earlier age.

Clinical features

- Lesions may be solitary, but are frequently multiple, and numbers increase with age (**Fig. 4.9**); ultimately, there may be many hundreds.
- Early lesions are often pale but become darker with time and may be very deeply pigmented, which may give rise to differential diagnostic difficulty with flat lentigines and actinic keratoses on the face and, for thicker lesions, with malignant melanoma.
- Individual lesions typically have a 'stuck-on' appearance and the surface may be 'greasy', but more commonly rather rough and warty, often marked by plugged follicular orifices.
- Lesions can be highlighted with gentle cryotherapy.
- Seborrhoeic keratoses often catch on clothing and may become inflamed and irritated.

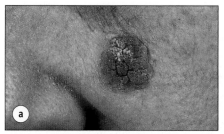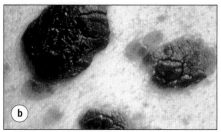

Fig. 4.9 *Seborrhoeic keratoses.* *These extremely common lesions vary considerably in size, number, and colour (see also Fig 2.2b). The degree of pigmentation varies widely — **(a)** pale brown; **(b)** much darker brown.*

Site(s) of predilection

These tumours can occur anywhere, but are more common on the head, neck, and trunk. In black skin, multiple small lesions may appear on the face. This is often termed dermatosis papulosa nigra (**Fig. 4.10**), but is essentially a variant of inherited seborrhoeic keratosis. On the limbs, lesions may be smaller and less pigmented. The so-called stucco keratosis is probably a variant.

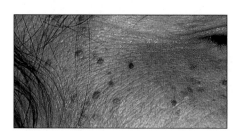

Fig. 4.10 *Dermatosis papulosa nigra.* *The histology of the lesions seen in this common inherited condition is that of a seborrhoeic keratosis.*

Pathology

There is irregular expansion of the epidermis with a variable degree of acanthosis and papillomatosis. The development of horn cysts is a characteristic feature.

Investigation and treatment

Most lesions can be left alone. However, if there is diagnostic doubt, a biopsy should be performed. If seborrhoeic keratoses are symptomatic, or if the cosmetic appearance is sufficiently annoying, they can be removed by curettage and cautery or treated with simple cryotherapy. They often recur.

Clear-cell acanthoma

Epidemiology and aetiology

This is an uncommon tumour, most often seen in the elderly.

Clinical features

The typical appearance is of a small, dome-shaped, red lesion, often compared to a cut strawberry (**Fig. 4.11**). There may be a wafer-like scale at the junction with normal skin. More than one lesion may be present.

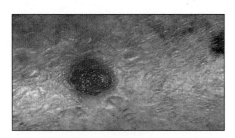

Fig. 4.11 *Clear-cell acanthoma (of Degos).*

Site(s) of predilection
Clear-cell acanthomas nearly always occur on the lower leg.

Pathology
There is thickening of the epidermis, with a remarkable, sudden transition from normal-staining keratinocytes to pale cells containing glycogen.

Investigation and treatment
Excision biopsy will help if there is diagnostic difficulty. Lesions also respond well to cryotherapy.

Epidermoid cysts

Epidemiology and aetiology
Epidermoid cysts, frequently called sebaceous cysts (as are trichilemmal cysts — *see* page 107), are common. They often follow acne or some trauma to the skin, or may arise apparently spontaneously.

Clinical features
Lesions may be solitary or multiple. Each lesion is a dermal, cystic lump which can be felt to move over the subcutaneous fat but with the overlying epidermis. A punctum is frequently visible over the surface. The cysts may become red, inflamed, and extremely painful.

Site(s) of predilection
The most common sites for epidermoid cysts are the head and neck (especially around the ears) and the upper trunk, but they can occur anywhere.

Pathology
The cyst is epithelial-lined and the contents consist of lamellated keratin. A few hairs may occasionally be found.

Investigation and treatment
Excision is usually curative assuming that the cyst is removed intact.

Milia

Epidemiology and aetiology
Milia are small keratin cysts which are seen in several different clinical situations:
- In newborn infants.

- As part of a familial trait.
- After physical trauma, blistering, or inflammation in the skin.
- Arising spontaneously for no apparent reason.

They may arise from immature sebaceous glands.

Clinical features

Milia are small, rarely exceeding 2 mm in diameter. They are usually white or pale cream (**Fig. 4.12**). Neonatal milia disappear spontaneously. Those seen in adults may do so as well, although many persist.

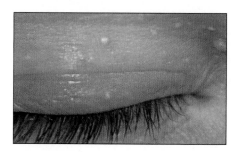

Fig. 4.12 *Milia in a typical site. This pattern is often familial.*

Site(s) of predilection

In neonates, the lesions are scattered across the face. In adults, milia secondary to trauma or blistering may appear anywhere. For example, milia are a prominent feature of porphyria cutanea tarda (*see* Chapter 8) and are mainly seen on the dorsa of the hands. Otherwise, by far the most common site for milia is the central face, especially around the eyes (*see* **Fig. 4.12**).

Pathology

The thin epithelial wall contains lamellated keratin.

Investigation and treatment

The diagnosis is usually straightforward. Although no treatment is necessary, the patient may wish the lesions to be removed, in which case they may be extruded following incision over the surface. A more practical solution for multiple milia may be the use of a fine needle and a hyfrecator.

Trichilemmal (pilar) cysts

Epidemiology and aetiology

These common scalp cysts are frequently familial.

Clinical features

There may be one or many (**Fig. 4.13**). The cysts are usually small initially, but may become very large and lobulated. Lesions may undergo inflammatory changes.

Site(s) of predilection

The scalp is by far the most common site.

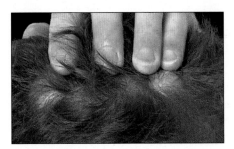

Fig. 4.13 *Two large trichilemmal cysts in a man who had already had several removed (his mother had also had them).*

Pathology

There are differences in the details of the wall of this cyst compared with that of an epidermoid cyst. In particular, there is no granular cell layer in the wall of a trichilemmal cyst.

Investigation and treatment

Lesions can be excised and often enucleate very easily following a superficial incision over the surface of the cyst.

Trichofolliculoma

Epidemiology and aetiology

Most, if not all, trichofolliculomas arise as malformations of pilosebaceous units.

Clinical features

The most characteristic feature is the presence of a small tuft of hair emerging from a small lump.

Site(s) of predilection

Trichofolliculomas are nearly always found on the face.

Pathology

Several hairs are seen within one large, abnormal, follicular canal. There may also be several attached aberrant sebaceous glands.

Investigation and treatment

The lesion is best excised.

Trichoepithelioma

Epidemiology and aetiology

Trichoepitheliomas are also malformations of the pilosebaceous apparatus.

Clinical features

There are two main presentations: multiple (or epithelioma adenoides cysticum) and solitary. The appearance of multiple trichoepitheliomas is an autosomal dominant disorder.

The individual lesions are usually papules of 3–5 mm diameter which have a translucent quality. Solitary lesions may be confused with basal cell carcinoma. Transformation to basal cell carcinoma has been reported.

Site(s) of predilection
Trichoepitheliomas nearly always occur on the face, although lesions may occasionally be seen on the upper trunk. When multiple, they are usually symmetrically distributed and tend to cluster around the eyes and nose.

Pathology
The dermis contains lobulated clusters of darkly staining cells which may be confused with basal cell carcinoma on superficial inspection.

Investigation and treatment
A biopsy is probably sensible unless there is already a positive family history. A solitary trichoepithelioma, or any troublesome lesion in the multiple form, should be excised.

Desmoplastic variant
Very occasionally, clinicians will encounter a solitary, annular lesion on the face which closely resembles a basal cell carcinoma but which, histologically, is composed of strands of darkly staining cells, connective tissue, and keratin-filled cysts. This lesion has been termed 'desmoplastic trichoepithelioma'.

Tricholemmoma

Epidemiology and aetiology
Tricholemmomas are hamartomas of the outer root sheath of the hair follicle. They are seen in patients with Cowden's syndrome, an inherited disorder in which the occurence of breast and pancreatic cancers is greatly increased in frequency.

Clinical features
Tricholemmomas are nondescript, flesh-coloured papules and nodules. They may be solitary or, in association with Cowden's syndrome, appear in clusters. Other changes may accompany the multiple form, notably a so-called cobblestone appearance on the lips of the mouth.

Site(s) of predilection
Lesions are seen on the head and neck, predominantly on the face around the nose, mouth, and ears.

Pathology
The histological features are somewhat similar to those of basal cell carcinoma in that there are columns of epithelial cells present, often with a lobulated appearance, and there may be some degree of peripheral palisading.

Investigation and treatment
Solitary lesions can be excised. The diagnosis of multiple tricholemmoma by biopsy should lead to a high degree of vigilance regarding breast and pancreatic malignancy and should involve appropriate specialist expertise.

Trichodiscoma

Epidemiology and aetiology

Trichodiscomas are thought to arise from a specialized receptor within the hair follicle. The occurrence may be familial.

Clinical features

Most reports have been of multiple, flat, flesh-coloured papules.

Site(s) of predilection

Trichodiscomas occur on the face.

Pathology

Each papule represents an area of altered dermal connective tissue, often with abnormal vasculature.

Investigation and treatment

A biopsy will be needed to establish the diagnosis.

Pilomatricoma (calcifying epithelioma of Malherbe)

Epidemiology and aetiology

Pilomatricomas are relatively common, with most tumours arising in childhood and adolescence. They may occur in patients with dystrophia myotonica.

Clinical features

The classical lesion is a relatively deep-seated nodule in a child or young adult. The tumour feels very hard, almost stone-like, on palpation. The surface will often reveal a faceted or tented appearance if the skin is stretched over the surface (**Fig. 4.14**).

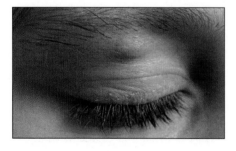

Fig. 4.14 *A pilomatricoma on the right eyelid.*

Site(s) of predilection

These tumours are usually found on the head and neck.

Pathology

The histopathological appearances are very striking. A dermal nodule, which may extend into the subcutis, is seen, along with an island of cells, some darkly staining and basophilic (towards the edge of the lesion), some pale pink and eosinophilic (towards the centre). In this latter group of cells, the nuclear outlines remain, resulting in the so-called shadow or ghost cell.

Investigation and treatment

X-ray of the lesion may reveal calcification. Most patients request excision of the nodule.

Inverted follicular keratosis

Epidemiology and aetiology

This relatively uncommon lesion may be a variant of a seborrhoeic keratosis (*see* page 104). The diagnosis is often only made on histology after removal.

Clinical features

Generally solitary, inverted follicular keratoses present as nondescript, scaly papules or nodules.

Site(s) of predilection

Most occur on the head and neck.

Pathology

The pathological changes are centred on a follicular opening. Features seen are acanthosis, a degree of disorganization and disarray among the keratinocytes, and a few mitoses. This may cause some concern regarding possible malignancy. Squamous eddies and keratin cysts are also found.

Investigation and treatment

Most inverted follicular keratoses are removed because of diagnostic uncertainty.

Fibrofolliculoma

Epidemiology and aetiology

The autosomal dominant condition known as the Birt–Hogg–Dubé syndrome is characterized by the presence of multiple fibrofolliculomas, as well as acrochordons and hidradenomas. Very occasionally, solitary lesions are found.

Clinical features

The lesions are smooth, yellowish papules.

Site(s) of predilection

Fibrofolliculomas occur on the face.

Pathology

Each papule represents a malformed pilosebaceous unit surrounded by connective tissue.

Investigation and treatment

A biopsy will help with the diagnosis.

Sebaceous adenoma and 'senile sebaceous hyperplasia'

Epidemiology and aetiology

These lesions are seen in older patients and presumably represent one form of cutaneous ageing.

Clinical features

There may be one or several lesions, each of which is initially a soft, yellowish papule. As it enlarges, a rim may begin to form, which can make the lesion difficult to distinguish from a very small, early, basal cell carcinoma (*see* Fig. 4.24a).

Site(s) of predilection

These are almost always found across the forehead and cheeks.

Pathology

There are otherwise normal sebaceous glands arranged in clumps or lobules in the dermis.

Investigation and treatment

Excision biopsy of a suspicious-looking lesion may be needed. Typical, multiple lesions may be either ignored or treated with simple destructive techniques, such as cautery, hyfrecation, or cryotherapy.

Syringoma

Epidemiology and aetiology

There remains some debate as to whether these tumours arise from apocrine or eccrine elements. They are more common in women. Most instances are sporadic, although familial cases have been described.

Clinical features

Typically, the lesions appear as multiple, flesh-coloured, flat-topped papules. They normally first arise in early adult life and gradually increase in size and number over the years.

Site(s) of predilection

Syringomas are most common around the eyes (**Fig. 4.15a**), but may also occur on the neck and face. Much less commonly, lesions may erupt over the lower abdomen (**Fig. 4.15b**) or upper trunk.

Pathology

The histopathological appearances are highly characteristic. There are collections of small ductal structures in the upper dermis, embedded in connective tissue. Many of these areas

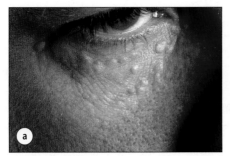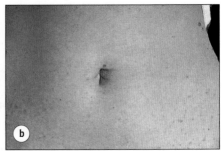

Fig. 4.15 *Syringomas — (a) in a typical site; (b) 'eruptive' syringomas on the lower abdomen.*

have small protrusions resembling the tail of a tadpole, or giving the overall look of a comma.

Investigation and treatment

No treatment is very satisfactory, although gentle hyfrecation or cautery can produce reasonable results.

Eccrine hidrocystoma

Epidemiology and aetiology

This is a rare tumour, usually seen in older women.

Clinical features

Small, apparently cystic, lesions are seen. They enlarge when the skin is hot.

Site(s) of predilection

Eccrine hidrocystomas are found on the eyelids and cheeks.

Pathology

There are ductal structures in the dermis.

Investigation and treatment

A biopsy will confirm the diagnosis, and the lesions respond well to cautery or hyfrecation.

Apocrine hidrocystoma

Epidemiology and aetiology

Apocrine hidrocystomas are relatively common and are derived from apocrine glands.

Clinical features

The characteristic lesion is a solitary, blue-black nodule.

Site(s) of predilection

These lesions almost always occur on the face, especially near the inner canthus. Lesions have been reported on other areas where apocrine glands are numerous.

Pathology

The tumour consists of cystic apocrine ducts.

Investigation and treatment

It is simple to excise the lesion.

Eccrine spiradenoma

Epidemiology and aetiology

This is an uncommon tumour derived from eccrine sweat glands.

Clinical features

The lesion is a solitary dermal nodule. There is often a bluish tinge and the lesion may be tender when knocked.

Site(s) of predilection

Most eccrine spiradenomas occur on the limbs.

Pathology

The histology is striking. There are dermal masses composed of two cell types: pale-staining, larger cells are found centrally and around ductal luminae, and darker-staining, smaller cells are found around the edges of the lobules.

Investigation and treatment

Excision, which is straightforward.

Eccrine poroma and eccrine-duct tumours

Epidemiology and aetiology

A number of lesions are thought to arise from the ductal portion of the eccrine sweat apparatus.

Clinical features

Eccrine poromas are usually pink, raised lesions with a 'moist' surface (**Fig. 4.16a**). Eccrine-duct tumours are usually nondescript dermal nodules.

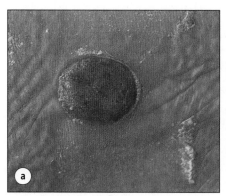 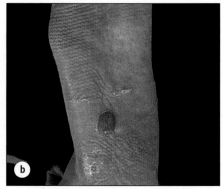

Fig. 4.16 *Eccrine poroma — (a) a typical example; (b) on the sole, a typical site.*

Site(s) of predilection

Eccrine poromas are most commonly found on the palms and soles (**Fig. 4.16b**). Eccrine-duct tumours may occur anywhere.

Pathology

Both types of tumour are composed of small cuboidal cells.

Investigation and treatment

Excision is the treatment of choice.

Hidradenoma

Epidemiology and aetiology
These rare tumours are derived from sweat glands.

Clinical features
Hidradenomas are dermal nodules, with few other distinguishing features. In some, however, the overlying epidermis becomes significantly thickened.

Site(s) of predilection
Most occur on the head and neck.

Pathology
Cuboidal cells form duct-like structures, around which there are larger masses of clear cells.

Investigation and treatment
These tumours are usually solitary and can be excised.

Syringocystadenoma papilliferum

Epidemiology and aetiology
These tumours/naevi arise from apocrine-derived tissue elements. They are not common, but are seen in association with sebaceous naevi (*see* page 101).

Clinical features
The tumour is a slow-growing mass that protrudes from the surface of the skin and often has a moist surface. There may be an underlying sebaceous naevus.

Site(s) of predilection
As with sebaceous naevi, most occur on the head and neck.

Pathology
The main histological feature is the presence of cystic spaces with an apocrine epithelial lining.

Investigation and treatment
The lesion is best excised.

Cylindroma (turban tumour)

Epidemiology and aetiology
These tumours are of uncertain histogenic origin.

Clinical features
Often there are multiple lesions, which are rounded, pink masses with a smooth surface.

Site(s) of predilection
Lesions are predominantly seen on the head and neck, particularly the scalp.

Pathology

There are two cell types: one large and one small. They are arranged in clumps and strands, separated by stroma.

Investigation and treatment

Large, troublesome lesions can be excised, but many are frequently found, and wide excision and grafting may therefore be required.

- Seborrhoeic keratosis is a common benign skin condition presenting mainly in the elderly with warty lesions on the head, neck or trunk.
- Epidermoid cysts are common lesions found on the head, neck and upper trunk and often follow acne or trauma to the skin.
- Milia are keratin cysts found most often in neonates but also in adults secondary to trauma or blistering.
- Trichilemmal or common scalp cysts are often familial and can be easily treated.

DYSPLASTIC AND MALIGNANT EPIDERMAL TUMOURS

Keratoacanthoma

Epidemiology and aetiology

Keratoacanthomas (often abbreviated to KA) are common, certainly as compared with some of the lesions discussed previously. They are mostly seen in the middle and later years of life, and chronic exposure to sunlight is likely to play a role in their pathogenesis. Other carcinogens, including tars and hydrocarbons, may be important causative agents in some patients.

Clinical features

Lesions present with several highly characteristic features:
- A short history of rapid growth, usually over 4–6 weeks.
- Initially, a small papule appears and is often dismissed by the patient as 'just a spot'.
- As the lesion grows, it becomes rounder, the edges become more rolled, and a keratotic plug develops in the centre (**Fig. 4.17**).
- If left alone, the lesion shrinks and disappears, often leaving a small, puckered area in its wake.

Mostly, keratoacanthomas reach a maximum diameter of 1–2 cm, but, very occasionally, may be much larger.

Keratoacanthomas are usually solitary, but there are rare situations in which multiple tumours arise.

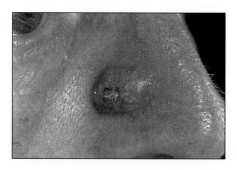

Fig. 4.17 *A typical keratoacanthoma.*

Site(s) of predilection

Keratoacanthomas occur on sun-exposed sites. They are most frequently encountered on the face, neck, and ears, but can occur on the limbs. Giant keratoacanthomas are usually found on the arms.

Pathology

Keratoacanthomas are symmetrical. There is a central tumour mass of proliferating squamous cells in which there is disorganization and loss of polarity. This extends deeply down into the dermis. Surmounting this mass is the clinically visible hyperkeratotic plug. At the edges, the epidermis appears to stretch and attenuate as it approaches the lesion and often seems to rise up to meet the tumour mass itself — an effect often described as resembling a shoulder.

Investigation and treatment

An early keratoacanthoma can be difficult to distinguish from several other lesions, such as a viral wart, hypertrophic actinic keratosis, and giant molluscum contagiosum. The main issue, however, is to avoid missing a squamous cell carcinoma (SCC), some of which may have features that closely resemble those of a keratoacanthoma (although SCC usually have a longer history). There are only two ways to be certain: one is to wait expectantly for spontaneous resolution; the other is to remove the lesion and submit it for histology. In the very elderly and frail, the former course may be reasonable. However, in most instances we would recommend formal excision. This probably produces the best cosmetic result, reduces anxiety and removes doubt from the minds of the patient and relatives, and provides useful histopathological information.

Actinic (solar) keratosis

Epidemiology and aetiology

Chronic exposure to solar and other ionizing radiation results in a number of changes in the skin. These include a tendency for the epidermis to produce hyperkeratotic patches called actinic keratoses. These lesions occur earlier in fair-skinned individuals and in those living in very sunny climates, such as Australia and the southern United States, where almost everyone develops some eventually. The appearance of actinic keratoses signals the fact that the skin has developed a significant degree of dysplastic change and that the patient is more likely to develop malignancy. Indeed, areas of actinic keratosis may progress to squamous cell carcinoma, although the potential for any individual patch to do this is low.

Clinical features

- Present as scaly patches (**Fig. 4.18 a** and **b**) often on an erythematous background.
- Single or multiple lesions, especially on a bald scalp.
- Most remain fairly flat and static in size, but some slowly spread laterally; this is especially true of a variant that becomes pigmented.
- Some become large, significantly elevated, and hypertrophic.
- Tend to wax and wane in presentation but occasionally may disappear spontaneously.

Site(s) of predilection

Actinic keratoses occur on any site that is chronically exposed to the sun: the face, ears (**Fig. 4.18c**) and neck, the skin of the bald male scalp, the arms and hands, the lower regions of the legs. Similar changes occurring on the lip are known as actinic cheilitis (**Fig. 4.18d**).

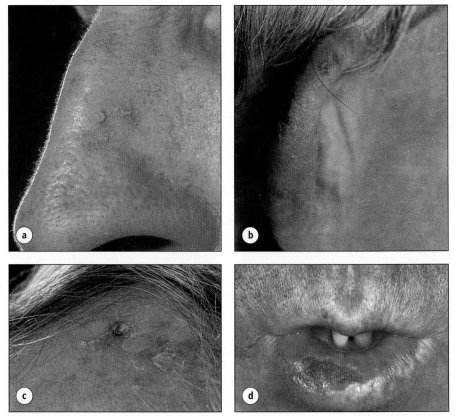

Fig. 4.18 *Actinic (solar) keratosis* — *(a) on the left side of the nose; (b) on the outer margin of the ear, a typical site; (c) multiple lesions on the forehead; (d) similar changes on the lower lip are known as actinic cheilitis.*

Pathology

Each area of keratosis is remarkably discrete, both clinically and histologically. A range of pathological changes are seen in these areas, which essentially represent a dysplastic 'field change' within the affected epidermis. There is a variable degree of hyperkeratosis and parakeratosis, and the epidermal cells are paler and somewhat disordered. There may be patchy dyskeratosis (*see* Darier's disease in Chapter 11) or changes indistinguishable from Bowen's disease (*see* below). Follicular orifices are often, but not always, spared.

Investigation and treatment

Although there is usually no problem with the diagnosis, this is not always the case. Thin, flat basal cell carcinomas, Bowen's disease, and lesions of discoid lupus erythematosus (*see* Chapter 5) can all look very similar. There have also been some recent reports of amelanotic lentigo maligna presenting as rather atypical-looking actinic keratoses. Furthermore, squamous cell carcinomas may develop in skin affected by actinic keratoses, and hypertrophic lesions may need to be investigated. In any of these situations, a skin biopsy will be helpful.

Actinic keratoses respond extremely well to cryotherapy. Large, hypertrophic lesions may be better curetted or even excised. An alternative to surgery is the use of the topical antimitotic agent 5-fluorouracil cream. This is quite irritant, but, if used correctly, is highly effective. A standard approach is to ask the patient to apply the cream to the affected area(s) of skin once daily for 3 weeks. A brisk irritant reaction usually develops during the treatment period, but this settles rapidly once treatment ceases. Repeat treatment cycles may be required to eradicate multiple keratoses.

Bowen's disease (intraepithelial carcinoma)

Epidemiology and aetiology

Bowen's disease, like actinic keratosis, is predominantly a disorder of sun-exposed skin (although, in the past, arsenic-containing medicines and tonics also induced Bowen's disease). It becomes much more common with advancing years.

Clinical features

- Red, scaly, and well demarcated patches (**Fig. 4.19**) which may be solitary or multiple.
- May closely resemble psoriasis but the scale (instead of being parakeratotic, flaky, and silvery) is thick and more adherent.
- Surface below (if lifted gently with a fingernail) is found to be moist but does not bleed.

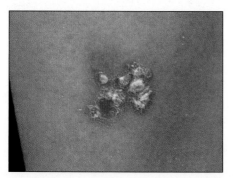

Fig. 4.19 *A typical patch of intra-epithelial squamous cell carcinoma (Bowen's disease) (see also Fig. 2.1b).*

Site(s) of predilection

Bowen's disease may appear on any sun-exposed area.

Pathology

Histologically, there is gross disorganization of the epithelium, with multiple mitoses. The basement membrane is, by definition, intact — any sign of invasion automatically converts the situation to that of invasive squamous cell carcinoma.

Investigation and treatment

It is appropriate, in most instances, to take a biopsy to confirm the diagnosis, following which there is a choice of therapeutic interventions: excision of small areas; cryotherapy; curettage; radiotherapy. The decision as to which is best relates to the size and site of the lesion, and the age of the patient. Lesions on the leg, in particular, need to be treated gently, especially in older patients, because of problems with healing.

- Keratoacanthomas are rapidly-growing skin lesions associated with chronic exposure to sunlight and can be easily confused with squamous cell carcinomas.
- Actinic keratoses are hyperkeratotic patches in the epidermis produced by chronic exposure to sunlight and other ionizing radiation and associated with dysplastic change in the skin and subsequent development of squamous cell carcinoma.
- Bowen's disease is a common premalignant condition developing on sun exposed skin and presenting with a psoriasis like-scale although thick and more adherent.

Bowenoid papulosis

This term has been used to describe the features seen in a group of patients who develop multiple lesions resembling flat seborrhoeic keratoses or plane warts, usually, but not exclusively, on the genitalia (**Fig. 4.20**). Histology shows the changes of Bowen's disease, but the lesions resolve in time without treatment. The cause is almost certainly infection with wart virus (especially HPV 16).

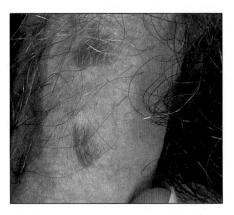

Fig. 4.20 *Bowenoid papulosis* — *two areas of lesions.*

Vulval intraepithelial neoplasia (VIN)

A full discussion of the occurrence of vulval *in-situ* squamous cell carcinoma will be found in most good gynaecology textbooks. However, such changes may present to the dermatologist. The clinical appearances may vary considerably, from a few flat lesions to gross epithelial irregularity and warty hyperkeratosis. The conventional classification, VIN I, II, and III, is based on the degree of histological 'atypia' present. Again, wart virus is probably involved in many cases. Any patient with such changes requires full investigation, including colposcopy and cervical smears.

Erythroplasia of Queyrat

Epidemiology and aetiology

This is the equivalent of Bowen's disease on the glans penis. There is no doubt that much dysplastic change on both male and female genitalia is associated with infection with HPV.

Clinical features

Red, well-demarcated patches develop on the glans. There is a variable amount of scale, but often very little in the uncircumcised. Instead, the surface is often said to be 'velvety', but may be quite shiny and moist-looking (Fig. 4.21).

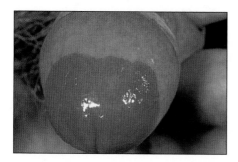

Fig. 4.21 *A well-circumscribed patch of squamous cell carcinoma* in-situ *(erythroplasia of Queyrat).*

Pathology

The changes are identical to those of Bowen's disease except that, being on the penis, there may not always be significant hyperkeratosis.

Investigation and treatment

The main differential diagnoses are non-specific balanitis (the equivalent of intertrigo), recurrent candidal infection, and Zoon's balanitis (*see* Chapter 5). A biopsy should be considered in any red patch on the penis, especially if it has not responded to topical anti-inflammatory or anti-infective agents. Small areas of erythroplasia can be treated with cryotherapy, but larger areas may require radiotherapy or, if the condition involves the prepuce as well, circumcision and radiotherapy. Some dermatologists recommend 5-fluorouracil cream or imiquimod.

Invasive squamous cell carcinoma

BOX 4.3

Squamous cell carcinoma
Malignant tumour derived from keratinocytes, usually arising in sun-damaged skin.

Epidemiology and aetiology

Like its *in-situ* counterpart, most areas of invasive squamous cell carcinoma (SCC) on the skin develop in older patients, particularly on skin exposed to high cumulative doses of ionizing radiation or other carcinogens. Particularly important are chronic exposure to radiation (e.g. ultraviolet radiation, X-rays) and to tar-derived compounds. A famous example of the latter is the occurrence of scrotal SCC in chimney-sweeps and oil-workers (**Fig. 4.22**), but tobacco smoking is associated with lip cancers, where heat may also play a role. SCC may also arise in areas of chronic injury, such as ulcers and scarred areas following burns or infections such as lupus vulgaris. Another, more recent, aetiological factor has been the extension of immunosuppression for transplant recipients. These patients not infrequently develop SCCs, especially on sun-exposed sites.

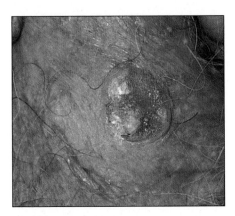

Fig. 4.22 *Scrotum squamous cell carcinoma in a man occupationally exposed to oils.* *Similar tumours used to occur in chimney sweeps.*

Clinical features

- May present with a number of clinical appearances:
  - small, scaly patches, very similar to actinic keratoses (**Fig. 4.23a**)
  - larger masses (**Fig. 4.23b**)
  - ulcers (**Fig. 4.23c**).
- May occasionally (as indicated on pages 116–17) be virtually indistinguishable from a keratoacanthoma.
- Presence of SCC must be suspected if any new change develops in chronically damaged skin — e.g. an ulcer or nodule arising in old scar tissue (**Fig. 4.23d**) or the elevation of the edge of an established leg ulcer.

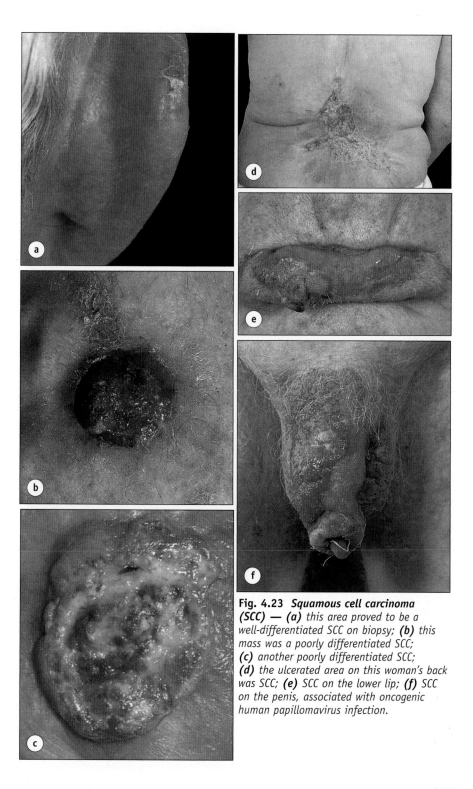

Fig. 4.23 *Squamous cell carcinoma (SCC)* — (a) this area proved to be a well-differentiated SCC on biopsy; **(b)** this mass was a poorly differentiated SCC; **(c)** another poorly differentiated SCC; **(d)** the ulcerated area on this woman's back was SCC; **(e)** SCC on the lower lip; **(f)** SCC on the penis, associated with oncogenic human papillomavirus infection.

Site(s) of predilection

Sun-exposed sites are the most common areas involved in clinical practice: the head and neck (especially the front and rim of the pinna and the lips — Fig. 4.23e), the arms and hands, the lower parts of the legs. In patients whose SCC is associated with occupational or other exposure to other ionizing radiation, lesions may appear in unusual sites. As indicated on page 123, genital SCC may be HPV-related (Fig. 4.23f).

Pathology

The epidermis is markedly disorganized, with dyskeratosis, hyperkeratosis, and numerous mitoses. The degree of such changes is very variable, both from one tumour to another and between different areas of tumours. In other words, SCCs may be very well differentiated (as is often the case in those arising in sun-damaged skin), or highly anaplastic and aggressive. The feature that distinguishes SCC from the pre-invasive conditions described above is the presence of fingers of epithelium stretching down into the dermis, breaching the basement membrane.

Investigation and treatment

A biopsy is essential if there is any doubt, but, if the lesion is reasonably small, the most appropriate action is an excision with primary closure. Larger lesions may require more extensive surgery with flaps or skin grafts. An alternative approach is to obtain a tissue diagnosis and then treat with radiotherapy. SCCs are capable of metastasis and, while cutaneous SCC is, fortunately, not associated with a high rate of spread, lesions of the lip and those induced by radiation and other carcinogens are more aggressive. It is important, therefore, to check for draining lymph nodes and to remove any that are enlarged, preferably at the initial procedure. Follow-up should include a check of the nodes, and also distant sites.

- Invasive squamous cell carcinoma (SCC) develops mainly in older patients on skin exposed to high cumulative doses of ionizing radiation or other carcinogens.
- SCC may also arise in ulceration or following burns or infections, or in transplant patients under immunosuppression.
- Cutaneous SCC does not commonly metastasize but lesions of the lip and those induced by radiation and other carcinogens are more aggressive.
- Treatment is by surgical excision or radiotherapy.

Carcinoma cuniculatum

A particularly indolent form of SCC is seen on the foot, especially the plantar surface. The lesion usually presents as a mass of keratotic tissue, often with sinuses opening on the surface. Histology is not always conclusive because the lesion is so well differentiated. The most appropriate management is wide excision once the nature of the problem has been recognized.

Basal cell carcinoma ('rodent ulcer')

BOX 4.4

Basal cell carcinoma
Malignant tumour arising from basal keratinocytes of the epidermis, most common in sun-damaged skin in 'fair' individuals.

Epidemiology and aetiology

Basal cell carcinoma (BCC), like other skin cancers, has become increasingly common over recent decades, especially in fair-skinned races. In some countries (including the United Kingdom), it is probably overall the most common single malignancy in both sexes. Some of this rise is due to the increasing frequency of BCC in older age-groups and the rise in the average age of all populations. However, another important factor is that excessive exposure to sunlight is clearly linked causally with BCC, as it is with the other two important epidermal skin cancers SCC and malignant melanoma. There also seems to be no doubt that some people are more prone to develop BCC than are others, and may develop multiple tumours. Rarely, too, BCCs may be seen as part of two genetically determined syndromes: Gorlin's (or the basal cell naevus) syndrome and Bazex syndrome, in which multiple BCCs occur along with follicular atrophoderma (*see* Chapter 11).

It is not entirely clear as to what the cell of origin of BCCs is, but it is clear that the epidermal component is intimately and pathogenetically linked with its adjacent connective tissue.

Clinical features

Most BCCs are rather indolent, slow-growing tumours. Some (especially the superficial variety) rarely, if ever, create more than a minor inconvenience. However, occasional tumours exhibit a much more aggressive growth pattern, with rapid extension and invasion. This is particularly troublesome in tumours arising around the eyes, nose, and ears.

A number of clinical patterns of BCC can be distinguished:

Solid/nodular
- Lesions begin as small papules with a translucent quality but frequently expand with a central depression resulting in an annular appearance (**Fig. 4.24a**).
- Telangiectatic vessels coursing over the surface of the lesion are highly characteristic (and of cystic BCCs).

Cystic
- Results in a lesion of particular translucence.

Morphoeic
- Lesions with much greater stromal, connective tissue element (*see* Pathology on page 127).
- Results in a flat or depressed area, closely resembling a scar or a small area of localized scleroderma (hence the name) (**Fig. 4.24b**).

- Can be extremely difficult to identify the edges of these tumours clearly.

Superficial
- Lesions (especially those occurring on the trunk) may exhibit a very superficial growth pattern (**Fig. 4.24c**).
- Present as indolent, reddish areas with a fine, serpiginous edge, often flecked with pigment.
- Area continues to expand for years, leaving irregular, roughened skin centrally, but larger nodular elements may occasionally arise in these tumours.

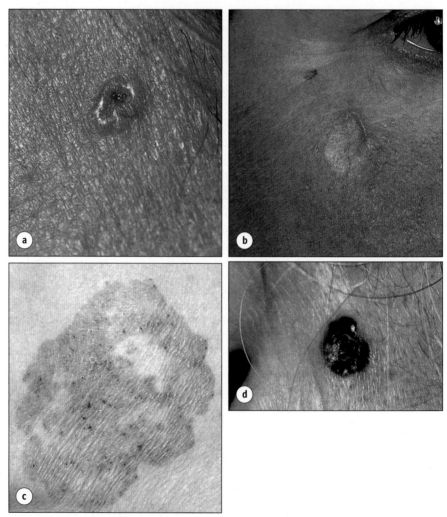

Fig. 4.24 **Basal cell carcinoma (BCC)** — **(a)** a typical, small, nodular BCC (a telangiectatic vessel can be seen on the surface); **(b)** this scar-like area is a morphoeic BCC; **(c)** a superficial BCC; **(d)** a pigmented BCC.

BCCs may also be pigmented (see **Fig. 4.24d**), sometimes markedly so, giving rise to diagnostic difficulties, particularly in distinguishing them from nodular melanomas.

Site(s) of predilection

Solid, cystic, and morphoeic BCCs typically affect the head and neck, specifically the face, the neck, and the ears and retroauricular area. However, lesions may occur in the scalp and on the limbs, and superficial BCCs are most prevalent on the trunk. They may even occur in the perineum, although this is very rare.

Pathology

BCCs present a striking histological picture. The cells are darkly staining and usually grouped in clumps or islands, with a tendency for the cells at the edges to produce a 'palisaded' effect. Initially, connections between these islands and the overlying epidermis are usually demonstrable, but later some islands appear to be entirely disconnected. In fixed specimens, there is often a gap between these clumps of cells and the very distinctive stromal tissue in the underlying or surrounding dermis that clearly forms an integral part of a BCC. Melanocytes and melanin granules may be prominently dispersed among the cells.

In superficial BCCs, there are often multiple foci of buds of tumour cells pushing downwards into the dermis.

In morphoeic BCCs, the pattern is different: the tumour cells are in much narrower strands and columns, often extending deep into the dermis and beyond, between stromal connective tissue.

Investigation and treatment

If there is any diagnostic uncertainty, an incisional biopsy can be performed. Small tumours are easily excised, although some practitioners use cryotherapy. Curettage and cautery or cryotherapy are useful in dealing with large superficial BCCs on the trunk. There was at one time a vogue for curettage and cautery for nodular and cystic lesions, but this is not now as favoured as it was. Recurrences are, perhaps, too common, and it can be difficult to define the extent when they do happen, because of the scarring following treatment. Larger lesions may require the attentions of a dermatologic or plastic surgeon, although radiotherapy is an alternative, especially in the very elderly. For very large lesions, for those adjacent to the nose, eyes, and ears, or for some morphoeic lesions, microscopically controlled surgery (Mohs' surgery) is appropriate. Here, horizontal slices are removed and processed immediately. Areas with residual tumour islands are excised and re-excised until demonstrably clear. The resulting defects may be left to heal by secondary intention or repaired by flaps or grafts.

- Basal cell carcinoma (BCC) is a common skin malignancy found in elderly and middle-aged patients, and is associated with excessive sun exposure.
- Most BCCs are slow growing but some exhibit a much more aggressive growth pattern, with rapid extension and invasion.
- BCC rarely metastasize.
- Incisional biopsy is recommended with any diagnostic uncertainty.

Paget's disease of the skin

Epidemiology and aetiology

Paget's disease of the skin is rare but important. It occurs on the breast (when it is always associated with an underlying intraductal carcinoma) or at extramammary sites (notably in the anogenital region, where underlying cancers may also be found).

Clinical features

- Unilateral disease on the breast.
- Fixed plaque of (usually) non-itchy skin over the nipple, or the areola, or both (**Fig. 4.25**).
- Surface may be scaly or glazed, or may resemble eczema.
- Gradually extends and may occasionally ulcerate.
- Unresponsive to topical steroids.
- Sometimes possible (but by no means always) to feel an underlying lump in the breast.
- Extramammary sites are less easily diagnosed clinically, largely because there are many more differential diagnoses.
- Changes on skin may be very similar to those described for breast disease, but the lesion may also resemble a superficial epidermal lesion such as a seborrhoeic keratosis.
- In vulval and perianal skin areas become moist and reddened and more often multifocal.
- Lesions may extend into the vagina and anus.

Pathology

Histology is diagnostic. The epidermis contains the characteristic Paget's cells — large, round cells with a clear cytoplasm which stain with para-aminosalicylic acid (PAS). The pathology can be confused with that of a superficial spreading melanoma.

Investigation and treatment

A biopsy is essential. A diagnosis of Paget's disease of the breast necessarily involves a mastectomy and it is crucial that the diagnosis is made as early as possible. The main differential diagnosis is of eczema (which is common on the nipples, but which is more often bilateral, itches, and responds to steroids). In extramammary Paget's disease, a search for underlying tumours should also be undertaken. These have included carcinomas of the rectum, cervix, vagina, and ovary, as well as rare skin tumours such as sebaceous and sweat gland carcinomas.

- Paget's disease of the skin is rare but important due to its association with various forms of breast cancer.
- Biopsy is essential as histology is diagnostic.
- Diagnosis necessarily involves a mastectomy.
- Eczema is the main differential diagnosis.

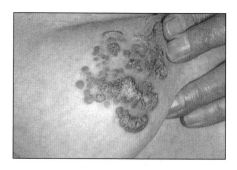

Fig. 4.25 *Paget's disease of the nipple.*

Sweat gland carcinomas

Epidemiology and aetiology

Malignant change may arise in some of the benign sweat gland tumours described on page 113, but some tumours present as primary malignancies of sweat-gland-derived tissue. Several entities are recognized, all of which are rare.

Clinical features and site(s) of predilection

Lesions may present in a variety of ways: the most common is a firm, sometimes tender, reddish nodule, essentially arising anywhere, but more commonly on the hands, feet, and head. One variant is seen on the upper lip, where the lesion is usually very non-specific, appearing simply as a flesh-coloured papule or plaque. Some lesions occur in the scalp.

Pathology

Most tumours show the features of an adenocarcinoma, with cytological atypia and invasion. Some are much more banal histologically.

Investigation and treatment

Lesions should be excised. Tumours may metastasize to lymph nodes and distant sites, and appropriate clinical examination and investigations should be performed.

Porokeratosis

Porokeratosis of Mibelli

Lesions classified under this heading may appear anywhere, although they are most common on the arms and legs. In some patients there is a clear autosomal dominant inheritance pattern. The initial individual area consists (as do the other forms of porokeratosis) of an annular lesion with a fine, slightly elevated margin (representing the cornoid lamella) (**Fig. 4.26**). The centre may be smooth, slightly atrophic, or scaly. The areas tend to extend and merge with adjacent lesions, often eventually involving the whole of a limb. Malignant transformation may occur at a later stage.

It is not usually possible to halt the progress of this type of porokeratosis, but individual dysplastic and malignant areas need to be excised. Oral retinoid therapy may reduce the tendency to malignancy.

Disseminated superficial porokeratosis

Patients are also encountered who have widespread, small porokeratoses, often on the arms and legs. The skin frequently shows signs of chronic sun damage (in which case the lesions

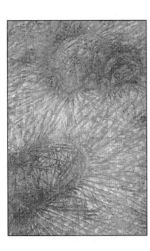

Fig. 4.26 *Porokeratoses, showing the disc around a slightly atrophic centre.* These were of the disseminated actinic variety.

are generally on the extensor surfaces of the limbs), and 'actinic' is often added to the diagnostic label. In other patients, the lesions appear on normal skin; this may be an inherited tendency.

Linear porokeratosis

Linear or zosteriform areas comprised mostly of porokeratoses are most likely to be variants of epidermal naevi (*see* page 98).

Epidemiology and aetiology

All forms of porokeratosis are associated with clonal expansion of keratinocytes. In some forms this appears to be genetically determined, while in others environmental triggers may be more important. There is a variable tendency to neoplastic transformation.

Pathology

The cardinal histopathological feature is of a column of parakeratotic cells at the edge of the area of porokeratosis, known as a cornoid lamella.

Sebaceous carcinoma

Epidemiology and aetiology

These rare skin cancers are composed of tissue thought to be of sebaceous gland origin.

Clinical features

Lesions are single, nodular, and often rather translucent. They may have a yellowish tinge.

Site(s) of predilection

Sebaceous carcinomas mostly arise on the head and neck.

Pathology

The tumour consists of clumps of atypical cells, often deep within the dermis, showing sebaceous differentiation.

Investigation and treatment

The lesion should be excised.

Merkel cell tumour

This very rare tumour arises as a nodule anywhere on the skin surface. The cells are derived from the neuroreceptor Merkel cell. Histologically, the tumour consists of cells that look rather poorly differentiated, and the definitive diagnosis may be difficult without electron microsopy.

The tumour should be widely excised and postoperative radiotherapy has also recently been advocated. Unfortunately, however, recurrence and metastasis are common.

NAEVI AND TUMOURS OF MELANOCYTES

NAEVI OF MELANOCYTES

BOX 4.5

Melanocytic naevi
Aggregations of melanocytes proliferating to produce discrete lesions, visible and palpable.

Melanocytes are derived from the neural crest. Chiefly, melanocytes are spread out along the dermo-epidermal junction, gainfully employed in melanin production. Nevertheless, in most of us, aggregations of melanocytes proliferate to produce discrete lesions that are visible to the naked eye and palpable to the probing finger. These aggregations are called melanocytic naevi. For the vast majority of people, this poses no problem apart from minor cosmetic inconvenience or discomfort. However, in a few people, the lesions have a greater significance, especially when they are precursors to malignant melanoma or are markers of a genetic tendency to malignant melanoma. Conventionally, these lesions are classified as congenital and acquired. There is some overlap here because, of course, birth is an event with no specific relation to melanocyte development. It is clear, for example, that some of the melanocytic naevi that appear in the early years of life are very similar to those that are present at birth — and may have the same significance. Conversely, some of those present at birth are small and behave in very much the same way as do those that arise later.

Congenital melanocytic naevi

Epidemiology and aetiology

Melanocytic naevi are present in approximately 1% of all live births. It is not known at what point they arise during intrauterine life. They are of significance because the giant type carries a substantial increase in the risk of malignant melanoma. Although it is hard to estimate the risk associated with smaller naevi, as many are excised relatively early in life, it is generally accepted that the larger they are, the greater the probability of malignant transformation. Some naevi arising in the first few years of life may have a similar potential, but this remains to be clarified.

Clinical features

Smaller naevi
- Well-circumscribed papules or plaques, which often feel rather deeper and thicker than the commoner congenital naevi (**Fig. 4.27**).
- Hair follicles are frequently found within the naevi. Surface may be smooth or rougher and quite verrucous.
- Several lesions may be present occasionally.

Larger naevi
- Can vary in size from a few centimetres across to the enormous giant melanocytic or bathing-trunk naevus (**Fig. 4.28**).
- Huge area of the body surface is involved in the latter and there may be multiple (sometimes thousands) smaller lesions present.

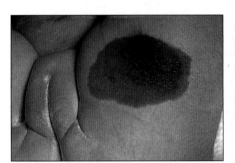

Fig. 4.27 *A congenital melanocytic naevus.*

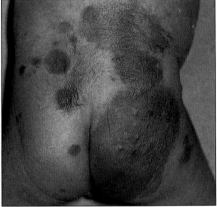

Fig. 4.28 *A giant melanocytic (bathing-trunk) naevus.*

Site(s) of predilection
Congenital melanocytic naevi may occur anywhere.

Pathology
The histology is essentially that of a compound melanocytic naevus (*see* page 134), but there is often a greater degree of separation between the epidermal component and the dermal nests, which usually lie more deeply within the dermis. Furthermore, there is a much greater tendency for there to be a degree of peri-adnexal involvement, particularly around hair follicles, than there is in acquired naevi. There may be quite significant epidermal hyperplasia.

Investigation and treatment

There is usually no doubt about the diagnosis. The problem is to decide what course of action to take. Paradoxically, the lesions that are of least threat to the patient (i.e. the small naevi) can usually be excised easily and with little cosmetic problem. The issue is how to tackle the larger lesions, particularly the giant type. One approach has been to dermabrade these lesions within the first few days of life. This can reduce the extent of the pigmentation, but whether it has any effect on the long-term outcome is unknown. A combination of serial excisions, grafting, and tissue expansion has also been used, but the cosmetic results can be poor.

In between these extremes are those naevi that are too large for easy excision but in which the risk of malignancy is not as great as with the giant type. It is probably good advice to monitor these lesions until puberty, removing any new or enlarging areas immediately. A controlled surgical approach in the teenage years undertaken by plastic and reconstructive surgeons may then be appropriate.

'Acquired' melanocytic naevi

Most melanocytic naevi appear well after birth — during childhood, adolescence, and early adult life. Lesions become much less common with advancing age.

The importance of these lesions lies in their relationship with malignant melanoma. It seems quite likely that similar genetic and environmental factors are involved in both melanocytic naevi and melanoma. For example, there is some evidence that increased exposure to the sun during childhood results in a larger than expected number of melanocytic naevi. Since childhood sun-exposure also appears to be linked to melanoma risk, and since the presence of a large number of melanocytic naevi is an independent risk-factor for melanoma, this may well indicate an important aetiological relationship.

Junctional, compound, and intradermal naevi

Epidemiology and aetiology

Conventional wisdom has it that all acquired melanocytic naevi represent abnormal collections of melanocytes and that they pass through the three sequential phases, junctional, compound, intradermal as the lesion matures (**Fig. 4.29**). This occurs at

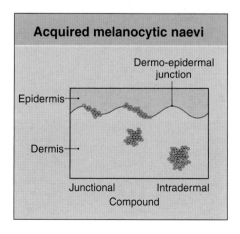

Acquired melanocytic naevi

Dermo-epidermal junction

Epidermis

Dermis

Junctional   Intradermal
Compound

Fig. 4.29 *The phases of acquired melanocytic naevi.*

different rates in different naevi. Mostly, the junctional phase is predominant in children, adolescents, and young adults, whereas compound and intradermal naevi are more evident in later life. Ultimately most, if not all, simple acquired melanocytic naevi disappear given long enough.

Clinical features

The clinical features seen in these lesions depend on the phase in their development at which they are examined.

Junctional naevi (Fig. 4.30)
- May be slightly raised, but are largely flat, brown or black marks.
- Vary in diameter from about 1 to 10 mm.
- Edge generally smooth and even but may be quite irregular.
- No matter how unusual the shape of the naevus, the normal skin markings on the surface are generally preserved unless it has been subject to abrasion or trauma.

Compound naevi
- Fleshier than their junctional predecessors (**Fig. 4.31**) and have an obvious dermal component on palpation.
- May retain their pigment but commonly lesions become progressively paler and more flesh-coloured.

Intradermal naevi (Fig. 4.32)
- Final phase in the maturation of acquired melanocytic naevus.
- Most common clinical appearance is of a flesh-coloured or pale-brown lesion that protrudes from the skin surface, sometimes to a significant extent.

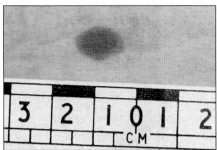

Fig. 4.30 *A junctional naevus.*

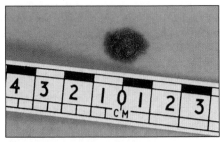

Fig. 4.31 *A compound naevus.*

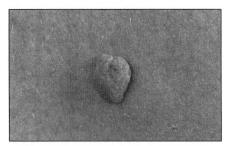

Fig. 4.32 *A pedunculated intradermal naevus.*

Site(s) of predilection

Melanocytic naevi may occur anywhere, although some sites are only involved relatively rarely: palms and soles, genitalia, ears. The presence of several naevi in unusual sites is another feature that marks the patient out as having 'atypical' features.

Pathology

Naturally, the histopathological changes are mirrored in the clinical appearances.

In the junctional phase, compact, distinct nests of melanocytes are present at the dermo-epidermal junction. The cells may be quite large and have abundant, clear cytoplasm.

Compound naevi contain melanocytes both at the dermo-epidermal junction and, because of continued proliferation and maturation, within the dermis. The dermal component is usually well ordered, with the small, darkly staining cells grouped together in columns. The cells may extend quite deeply and may surround appendages. They appear to push through the connective tissue rather than invade and divide it.

Finally, in the true intradermal naevus, the junctional element is lost (although small residual areas may be found on multiple sectioning). The cells are located, therefore, entirely within the dermis, but are, again, grouped in orderly columns.

In both compound and intradermal naevi, the dermal melanocytes are round, oval, or angular in shape (these are sometimes called type-B cells), or, especially deeper in the dermis, may be spindle-shaped (so-called neural or type-C cells).

Investigation and treatment

Excision of an acquired melanocytic naevus is only justified on pathological grounds if there is any suggestion of malignancy.

'Atypical', or 'dysplastic', naevi

Epidemiology and aetiology

There is, as yet, no true consensus as to the status of melanocytic naevi that fulfil the criteria laid down by various authorities under these headings. Lesions described as either 'atypical' or 'dysplastic' are seen:

- Sporadically, as single lesions, in otherwise entirely normal people.
- In large numbers in people with a strong family history of melanoma, and in whom melanomas occur with enormously increased frequency. This is variously termed the 'familial atypical mole melanoma syndrome', the 'dysplastic naevus syndrome', and the 'BK mole syndrome'.
- In large numbers in people with, at the time of presentation, no other significant problems (and in particular with no personal or family history of melanoma). This is known as the 'atypical mole syndrome phenotype'.

Clinical features

Naevi are generally considered to be 'atypical' if they are over 5 mm in diameter and have an irregular outline (**Fig. 4.33**). As indicated previously, some people have several naevi that would fit this description and, indeed, often have large numbers of relatively banal melanocytic naevi as well. Such patients may also have naevi in relatively unusual places, such as the scalp, buttocks, and hands and feet, and melanocytic lesions in the iris. This phenomenon was first noticed when it was realized that these changes represent a cutaneous marker for a genetically determined tendency to melanoma, in the so-called BK mole, familial atypical mole melanoma, or dysplastic naevus syndromes.

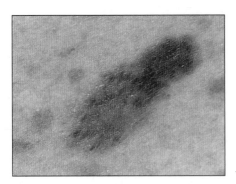

Fig. 4.33 *A clinically 'dysplastic' naevus.*

More recently it has become apparent that the same clinical features occur without a family or personal history of melanoma, and, for such individuals, the concept of the 'atypical mole syndrome phenotype' has been promulgated. It is important to be aware of this because it is becoming clearer that this phenotypic appearance is associated with an increased risk of malignant melanoma.

Site(s) of predilection
Atypical naevi can occur anywhere.

Pathology
There is some controversy about the histological appearances of these lesions. Some authorities are reluctant to accept the concept of histological 'atypicality' at all, arguing that the same appearances occur from time to time in clinically quite banal naevi. Furthermore, naevi that are 'atypical' clinically may present a very bland histological picture. In other words, the clinical and histological appearances that are associated with 'atypicality' are not always in concert. However, the changes that are most frequently described in this context are:
- The melanocytes at the dermo-epidermal junction are seen to spread laterally rather than remaining in 'nests', a change often called lentiginous melanocytic hyperplasia.
- There is bridging between adjacent nests of junctional melanocytes.
- There is elongation of epidermal rete ridges.

Investigation and treatment
Once again, there are some disagreements about how to manage the individual with atypical naevi. When only one or two are present, removal under local anaesthesia is probably the simplest way of providing reassurance and, of course, eliminates the problem. It is the management of patients with multiple lesions, however, that raises the questions. Based on current knowledge, the most practical solution would seem to be to excise some representative naevi to establish whether they show histological, as well as clinical, 'atypia'. The patient can then be counselled about the situation and followed up. They should be asked to look out for new lesions between visits. In addition, it is probably best practice to take an initial set of good clinical photographs and examine these at each successive visit, alongside the patient. The reason for this is the need to look out for the development of malignant melanomas. These appear not only within the naevi (indeed, this is relatively rare) but also in otherwise completely normal skin. A review of clinical photographs will therefore allow a comparison of the pigmented lesions extant at the outset and those present on the day of the review.

Sutton's halo naevus (leucoderma centrifugum acquisitum)

Clinical features

- Ring of white skin appearing around a melanocytic naevus (**Fig. 4.34**).
- Depigmented area is indistinguishable from a patch of vitiligo (see Chapter 10) with which this phenomenon may also be associated.
- May occasionally have several moles that behave in this way.
- Different courses are possible:
  - Pale patch may persist for a few months and then disappear.
  - Central naevus may diminish in size and thickness, and even disappear completely, following which the area usually repigments.
  - Changes may persist indefinitely.

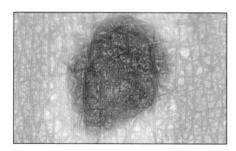

Fig. 4.34 *A halo naevus.*

Site(s) of predilection
Any naevus may be affected, anywhere on the body surface.

Pathology
Histology shows a naevus surrounded by an inflammatory reaction.

Investigation and treatment
No specific treatment is required. Some parents and patients request removal of the mole. The authors have, on occasion, complied with this for naevi in certain sites whereupon the disease process has ceased, with complete repigmentation occurring. In an adult, however, it should be noted that a similar phenomenon may occur around a malignant melanoma.

Naevus 'en cockarde'

Clinical features
Some melanocytic naevi have rings of different colours, said to resemble the 'cockarde' adopted as a symbol during the French revolution (**Fig. 4.35**). They may be seen as single lesions or in among the rather odd-looking naevi described as 'atypical' or 'dysplastic' (*see* page 138).

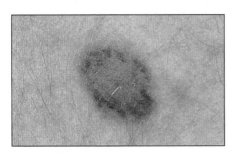

Fig. 4.35 *A naevus 'en cockarde'.*

Site(s) of predilection
These naevi may occur anywhere.

Pathology
There is nothing unusual histologically in the vast majority of these naevi.

Investigation and treatment
No specific treatment is required.

Spitz naevus

Epidemiology and aetiology
The so-called Spitz naevus is seen relatively often in dermatology clinics, especially in children. In older texts and papers, these lesions were sometimes labelled benign juvenile melanomas.

Clinical features

- Classical presentation brick-red, elevated, and firm (**Fig. 4.36**).
- Pressure results in a degree of blanching, but not to the same degree as seen in vascular lesions.
- Usually solitary but multiple lesions may occur and (rarely) a group may be found (situation known as 'agminate').

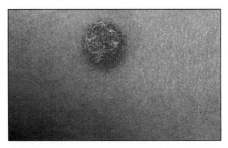

Fig. 4.36 *A Spitz naevus.* The typical 'brick-red' colour is well illustrated.

Site(s) of predilection
Spitz naevi are commoner on the head, neck, and upper trunk, but may occur virtually anywhere.

Pathology
The characteristic histological features associated with these lesions are:
- Junctional melanocytic cells that are larger than usual.
- A dermal component, comprising a mixture of epithelioid and spindle-shaped morphologies, the balance of which varies from lesion to lesion.
- Dermal vessels that are unusually prominent.
- On first inspection, Spitz naevi may be misinterpreted as malignant melanomas. However, on closer examination, the constituent cells can be seen to be relatively uniform, and to mature towards the base of the lesion. The overall architecture is also important: Spitz naevi are narrower at the base than at the surface and are symmetrical — a feature that would be unusual in an invasive melanoma. Although mitoses are seen (as in any proliferating lesion), they are usually few in number and appear normal.

Investigation and treatment
If the diagnosis is certain clinically, no further action is needed.

Spindle cell naevus of Reed

Epidemiology and aetiology
This is a rare variant of the melanocytic naevus, usually seen in adolescent and young adult females.

Clinical features
Spindle cell naevi are small, firm, and deeply pigmented (**Fig. 4.37**).

Site(s) of predilection
The lesions are most commonly found on the thighs.

Pathology
At first sight, the histology can look rather alarming. There is a marked junctional change, with a dermal component of spindle-shaped cells, giving rise to an appearance suggestive of melanoma. The lesion is, however, generally symmetrical and narrows towards the base.

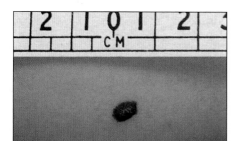

Fig. 4.37 A spindle cell naevus of Reed.
This rather worrying lesion proved, histologically, to be a pigmented spindle cell naevus.

Investigation and treatment

These lesions are often excised because of their dark pigmentation and, thus, uncertainty about them being benign.

Blue naevus

Epidemiology and aetiology

Blue naevi are relatively common and consist of circumscribed collections of functioning melanocytes within the dermis.

Clinical features

The lesion has a highly characteristic dusky-blue/black colour, with a smooth surface (**Fig. 4.38**); it is rarely more than a centimetre in diameter.

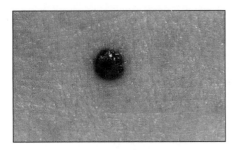

Fig. 4.38 *A blue naevus.*

Site(s) of predilection

Although they may occur anywhere, blue naevi are most common on the extremities (feet, hands), the buttocks and the scalp.

Pathology

Most commonly, there are spindle-shaped, dendritic melanocytes scattered in the dermis, often around appendages, and usually accompanied by a number of melanophages containing clumps of melanin. Less often, there are masses of larger cells present as well, known as a cellular blue naevus.

Investigation and treatment

The most important problem is the potential confusion between the blue naevus and malignant melanoma. Clinical diagnosis is usually straightforward, but excision and pathological examination may be a sensible approach if there is any doubt.

Speckled lentiginous naevus (naevus spilus)

Once in a while, one sees patients in whom multiple melanocytic lesions affect a localized area of skin. In some, this occurs in skin of otherwise normal colour and texture. In others, there is a background café-au-lait pigmentation. Occasionally, the area is linear or pseudo-dermatomal (**Fig. 4.39**); these lesions presumably represent more complex melanocytic malformations.

There is a degree of confusion about the best nomenclature for these lesions, but 'speckled lentiginous naevus' seems to avoid most of the pitfalls associated with other terms. Malignant change has been reported in such lesions.

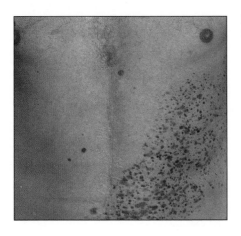

Fig. 4.39 *A pseudo-dermatomal speckled lentiginous naevus.*

DERMAL MELANOCYTOSIS

Mongolian blue spot

Epidemiology and aetiology

The 'Mongolian' blue spot occurs in over 90% of children of Mongolian extraction, but is also seen quite commonly in Indo–Asian and Afro–Caribbean infants. It is rare, however, in white European babies.

Clinical features

A bluish-grey patch of skin with otherwise entirely normal surface markings is present (**Fig. 4.40**). The area may be quite small or may be very extensive; it normally fades during the early years of life, but may persist.

Site(s) of predilection

The most common sites by far are the lower back and buttocks. However, very extensive lesions may cover large parts of the torso.

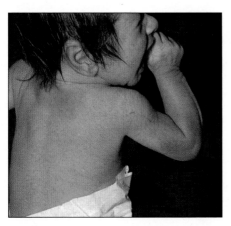

Fig. 4.40 *Dermal melanocytosis of an unusual extent and distribution.* It more commonly affects the sacral area.

Pathology

There are strands of dermal melanocytes present within the dermis, particularly around the neurovascular bundles.

Investigation and treatment

Nothing needs to be done apart from reassurance that all is well. As it is, most affected families are familiar with the appearance and do not present for medical attention.

Naevus of Ota and naevus of Ito

Epidemiology and aetiology

Both naevus of Ota and naevus of Ito are rare in white Europeans, but are seen more commonly in Asians, and in the Japanese in particular.

Clinical features and site(s) of predilection

Naevus of Ota affects the head and neck. The most obvious feature is dark, bluish pigmentation, usually affecting the cheek and eye (**Fig. 4.41**). Some areas may appear browner. Naevus of Ito affects the shoulder region.

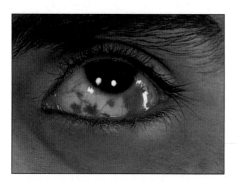

Fig. 4.41 Naevus of Ota. *Pigmentation of both cheek and sclera can be seen.*

Pathology

The histological features are essentially the same as those seen in the Mongolian blue spot.

Investigation and treatment

No specific therapy is required, although malignant melanoma has, very rarely, been reported to arise in these naevoid malformations. Advice on cosmetic camouflage may be useful.

BENIGN ACQUIRED MELANOCYTIC LESIONS

There is some overlap between what is congenital, naevoid, inherited, and acquired in the classification of melanocytic lesions.

Freckle (ephelis)

Epidemiology and aetiology

A freckle is an area of skin in which the melanocytes are more active and responsive to ultraviolet stimulation than in 'normal' neighbouring skin. They are seen particularly in young people, and are associated with the genetic skin-colour type that produces fair or reddish hair and fair skin.

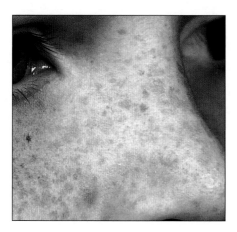

Fig. 4.42 *Typical freckles* *(the observant will have noticed the small naevus for which this photograph was actually taken).*

Clinical features

Freckles are usually 1–5 mm in diameter, always flat (**Fig. 4.42**), and vary in the depth of pigmentation from individual to individual and from season to season during the year. They darken in summer and fade in winter.

Site(s) of predilection

Freckles occur on the face, across the cheeks and nose, and on the upper trunk and arms.

Pathology

Histologically, the skin is essentially normal. Significantly, there is no increase in the number of melanocytes.

Investigation and treatment

No treatment is required.

Lentigo (pl. lentigines)

Epidemiology and aetiology

Lentigines collectively occur most frequently as an isolated phenomenon, but are occasionally a feature of some rare genetic disorders, such as the LEOPARD and the Peutz–Jeghers syndromes (*see also* Chapter 10). Some lentigines are seen in patients with sun-damaged skin and are termed solar lentigines.

Clinical features

Lentigines, like freckles, are flat (i.e. macular) and are much the same size (from one to a few millimetres across). However, the pigmentation is generally rather darker than in a freckle and does not vary with sun exposure.

Site(s) of predilection

Lentigines may occur anywhere. Large numbers may indicate one of the rarer syndromes mentioned above. Very occasionally, they may be arranged in a zosteriform pattern.

Pathology

Histologically, there is an increase in basal layer melanocytes, but without the nesting seen in junctional naevi.

Investigation and treatment

Investigation for lentigines is only required in the following circumstances:
- If there is any diagnostic doubt, particularly if lentigo maligna is a possibility, in which case a biopsy should be taken.
- If there are a large number present, then the possibility of associated abnormalities must be considered and investigated accordingly (*see* Chapter 10).

Labial melanotic macule

Epidemiology and aetiology

The cause of these lesions is unknown.

Clinical features and site(s) of predilection

Labial melanotic macules are what their name suggests: flat, pigmented areas on the lips (**Fig. 4.43**). They can be quite large. Similar lesions have been reported on the genitalia.

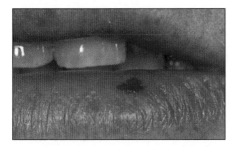

Fig. 4.43 *This flat, labial freckle is benign.*

Pathology

There is an increase in basal layer melanosis, but only a slight increase, if any, in the number of melanocytes.

Investigation and treatment

The major differential diagnosis is malignant melanoma, therefore removal — or at least biopsy — is often appropriate.

- Congenital melanocytic naevi are present at birth; large or 'giant' forms are associated with an increased risk of malignancy.
- Most melanocytic naevi are 'acquired' after birth and pass through three sequential phases junctional, compound, and intradermal.
- Excision of an acquired melanocytic naevus is only justified if there is suggestion of malignancy.
- Naevi are generally considered to be 'atypical' if over 5 mm in diameter and irregular in outline and thus justify histological investigation as there is risk of developing malignant melenoma.
- Halo naevi show a surrounding ring of depigmentation similar to vitiglio.
- Spitz naevi and blue naevi can easily be confused with malignant melanoma.
- 'Mongolian' blue spot occurs in over 90% of children of Mongolian extraction and also in Indo–Asian and Afro–Caribbean infants; naevus of Ota and naevus of Ito occur more commonly in Asians.
- Freckles darken on sun exposure; lentigines do not darken and are more common on sun-exposed elderly skin.

DYSPLASTIC AND MALIGNANT MELANOCYTIC LESIONS

BOX 4.6

Malignant Melonama
Malignant proliferation of melanocytes, usually arising in the epidermis, and most lethal of main skin tumours.

Malignant melanoma

Epidemiology and aetiology

There has been a dramatic increase in the incidence of malignant melanoma (MM) in white populations over the last 40 years. In many countries (e.g. Australia), MM is now one of the major cancers, accounting for a very significant morbidity and mortality. It is now the most common cancer of younger adults in the United Kingdom, although it is, in fact, numerically more common in older age groups. In the United States it has been estimated that by the year 2010, the individual lifetime risk of MM will be 1 in 50.

It is generally agreed that much of this increase is due to exposure to sunlight, and there is a large body of epidemiological evidence supporting this hypothesis. In particular, it seems that childhood sun-exposure and a pattern of intermittent bursts of sun, accompanied by sunburn, may be important. There are also a number of individual risk factors that may determine any one person's chance of developing an MM in their lifetime:

- Heredity — there are some rare families with a vastly increased risk (*see* atypical/dysplastic naevi on page 135). A family history of MM also increases an individual's risk independently.

- The presence of large numbers of melanocytic naevi (whether 'atypical' or not) — this may also be linked to heredity and to childhood sun-exposure.
- Skin colour/type (*see* Chapter 10) — those with very fair skin, especially with red hair and freckles, are at an increased risk, whereas those with genetically brown or black skin have a very low risk.

The prognosis of an individual tumour is closely related to its initial cross-sectional area and its level of invasion at first excision. Most pathology laboratories will provide a report indicating both the 'Clark's level' (**Fig. 4.44**) and a measurement (in millimetres) of the depth of tumour from the granular cell layer to the deepest visible point in the dermis (known as the 'Breslow' depth or thickness — **Fig. 4.45**). **Figure 4.46** gives the approximate predicted 5-year survival figures for various Breslow depths.

Although some authors debate the value of subclassifying MM, preferring instead to refer to the invasive level, there are two reasonably distinct preinvasive forms and four recognizable 'histogenic' types of MM that are seen in clinical practice:

- Lentigo maligna.
- Lentigo maligna melanoma.
- *In-situ* superficial spreading melanoma.
- Invasive superficial spreading melanoma.
- Nodular melanoma.
- Acral, lentiginous melanoma.

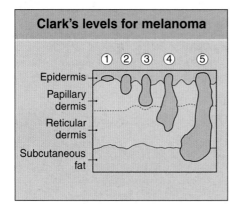

Fig. 4.44 Clark's levels of invasion.

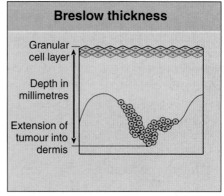

Fig. 4.45 A diagrammatic representation of the Breslow thickness.

A guide to Breslow thickness and 5-year survival of invasive melanoma	
Breslow depth	**5-year survival**
>0.75mm	>95%
0.76–1.5mm	>80%
1.6mm–3.5mm	>60–70%
>3.5 m m	<40%

Fig. 4.46 A guide to the Breslow thickness and 5-year survival guide of invasive melanoma.

Lentigo maligna

Lentigo maligna is seen in sun-damaged skin. It is therefore predominantly found in older patients, although the lower end of the age range is reducing.

Clinical features

The lesion begins as a small, brown smudge and gradually extends to produce an irregular-edged area of unevenly distributed pigmentation (**Fig. 4.47a**), often reaching a considerable size (**Fig. 4.47b**).

Site(s) of predilection

Most lesions occur on the face (**Fig. 4.47c**). Exceptionally sun-damaged skin on the upper arm or trunk may also be affected.

Pathology

Atypical melanocytes proliferate along the dermo-epidermal junction. Similar changes are seen around hair follicles. There is almost always a significant degree of elastosis in the underlying dermis.

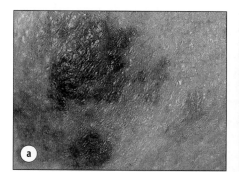
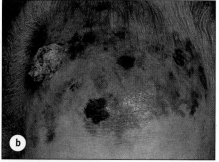
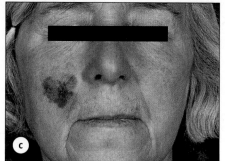

Fig. 4.47 Lentigo maligna — (a) close up of an area of lentigo maligna; **(b)** an enormous area of lentigo maligna on the head, in which thickened areas represent invasive lentigo maligna melanoma; **(c)** lentigo maligna on the cheek, perhaps the most typical site.

Investigation and treatment

An incisional or punch biopsy will confirm the diagnosis. Although lentigo maligna can be eradicated clinically by the use of cryotherapy, excision should be advised for all but the largest lesions because of the risk of recurrence and the development of invasive change. It may also be reasonable to be less draconian in a very elderly patient.

Lentigo maligna melanoma

This term is used for invasive melanoma developing within a lentigo maligna.

Clinical features

A nodular or thickened area develops within a pre-existing lentigo maligna (*see* **Fig. 4.47b**).

Pathology

Histology reveals an invasive component in addition to the surrounding changes of lentigo maligna.

Investigation and treatment

The whole lesion should be excised and sent for histology and assessment of the level of invasion (*see* page 146).

Superficial spreading melanoma

Superficial spreading malignant melanoma (SSMM) represents the most common 'type' seen in white-skinned individuals in most countries. SSMM begins with a phase of gradual extension along the dermo-epidermal junction, in a manner similar to lentigo maligna, before invasion into the underlying dermis occurs. This so-called radial growth phase may last for some years.

Clinical features

- Varies in size from a few millimetres to (rarely) several centimetres across (*see* **Fig. 4.48**); lesion will typically be a centimetre or so in diameter by the time the patient presents to a physician.
- Most lesions have a degree of irregularity in their edge, and this feature is often marked (*see* **Fig. 4.48a**).
- Irregularity of pigmentation is also a cardinal feature, often accentuated by areas of spontaneous regression, which are common in SSMM (*see* **Fig. 4.48c**).
- *In-situ* lesions (i.e. no dermal invasion at all) are macular or virtually impalpable.
- Lesion may become more raised and surface characteristics may alter (scaling, bleeding, or ulceration) in invasive SSMM or when a nodular component has developed within SSMM.

Various groups have produced checklists, or scoring systems, to try to assist in the diagnosis of SSMM. The two most widely quoted are illustrated in **Figures 4.49** and **4.50**.

Site(s) of predilection

SSMM is most commonly seen on the legs in women (*see* **Fig. 4.48d**). When it occurs in men, it is most common on the trunk, particularly the back. Lesions, however, may arise anywhere.

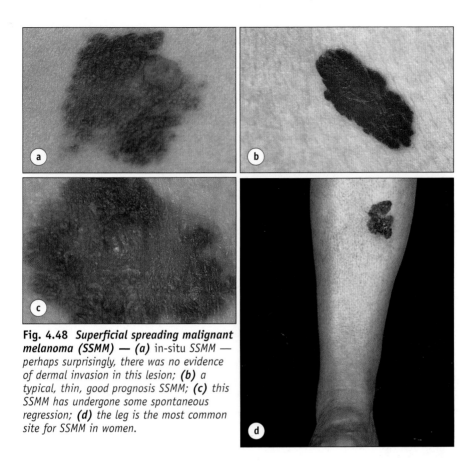

Fig. 4.48 *Superficial spreading malignant melanoma (SSMM) — (a)* in-situ *SSMM — perhaps surprisingly, there was no evidence of dermal invasion in this lesion; (b) a typical, thin, good prognosis SSMM; (c) this SSMM has undergone some spontaneous regression; (d) the leg is the most common site for SSMM in women.*

The 'ABCD(E)' method

'A' = Asymmetry
'B' = Border (irregular)
'C' = Colour variation
'D' = Diameter (over 6 mm)
'E' = Enlargement*
*Added recently and not used by all authorities

Fig. 4.49 *The 'ABCD(E)' method for the diagnosis of superficial spreading malignant melanoma*

149

The 'seven-point check list'	
Major features	**Minor features**
Change in size	Diameter >7 mm
Change in shape	Inflammation
Change in colour	Itching, oozing or bleeding

Fig. 4.50 *The 'seven-point check list'* for the diagnosis of superficial spreading malignant melanoma

Pathology

In-situ lesions show a proliferation of atypical melanocytes within the epidermis. The cells are often arranged in clumps, although there are also many single cells, some of which may be found in the upper layers of the epidermis. Invasive SSMM has these features together with extension of malignant cells into the underlying dermis.

Investigation and treatment

Any lesion suspected of being SSMM should be excised with a clear margin. There is a considerable debate about the necessity for wide excision, which some surgeons still advocate, especially for thicker lesions with deeper invasion. However, the most important treatment is an adequate primary removal. A debate on further surgery can be held once this has been achieved. All pathology reports, should, therefore, contain an indication of the depth of invasion, usually using both 'Clark's levels' and 'Breslow thickness' (*see* page 146). The role of sentinel node mapping as a guide to prognosis and further treatment is as yet uncertain. No chemotherapeutic agent has yet been proven to improve the long-term survival of patients with melanoma.

Some dermatologists advocate special techniques for aiding the diagnosis of MM, and SSMM in particular. These include use of the 'dermatoscope' and epiluminescence microscopy (*see* Chapter 2).

Nodular melanoma

Clinical features

- Lesions present as nodules, sometimes smooth and dome-shaped (**Fig. 4.51a**), sometimes more irregular, and sometimes quite crusty and verrucous (**Fig. 4.51b**).
- Nodular melanoma is not always pigmented, and a small halo of pigment can often be seen around the base of the tumour (**Fig. 4.51c**).
- Lesions usually arise and grow rapidly, and may be quite large at presentation.

Site(s) of predilection

Although nodular MM is said to be more common on the upper back, the lesion may arise anywhere.

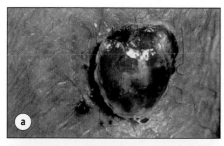

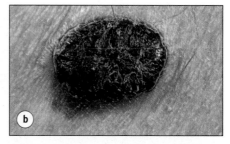

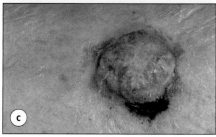

Fig. 4.51 *Nodular malignant melanoma (MM) — (a)* a smooth-surfaced nodular MM; *(b)* a verrucous nodular MM; *(c)* a largely amelanotic nodular MM — a small area of pigmentation is visible around the base of the lesion.

Pathology

A mass of tumour cells invades and, often, replaces the dermis. There is a malignant component within the epidermis, but no lateral spread — which would, by definition, result in the tumour being classified as SSMM.

Investigation and treatment

Treatment consists of immediate excision and histopathology, including depth of invasion (page 146).

Acral melanoma

Epidemiology and aetiology

This is the rarest form of MM in white-skinned populations, However, it is relatively more common in Asians and in Afro–Caribbeans. Although originally subclassified to account for lesions on the palms and soles and under the nails, it has been pointed out that MM of oral, anal, and genital epithelia present similar histological features.

Clinical features and site(s) of predilection

The most typical presentation is of a flat, pigmented area on the palm or sole (**Fig. 4.52a**) or a pigmented area under a fingernail or toenail (**Fig. 4.52b**). One of the more difficult diagnoses in dermatology is to distinguish between a subungual haematoma and an early acral MM. If there is pigment in the nail fold (Hutchinson's sign — see **Fig. 4.52b**), MM is more likely, but often the only way to tell is to take a biopsy, either by lifting the nail plate and sampling the underlying nail bed, or by performing a full-thickness nail biopsy (*see* Chapter 2).

Pathology

Histology shows a proliferation of malignant and atypical melanocytes within the epidermis. A notable feature is that acral MM may appear to be multifocal microscopically, with 'skip' areas of completely normal tissue between tumourous areas.

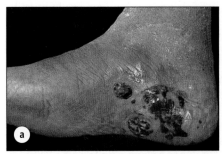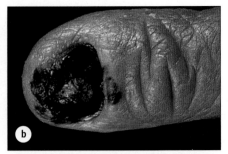

Fig. 4.52 *Acral malignant melanoma (MM)* — *(a)* nodules and metastatic spread have already developed in this long-standing acral MM; *(b)* an acral lentiginous MM showing the classical 'Hutchinson's sign'.

Investigation and treatment

A biopsy is essential. If the diagnosis is confirmed, adequate excision is required. This may involve the amputation or partial amputation of a digit.

Prevention of death from MM

Efforts have been made in many countries to educate the populace about the links between sun exposure and skin cancer, especially MM. The pioneers in this area have been the Australians, who have been very successful in altering sun-exposure behaviour. Similar efforts will no doubt continue over the coming decades in all countries with fair-skinned people which have the resources to do so.

Primary prevention, however, will take time. Meanwhile patients with MM must receive treatment as promptly as possible because, as indicated previously, the prognosis is related to the depth of invasion and, therefore, the sooner the tumour is excised the better. Education campaigns on early diagnosis have been run in several countries, with some apparent success in bringing patients forward earlier than would otherwise have been the case.

Treatment of late-stage, recurrent MM

MM is capable of metastasis to local lymph nodes and to distant sites, such as bone, brain, lungs, and liver. Most dermatologists and surgeons keep patients with primary MM under surveillance for a period of time (usually a minimum of 5 years) and monitor their progress. Enlargement of nodes or the appearance of other symptoms should initiate appropriate surgery or investigations. For example, some patients appear to benefit from lymph node clearance.

Distant metastases are more difficult to treat because MM is not particularly radiosensitive and is notoriously resistant to most chemotherapeutic regimens. However, there have been some remarkable apparent successes and most specialists can recall the occasional case where a patient has lived for long periods after therapeutic intervention. Immunotherapy has had its advocates and has recently been revisited, again with claims of success.

However, the clue to 'curing' MM must remain its early surgical excision if at all possible.

- Dramatic increase in the incidence of MM in white populations over the last 40 years.
- Most common cancer of younger adults in the UK.
- Prognosis closely related to initial cross-sectional area and level of invasion at first excision.
- MM is capable of metastasis.
- Early lesion 'cured' by surgical excision.

NAEVI OF DERMAL COMPONENTS

NAEVI

Connective tissue naevi

As with other components of the skin, malformations and hamartomas may occur in the dermal connective tissue. Some of these are seen as one feature of multisystem syndromes (e.g. tuberous sclerosis, pseudoxanthoma elasticum, Buschke–Ollendorff syndrome). These lesions are generally predominantly composed of either collagen or elastin.

Collagen naevi

Epidemiology and aetiology

The shagreen patch of tuberculous sclerosis is a collagen naevus (*see* Chapter 11). Collagen naevi may also be seen either as part of a rare familial syndrome, sometimes in association with cardiac defects, or as a sporadic feature without associated abnormalities.

Clinical features

Familial and sporadic eruptive collagen naevi are usually multiple, and are flesh-coloured, dermal nodules.

Site(s) of predilection

Lesions are more common on the limbs, but may occur on the trunk.

Pathology

Histology reveals condensations of coarse bundles of collagen.

Investigation and treatment

A biopsy may be required. It is usually prudent to obtain radiographs to exclude the presence of the osteopoikilosis seen in the Buschke–Ollendorff syndrome (see below). In the familial form, the advice of a cardiologist is needed.

Elastic naevi

Very similar lesions to those described for elastic naevi are, on histological examination with special stains, found to contain abnormal elastic fibres. These are known as juvenile elastomas and most commonly occur on the upper thighs and trunk. Sometimes they coalesce into larger plaques. When such lesions are associated (as they often are) with some stippling and opacities — best seen in the epiphyses and metaphyses of the long bones, in the pelvis, and in the carpal and tarsal bones — the condition is known as dermatofibrosis lenticularis disseminata, or the Buschke–Ollendorff syndrome. The bony changes are of no consequence functionally and a good prognosis can always be assured. However, the changes are often not seen until after puberty and it is important to warn parents that this is the case.

- Connective tissue naevi are flesh-coloured, dermal nodules predominantly composed of either collagen or elastin.
- Shagreen patch of tuberculous sclerosis is a collagen naevus.

VASCULAR NAEVI

> **BOX 4.7**
>
> **Vascular naevi**
> Vascular blemishes due to dilated and tortuous vessels either superficially or deep within the dermis.

Vascular blemishes are very common indeed. Most cause no trouble or present relatively minor cosmetic problems, but some are very disfiguring and a few cause major difficulties. The classification of vascular birthmarks is by no means uniform and we are adopting a relatively simple approach, based on both clinical and histological parameters.

TELANGIECTATIC NAEVI
There are two main forms of these lesions, which are both composed of dilated and tortuous, but otherwise essentially normal, vessels:
- The superficial capillary type.
- The deep capillary type (port-wine stain).

The superficial capillary type
Approximately 50% of all neonates have a salmon patch (at the nape of the neck), a stork mark (at the nape of neck or on the forehead), or angel's kisses (on the eyelids). It is often stated that lesions on the neck disappear, but, in fact, many persist, hidden by hair. Lesions on the face usually fade quite quickly and cause no further problems.
- The pathology shows abnormal, dilated vessels within the superficial dermis.
- No investigation or treatment is needed.

The deep capillary type (port-wine stain)
Here there are vessels much deeper in the dermis and the vascular abnormalities may extend further, and deeper, during life. These lesions are permanent and are often very unsightly. They may also be associated with intracranial vascular malformations (the Sturge–Weber syndrome).

Lesions may vary in size from a few millimetres to many centimetres in diameter (Fig. 4.53a and b), and, very occasionally, may cover whole limbs or more. The colour also

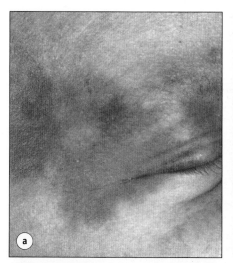

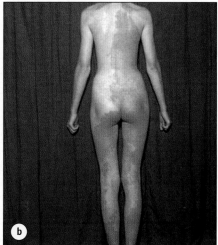

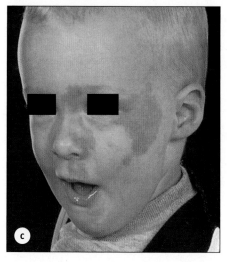

Fig. 4.53 *The deep capillary type (port-wine stain) of telangiectatic naevus —* *(a)* *a capillary naevus on the eyelids — care needs to be taken in case this child develops glaucoma;* *(b)* *an extraordinarily extensive port-wine birthmark;* *(c)* *this child with a port-wine stain in the area of the trigeminal nerve, presented with fits.*

varies: some are a relatively pale pinkish-red, whereas others are very dark purple. All port-wine stains tend to darken as the years pass, and lesions may also become thicker with time. Lesions on or near the eyelid may be associated with glaucoma.

Many port-wine stains affect the head and neck, but (*see* **Fig. 4.53a**) other parts of the body may be involved as well or alone. When a port-wine stain involves the area supplied by the trigeminal nerve, there may be an ipsilateral intracranial vascular malformation, and this can result in mental retardation and long-tract neurological signs (**Fig. 4.53c**).

Regarding the pathology, dilated vessels are seen in the superficial dermis and, increasingly, in the deep dermis. The number and extent of these vessels gradually increase over the years.

Any child with a facial port-wine stain should be assessed neurologically. Any child with a persisting vascular blemish on or near the eyelid should be referred for an ophthalmic opinion because of the risk of glaucoma. The treatment of choice is obliteration of the aberrant vessels using one of the modern lasers. By the time this book appears, there will no doubt be a new type of therapy available that is claimed to be better than any previously used.

Deep arteriovenous malformations

Aberrant vascular development may also occur within subcutaneous tissues, with or without cutaneous involvement. The area is usually soft and warm. Many of these lesions are small and of no real consequence, but others lead to significant distortion of normal architecture and may need surgical correction.

Haemangiectatic hypertrophy

Occasionally, a patient presents with a vascular port-wine-type birthmark or deep arteriovenous malformation associated with hypertrophy of the affected area, usually a whole limb, but occasionally a digit.

Angiomatous naevi (cavernous haemangiomas)

Epidemiology and aetiology

These vascular tumours are seen in infancy and are said to occur in up to 10% of children by the age of one. They are slightly more common in premature babies. Some lesions are relatively superficial (superficial angiomatous naevi; strawberry naevus or mark), while others are deeper, involving the subcutis (deep angiomatous naevi). Very rarely, a child develops multiple lesions, sometimes in association with angiomas in internal organs (diffuse neonatal angiomatosis).

Clinical features

The most common presentation is of a rapidly growing, obviously vascular swelling in a baby a few days or a few weeks old (**Fig. 4.54a**). Most superficial angiomatous naevi are relatively soft, and somewhat irregular in outline. The deeper type presents as rather more diffuse swellings, and can be seen to have relatively normal skin overlying part of the area,

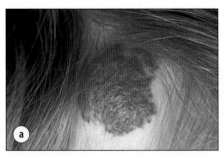

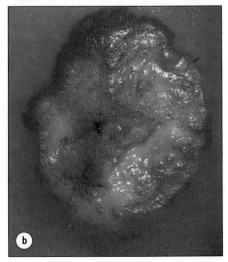

Fig. 4.54 *Strawberry naevi: (a) a typical strawberry naevus on the scalp; **(b)** a strawberry naevus undergoing spontaneous necrosis.*

at least at the outset. However, in many children, a deep component is accompanied by a superficial element on the surface. Some authors prefer the term 'mixed' angiomatous naevi for such lesions. The size and extent are extremely variable, with some lesions reaching their maximum size quite quickly, but with others (especially those with a significant deep component) continuing to grow and becoming very large. In the case of the deep type, large lesions may grossly distort normal anatomy.

Both types continue to grow for a few months (generally no more than six) and then stabilize. The majority also undergo spontaneous regression and may resolve completely. In superficial angiomatous naevi, this process often results in areas of necrosis within the lesion, which can look quite alarming (**Fig. 4.54b**). Just as lesions grow at different rates, the time taken for resolution to occur is also very variable. Superficial naevi usually start to resolve more rapidly than deeper lesions, but either type may last for some years. An oft-quoted rule of thumb is probably not far out: 40% gone by the age of 4 years; 50% by 5 years; 70% by 7 years; and 90% by 9 years. Resolution may be complete, but larger lesions, in particular, often leave a significant cosmetic abnormality, either as a result of residual atrophic areas, or loose, redundant skin over the affected area, or a combination of both.

Site(s) of predilection

Both superficial ('strawberry') and deep naevi may occur anywhere on the body surface, but the former seem to occur more frequently on the head and neck and on the buttocks and perineal area than elsewhere.

Complications

Several complications may arise in association with these naevi (**Fig. 4.55**). Superficial lesions often ooze, especially after trauma. Ulceration is also common and, as indicated above, may be part of the process of regression. Occasionally, this is complicated by infection, and there are cases of severe, life-threatening infections that have arisen in such naevi. If bleeding occurs within the angiomatous mass itself, coagulation factors and platelets may be sequestered, leading to full-blown consumption coagulopathy.

Lesions on the face may obstruct breathing or feeding, by distortion of the nose and mouth. Angiomatous naevi may also interfere with vision. If this happens, and the eye is deprived of visual signals for more than a few weeks, complete amblyopia will result. Angiomatous naevi overlying the lower back, sacrum, and buttocks may be associated with tethering of the spinal cord.

Complications of angiomatous naevi
Bleeding
Ulceration
Infection
Interference with feeding, breathing, or vision
Amblyopia
Systemic involvement by angiomatosis
Spinal tethering
Consumption coagulopathy (Kasabach–Merritt syndrome)

Fig. 4.55 *Complications of angiomatous naevi.*

Investigation and treatment

In most instances, nothing needs to be done apart from reassuring the parents and keeping a watchful brief. It is helpful to have available a picture or two of a child whose naevus has disappeared. However, many authorities now recommend that a scan be performed in a child with an angioma overlying the lower back or sacrum.

The main indications for immediate intervention are: uncontrolled bleeding; excessive size; interference with feeding, breathing or vision. The Kasabach–Merritt syndrome, formerly associated with all haemangiomas, has now been shown to be caused by Kaposiform haemangioendothelioma and tufted angiomas. These can be distinguished by the stain GLUT1.

The treatment of first choice is a short course of systemic steroids (at no less than 2 mg/kg/d, and possibly up to 4 mg/kg/d) following which many lesions will shrink dramatically. The treatment must not be tailed off too quickly and care must be exercised in watching for systemic side-effects. Injected steroids may be an alternative for smaller but troublesome lesions affecting, for example, the eyelids. Other options include sclerosant injections, embolization, and laser therapy. Vincristine has also been found helpful in rapidly expanding lesions.

Some patients will require surgical attention to correct deformities.

- Vascular naevi are common and most present only minor cosmetic problems, such as Salmon patches at the nape of the neck.
- Port wine stains (deep capillary vascular naevi) are deeper, more disfiguring lesions.
- Children with facial port-wine stain should be assessed neurologically.
- Angiomatous naevi (e.g. Strawberry naevi) are common in infancy (10% by age one).
- Indications for intervention in angiomatous naevi included uncontrolled bleeding, excessive size, and interference with feeding, breathing or vision.

DISORDERS IN WHICH ANGIOMAS AND VASCULAR MALFORMATIONS ARE A FEATURE

Vascular malformations and angiomas are also a feature of a number of disorders and syndromes. Some of these are listed in **Fig. 4.56.**

ANGIOKERATOMAS

Some angiomatous malformations are associated with a variable degree of overlying epidermal acanthosis, papillomatosis, and hyperkeratosis. These are known as angiokeratomas.

There are four well-recognized forms of angiokeratoma:
- Angiokeratoma circumscriptum.
- Angiokeratoma of Mibelli.
- Angiokeratoma of Fordyce.
- Angiokeratoma corporis diffusum (Anderson–Fabry disease).

Disorders in which angiomas and vascular malformations are a feature	
Sturge–Weber syndrome	Facial port-wine stain and cranial angioma.
Maffucci syndrome	Cavernous haemangiomas, dyschondroplasia.
Blue rubber bleb naevus syndrome	Venous malformations of the skin, gastrointestinal tract, and other organs.
von Hippel–Lindau syndrome	Retinal angiomas, cerebellar or medullary haemangioblastoma, port-wine stain (occasionally).
Proteus syndrome	Asymmetrical hypertrophy of the face and limbs, angiomas and angiokeratomas, epidermal naevi, subcutaneous masses.

Fig. 4.56 *Disorders in which angiomas and vascular malformations are a feature.*

Angiokeratoma circumscriptum

Clinical features
This type of angiokeratoma is a solitary, purplish plaque with a verrucous surface (Fig. 4.57).

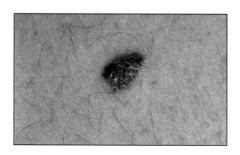

Fig. 4.57 *Angiokeratoma circumscriptum.*

Site(s) of predilection
The most common site is on the lower limb, but lesions may occur on the buttocks and occasionally elsewhere.

Investigation and treatment
Smaller lesions can be excised easily, although some authorities recommend diathermy or hyfrecation. Lasers have also been used more recently. Larger lesions may require the attention of a plastic surgeon.

Angiokeratoma of Mibelli
This form of angiokeratomatosis is thought to be provoked by cold and is often associated with a tendency to cold fingers and toes, acrocyanosis, and chilblains.

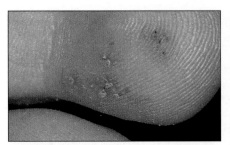

Fig. 4.58 *The small papular lesions of angiokeratoma of Mibelli in a classical site.*

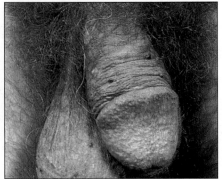

Fig. 4.59 *Angiokeratomas of Fordyce. These usually become more numerous with time.*

Clinical features

There are multiple, small lesions up to 5 mm in diameter. They most commonly begin during adolescence.

Site(s) of predilection

Angiokeratoma of Mibelli is most commonly seen on the fingers and toes (*see* **Fig. 4.58**).

Investigation and treatment

Individual lesions can be treated with diathermy, hyfrecation, or a laser.

Angiokeratoma of Fordyce

These lesions are extremely common in older men and women and often pass unnoticed until one bleeds.

Clinical features and site(s) of predilection

Small, verrucous, purple papules appear on the penis, scrotum, or vulva (**Fig. 4.59**). They gradually increase in number and persist indefinitely.

Investigation and treatment

Lesions can be treated by cryotherapy, diathermy, hyfrecation, laser, or excision.

Angiokeratoma corporis diffusum (Anderson–Fabry disease)

This is a rare, genetic disorder in which multiple cutaneous angiokeratomas are associated with a number of systemic abnormalities (*see* Chapter 11).

Lymphangioma circumscriptum

Epidemiology and aetiology

This birth defect can be particularly troublesome. The lesion is largely derived from lymphatic vessels, although other vascular components may be involved. Lymphangiomas have a complex structure, with a visible superficial component connected to a deeper 'cistern' by a network of lymphatic channels.

Clinical features

Lesions may be quite small or cover significant areas of skin. The most noticeable change is of a number of small vesicles, often said to resemble frog-spawn, which may be present at birth or appear within the skin in early childhood. These may extend and may become pinkish, due to a small amount of blood within the vascular spaces.

Site(s) of predilection

The shoulders and hips are common sites, but lesions can affect other parts of the body, including the limbs, the perineum, and the mouth.

Pathology

The dermis contains dilated lymphatic channels.

Investigation and treatment

Because of the deep component that is usually present, it is normally recommended that lymphangiomas are left alone unless there are compelling reasons to intervene. Unfortunately, inadequate excision is frequently followed by recurrence, and the situation may be worse than before, with new channels oozing sticky fluid replacing the blebs.

Mast cell naevi

Epidemiology and aetiology

The term cutaneous mastocytosis is used to describe any infiltration of the skin by abnormal quantities of mast cells (*see also* Chapter 6) and, as with any other tissue, there may be developmental abnormalities. A solitary collection of mast cells is known as a mast cell naevus or a mastocytoma.

Clinical features

Mast cell naevi vary in size and quite often exceed 1 centimetre in diameter. They are usually solitary, but may be multiple (at which point a semantic discussion could begin over whether the most appropriate label would be multiple mast cell naevi or urticaria pigmentosa — *see* Chapter 6). However, the individual mast cell naevus is usually a reddish papule or nodule that urticates when rubbed (**Fig. 4.60**).

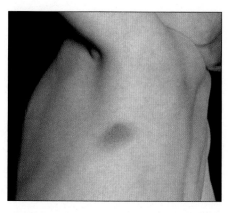

Fig. 4.60 *Mast cell naevus* — *this lesion urticated when rubbed — a classical sign of a solitary mastocytoma.*

Site(s) of predilection

These lesions may appear anywhere.

Pathology

The dermis is occupied by large numbers of mast cells.

Investigation and treatment

There is no need to remove a mast cell naevus unless it is causing significant symptomatic problems.

ACQUIRED BENIGN DERMAL TUMOURS

Dermatofibroma (histiocytoma, sclerosing haemangioma)

Epidemiology and aetiology

It is not clear how or why these extremely common tumours arise, although many authorities still cling to the notion that they may occur following minor scratches or insect bites.

Clinical features

- May be little to see on inspection apart from a degree of surface elevation and some discolouration (varying from a light-brown colour to quite deep pigmentation — see **Fig. 4.61**).
- On palpation a small, dermal mass, shaped like a lentil is found, which moves with the overlying epidermis; gentle squeezing often evokes an apparent 'dimple' on the surface.
- Not uncommon to see patients with several of these lesions.
- Less commonly, the tumour protrudes from the surface and very occasionally may be polypoid.

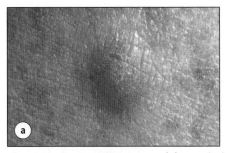 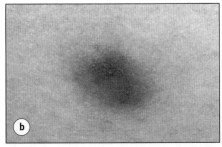

Fig. 4.61 *Dermatofibromas* — *(a)* a typical dermatofibroma (histiocytoma); *(b)* some of these lesions are pigmented.

Site(s) of predilection

Dermatofibromas are much commoner on the limbs, especially the lower legs. Women are particularly affected.

Pathology

A mild degree of epidermal hyperplasia usually overlies the main tumour in the dermis, where there is a mixture of elements: fibroblasts; histiocytes; proliferating, immature collagen; pigment (haemosiderin); and vascular proliferation. The balance of these components varies from lesion to lesion and explains some of the observed clinical differences in the degree of pigmentation. It also explains the somewhat confused, older nomenclature: histiocytoma being applied to more obviously histiocyte-predominant lesions; sclerosing haemangioma being used for those lesions with very marked vascular change.

Investigation and treatment

Very dark lesions may need to be excised because of concern that they may be malignant melanomas. However, most lesions are innocuous and can safely be left alone.

Fibrous papule of the nose

These small, firm, dome-shaped papules are nearly always found, as their name suggests, on the nose. They consist of a mixture of abnormal connective tissue and cells, some of which resemble naevus cells. They may bleed on contact and are often confused with cellular naevi and basal cell carcinomas.

Acrochordons (skin tags)

Epidemiology and aetiology

Skin tags are very common, increasingly so from middle-age onwards, and affect both sexes. They are more prevalent in the obese and may arise during pregnancy. Skin tags are also seen in association with acanthosis nigricans (*see* Chapter 8).

Clinical features and site(s) of predilection

Small, pedunculated, fleshy outgrowths are seen around the axillae, groin, and the side of the neck.

Pathology

Individual lesions consist of a tube of loose connective tissue surrounded by a rather atrophic epidermis.

Investigation and treatment

Tags can be removed easily by diathermy or hyfrecation.

Acquired digital fibrokeratoma

Epidemiology and aetiology

It is thought that digital fibrokeratomas may be the result of minor trauma to the digit on which they arise.

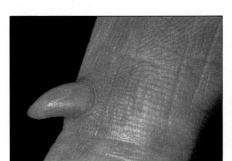

Fig. 4.62 *An acquired digital fibrokeratoma in a classical site.*

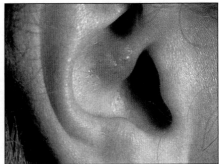

Fig. 4.63 *This small papule is an example of angiolyphoid hyperplasia with eosinophils.*

Clinical features and site(s) of predilection

The lesion is firm and may be papular or elongated. It often overlies an interphalangeal joint (**Fig. 4.62**) and may be tender if squeezed or knocked.

Pathology

Histologically, there is increased vascularity within a 'pseudo-dermis'. The overlying epidermis is generally normal for the area concerned.

Investigation and treatment

It is simple to remove the lesion under local anaesthesia.

Acquired benign angiomas and angiokeratomas

Acquired simple angiomas and angiokeratomas are relatively common. Some rare angiomatous tumours should also briefly be mentioned here:

- Simple angioma — a reddish or purple papule that may appear anywhere on the body surface. It may be dark enough to be confused with malignant melanoma.
- 'Cherry' angioma — red or purple in colour, it is strictly speaking, an angiokeratoma.
- It appears with advancing years and is often known as Campbell de Morgan spot. It has no sinister significance.
- Angiolymphoid hyperplasia — clusters of vascular lesions appear on the head and neck, often around the ears (*see* **Fig. 4.63**). The blood count may reveal eosinophilia.
- Pseudo-Kaposi's sarcoma — multiple, violet/purple papules are seen over the lower legs and feet, often in elderly women. There may be evidence of venous stasis.

Pyogenic granuloma

Epidemiology and aetiology

The term pyogenic granuloma is a misnomer. The lesion is essentially a rapidly growing mass of capillaries enmeshed in connective tissue. Pyogenic granulomas are most common in childhood, adolescence, and early adulthood, but may occasionally occur in later life. Trauma may be an important initiating factor.

Clinical features

- Lesion arises suddenly, often beginning as a small red spot but quickly enlarging into a lump some millimetres across (**Fig. 4.64**).
- Surface is initially smooth but often becomes eroded and bleeds easily on contact.
- Many pyogenic granulomas may appear to arise on a short stalk, with a collarette of hyperplastic epidermis around the base.
- Many begin to organize if left alone, with an epithelium spreading over the surface.

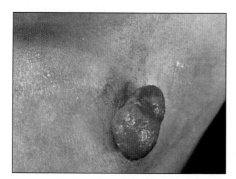

Fig. 4.64 *A pyogenic granuloma arising on a young woman's chin.*

Site(s) of predilection

Pyogenic granulomas are most common on the digits, but may appear anywhere. Multiple pyogenic granulomas around the nail folds and on the upper trunk occasionally occur in patients with acne who are treated with retinoids.

Pathology

The tumour consists of a mass of small, proliferating capillaries embedded in a loose, fibrous-tissue stroma. A significant inflammatory infiltrate is often present.

Investigation and treatment

Although pyogenic granulomas can be destroyed in a variety of ways, the simplest approach is to remove the lesion by curettage and cautery. By doing this, some tissue can be preserved for histology, which may be important if there is any diagnostic doubt. Lesions sometimes recur.

Neurofibroma

Epidemiology and aetiology

Neurofibromas are the main cutaneous feature of von Recklinghausen's neurofibromatosis (*see* Chapter 11). However, patients without this multisystem genetic disorder occasionally present with solitary lumps that prove, on histology, to be neurofibromas.

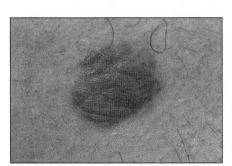

Fig. 4.65 *A solitary neurofibroma.*

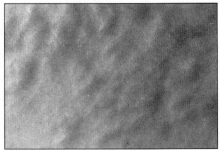

Fig. 4.66 *A cluster of cutaneous leiomyomas.*

Clinical features

Solitary neurofibromas usually present as flesh-coloured, dermal or subcutaneous nodules (**Fig. 4.65**). They may appear anywhere.

Investigation and treatment

Simple excision and pathology are all that is required.

Leiomyoma

Epidemiology and aetiology

Leiomyomas are tumours derived from smooth muscle and may be solitary, arising in the nipple or on the genitalia, or, as the so-called angioleiomyoma, on a limb. The commonest form, however, produces multiple lesions and derives from the arrector pili muscle (*see* Chapter 1).

Clinical features

Cutaneous leiomyomatosis produces a nodule or, more commonly, a cluster or plaque of smooth, firm, pink or reddish nodules (**Fig. 4.66**). The lesions may contract and often are painful in cold weather.

Site(s) of predilection

These are said to be common on the extremities, although the trunk may also be involved.

Pathology

There are numerous spindle cells in the dermis that, with special stains, can be shown to be of smooth muscle origin.

Investigation and treatment

Individual nodules can be excised, but larger areas present greater dilemmas. Plastic surgery may be required for extensive areas, but recurrence is quite common. Some female patients also develop uterine myomas (fibroids).

- Dermatofibromas present as small darkened dermal masses found mainly on the lower legs in women and may be mistaken for malignant melanoma.
- Skin tags are pedunculated fleshy outgrowths common in the middle-aged to elderly and, if necessary, can be removed by diathermy or hyfrecation.
- Pyogenic granulomas (red nodule, common childhood to early adulthood) require excision and histological examination to exclude malignant melanoma.
- Neurofibromas (cutaneous feature of von Recklinghausen's neurofibromatosis) usually present as flesh-coloured, dermal or subcutaneous nodules; require simple excision and pathology.

DYSPLASTIC AND MALIGNANT DERMAL TUMOURS

Dermatofibrosarcoma protruberans

Epidemiology and aetiology

Dermatofibrosarcoma protruberans (DFSP) is an indolent malignant tumour of fibrous tissue. It has local invasive potential, but hardly ever metastasizes.

Clinical features

Patients usually present with a nodule in the skin with an indeterminate history. The area may be reddish-brown (**Fig. 4.67**) or flesh-coloured, and gradually extends, often producing quite a large, irregular area. It is certainly possible to suspect the diagnosis in a large lesion, especially if it has a long history, but in the early stages, DFSP may closely resemble benign tumours, such as dermatofibromas, or a hypertrophic scar.

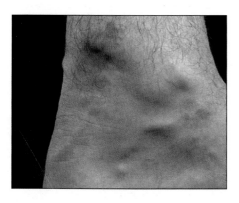

Fig. 4.67 *A dermatofibrosarcoma protruberans.*

Site(s) of predilection

The most frequent site is the trunk, although lesions may occur on the limbs.

Pathology

A mass of fibroblasts occupies the dermis. The tumour stains dark-blue as, unlike a dermatofibroma, it contains very little collagen. The cells are arranged in a so-called storiform pattern (which means 'like a rush mat'). The cells also extend widely, both laterally and deep into the subcutis, a feature that also distinguishes DFSP from a benign dermatofibroma.

Investigation and treatment
After a diagnostic biopsy, the tumour should be widely excised, including a large margin. Local recurrence is, however, very common.

Atypical fibroxanthoma

Epidemiology and aetiology
This is a rare tumour that occurs on the sun-exposed skin of the elderly. Despite its histological appearances, the tumour seldom metastasizes.

Clinical features and site(s) of predilection
The typical tumour appears, and grows rapidly, on the head and neck of a patient in their eighth decade or beyond. There may be ulceration and bleeding, and the tumour may reach a considerable size.

Pathology
The histological appearances are alarming, with a pleomorphic tumour mass containing large numbers of mitoses, closely resembling a highly malignant soft-tissue tumour.

Investigation and treatment
Excision is usually curative.

Malignant fibrous histiocytoma

Epidemiology and aetiology
Malignant fibrous histiocytoma is a much more aggressive tumour than DFSP. Some have been reported to occur in old injuries or areas of scarring.

Clinical features
These tumours are very variable. Some cutaneous presentations represent extension from deeper tissues, but some appear to arise within the dermis itself. It would be most common to find either an irregular, nodular mass or an eroded, ulcerated tumour.

Site(s) of predilection
Many of the reported cutaneous malignant fibrous histiocytomas have occurred on the limbs (**Fig. 4.68**), but they can arise anywhere.

Pathology
The pathology is variable, five different histological patterns having been described. The opinion of an experienced soft-tissue pathologist should be sought if there is any diagnostic doubt.

Investigation and treatment
Wide excision is the best hope of a cure, but these tumours metastasize and are frequently fatal.

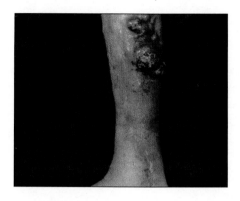

Fig. 4.68 *A malignant fibrous histiocytomas arising on the lower leg.*

Neurofibrosarcoma

Malignant change may occur in a neurofibroma in von Recklinghausen's disease (*see* Chapter 11). The tumour behaves as a malignant soft-tissue sarcoma.

MALIGNANT BLOOD-VESSEL TUMOURS

Angiosarcoma

These highly malignant tumours arise most commonly in the elderly. The site of predilection is the face or scalp, but some arise elsewhere. The lesions often begin as innocuous-looking vascular blemishes, but gradually extend, become thicker and more indurated, and finally ulcerate, or invade deeper structures, or both. Histological diagnosis can be very difficult as the early stages are also very nondescript microscopically. However, there are usually some areas found with the classical intravascular endothelial protrusions or 'buds'.

A very rare form of angiosarcoma affects children.

Lymphangiosarcoma of Stewart and Treves

In this rare disorder, multiple, reddish or purple papules and nodules develop in a lymphoedematous limb (often, but not exclusively, in the arm after mastectomy). The tumours grow quickly and disseminate rapidly.

Kaposi's sarcoma

Epidemiology and aetiology

Kaposi's (haemorrhagic) sarcoma was first described in elderly Jewish patients. However, this tumour has now been described in several different settings:

- The 'classical' form, largely restricted to elderly Ashkenazi Jews and northern Italians.
- As a primarily cutaneous disease in sub-Saharan Africa, but in much younger patients.
- As a lymphadenopathic disease in African children.
- In patients with AIDS.
- As a complication of immunosuppressive therapy, especially in patients with organ transplants.

It seems highly likely that at least some of the cases described in the second and third groups above were HIV-related, but the virus was unrecognized at the time.

Clinical features and site(s) of predilection

'Classical form'
- Purplish-brown patches appear on the extremities, particularly the feet, and very slowly grow into small, vascular tumours (**Fig. 4.69a**).
- Lesions may gradually extend up the leg and can become quite widespread but this normally takes years.
- Tumour may involve internal organs in a very few patients.

African endemic forms
- Patients are much younger and can include children.
- Cutaneous lesions may be juicier and less obviously vascular than in the classical disease (**Fig. 4.69b**) and spread more rapidly.
- Systemic involvement occurs much earlier; in some cases, the disorder appears to commence as a systemic disease, with prominent lymphadenopathy and hepatosplenomegaly.

Immunosuppressed patients (chemotherapy or AIDS)
- Lesions crop almost anywhere but often occur on the head and neck, and in the mouth.
- May resemble lesions seen in the classical form but can begin as very subtle, dusky, purplish patches similar to bruises, only later becoming thicker and more indurated.

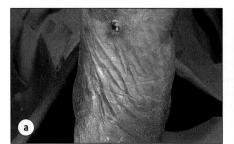 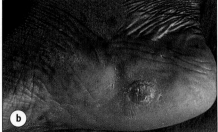

Fig. 4.69 *Kaposi's sarcoma — (a) an example of the classical form, on the foot of an elderly Jewish woman; (b) arising on the foot of a young West African.*

Pathology

The lesions are a mixture of vascular spaces, spindle cells, extravasated red cells, and haemosiderin within macrophages, with a variable inflammatory infiltrate.

Investigation and treatment

Localized areas respond well to radiotherapy. More widespread disease requires chemotherapy. Any young patient presenting with lesions of Kaposi's sarcoma must be screened for HIV infection. Further radiology may be required to look for multi-organ involvement.

LYMPHOMAS

The skin may be the primary site of a lymphoma, which, in almost all cases, is of T-cell origin, or be infiltrated by various haematological malignancies, including B-cell lymphomas (*see also* Chapter 6).

CUTANEOUS T-CELL LYMPHOMA (MYCOSIS FUNGOIDES)

Epidemiology and aetiology

A huge array of terms has been applied over many years to early phases in the evolution of this disorder (e.g. parapsoriasis-en-plaque, parakeratosis lichenoides, poikiloderma atrophicans vasculare), with the later stages often being called mycosis fungoides (MF) — the name given to it by Alibert, who is credited with its first description. Some of the earlier phases may also be referred to as pre-mycotic. Many authorities now prefer the term cutaneous T-cell lymphoma (CTCL) to cover all the different manifestations of the disease, but the other terms are still in common use around the world.

In essence, all the clinical appearances described below can be caused by the proliferation, within the skin, of an abnormal clone of skin-homing (or epidermotropic) T cells. It is not known why this process begins, and it can take years to evolve.

Clinical features

In the early years, there are essentially two common clinical appearances: slightly raised, fixed, eczematous and scaly plaques (**Fig. 4.70**) and a more atrophic change associated with increased vascularity and pigmentary disturbance, often still called poikiloderma atrophicans vasculare (**Fig 4.71**). The reader is referred also to Chapter 5, where the entity known variously as chronic superficial scaly dermatitis, xanthoerythrodermia perstans, or digitate dermatosis is illustrated (*see* Fig 5.40). This disorder can look very similar to plaque-type, early CTCL, and may need to be assessed with care. One useful sign is that CTCL is often itchy, while the 'benign' look-alike may not be.

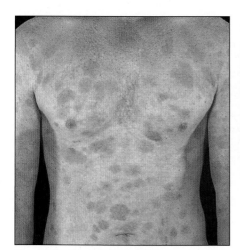

Fig. 4.70 *Mycosis fungoides.*

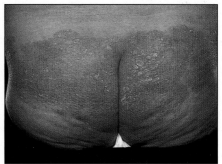

Fig. 4.71 *Poikiloderma atrophicans vasculare.*

In later phases of the disorder, tumours and ulceration may develop. This may be accompanied by, or precede, systemic involvement, with lymphadenopathy and hepatosplenomegaly being prominent features.

CTCL is also an important cause of follicular mucinosis (*see* Chapter 6).

Site(s) of predilection

No areas of the body are exempt from CTCL, although lesions are probably seen more often on covered sites (early lesions respond well to ultraviolet radiation — *see* below).

Pathology

The histological changes in early lesions may be very subtle and, indeed, it may not always be possible to make a definitive diagnosis on simple light microscopy alone. There is, however, a lymphocytic infiltrate present, which is usually, but not always, closely applied to the epidermis. A cardinal feature is the presence of lymphoid cells migrating into the epidermis and forming, in places, aggregates known as Pautrier micro-abscesses. In the poikilodermatous form of the disease there is often a loss of the basal cell layer, similar to that seen in the lichenoid dermatoses (*see* Chapter 5), but without the vacuolar degeneration. As lesions become more established, increasing numbers of grossly abnormal, darkly staining lymphoid cells appear. The infiltrating cells bear the surface markers of the T cell and are largely CD4+ve.

Investigation and treatment

Any patient with lesions suggestive of CTCL should have a skin biopsy. If the diagnosis is not confirmed at the first attempt, the patient should be observed; if the lesions remain characteristic, a further biopsy should be taken. There is no consensus on whether a full staging process is appropriate. Since many patients live for very long periods with limited disease progression, it is often perfectly reasonable to adopt a 'wait-and-see' policy.

Treatment depends on how advanced the CTCL has become. Early lesions often respond satisfactorily to a combination of topical steroids and UVB phototherapy or PUVA. Later lesions that appear to be confined to the skin can be managed with radiotherapy (for localized lesions) or electron-beam therapy (for widespread disease). There have also been encouraging reports of the use of extracorporeal photophoresis, and of bexarotene for later stages of the disease. The management of systemic disease with chemotherapy is the province of the clinical oncologist.

Special variants of CTCL

There are two rare, but distinct, clinical and histological states that are associated with CTCL.

One is the very unusual 'intra-epidermal' form known as pagetoid reticulosis or Woringer–Kollopp disease. This usually presents as a slowly growing plaque in which nests of lymphoid and histiocytic cells occupy the epidermis.

The other is the Sézary syndrome, which may be caused by other cutaneous inflammatory processes, but which must be treated as CTCL until proved otherwise. This disorder is a form of exfoliative dermatitis (*see* Chapter 5) in which both skin and peripheral blood contain numbers of large, darkly staining lymphoid cells known as Sézary cells.

B-cell lymphomas

As indicated on page 171, the skin may be infiltrated by B-cell lymphomas and other haematological malignancies (*see* Chapter 6).

PSEUDOTUMOURS

A number of swellings may occur within the skin or the subcutis that are not true tumours — the so-called pseudotumours.

Chondrodermatitis nodularis helicis (or antihelicis) chronicus

Epidemiology and aetiology
This very common lesion affects mostly older patients. It is thought to result from a degenerative and inflammatory process of the ear, probably with pressure acting as an initiating factor or as a co-factor.

Clinical features and site(s) of predilection
Chondrodermatitis affects the ear. The individual lesion is a papule, often with a central plug (**Fig. 4.72**), which is tender on pressure. Men are affected much more often than women. It is most common for the lesion(s) to appear on the rim of the helix, but they can also occur on the antihelix if this is particularly prominent.

The main problems with these lesions are the pain they cause and the fact that they can be confused with dysplastic lesions such as basal or squamous cell carcinomas.

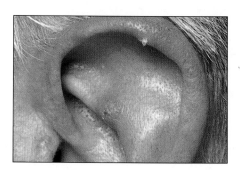

Fig. 4.72 *Chondrodermatitis nodularis helicis chronicus.*

Pathology
Histology reveals a marked inflammatory reaction in both skin and cartilage.

Investigation and treatment
Reasonable results can be obtained with injected steroids and cryotherapy. If there is any diagnostic doubt, however, the simplest approach is to excise the area under local anaesthesia.

Keloids and hypertrophic scars

Epidemiology, aetiology, and site(s) of predilection
Both of these conditions represent abnormally proliferative scar tissue. There is a degree of confusion about what differentiates a hypertrophic scar from a keloid scar. One authoritative textbook considers that the defining point is that a hypertrophic scar remains confined to the original dimensions of the injury, whereas a keloid extends beyond it. Another considers that the term hypertrophic scar is appropriate if the lesion ultimately

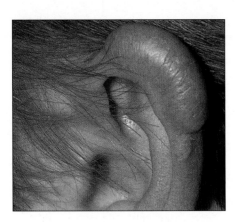

Fig. 4.73 *A keloid on the rim of the ear.*

undergoes a degree of spontaneous resolution. Use of either definition therefore means that the diagnostic distinction can only be made with a degree of retrospection and most lesions have to be treated *ab initio* as one and the same.

Hypertrophic and keloid scars usually follow some form of trauma (which may be remarkably trivial) or be a sequel to inflammation, such as that accompanying acne (*see* Chapter 5). Some keloids appear to arise without any preceding trigger.

Young people are much more prone than the middle-aged or elderly to hypertrophic and keloid scar formation. Certain anatomical sites are particularly susceptible: the chest, the upper back, the shoulders and upper arms down to the insertion of deltoid, the suprapubic region, and the ears (**Fig. 4.73**). Afro-Caribbeans are particularly predisposed to keloid formation, although any ethnic group may be affected.

Clinical features

- Present as smooth swellings in the line of a previous scar, injury, or inflammatory episode.
- Often itchy.
- May become quite red and livid and continue to expand over many weeks or months until, in most instances, the process becomes quiescent.
- Large keloids, such as those following burns, may also produce significant contractures and deformity.

Pathology

Whorls of connective tissue, and fibroblasts arranged in a haphazard fashion, are seen. Mast cell numbers are reported to be increased.

Investigation and treatment

The most satisfactory solution is to do as little as possible. Certainly, excision is highly likely to result in a recurrence, often larger than before. Some surgeons, however, maintain that postoperative radiotherapy or intralesional steroid injections produce better results. A more conservative approach involves the use of intralesional steroid injections with or without cryotherapy. Furthermore, application of silicon sheets to the area sometimes seems to reduce the size and firmness of the scars.

SUBCUTANEOUS TISSUE TUMOURS

Lipomas

Epidemiology and aetiology

Solitary lipomas are extremely common. Occasionally, multiple lesions are inherited as an autosomal dominant trait (**Fig. 4.74**).

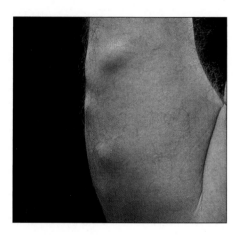

Fig. 4.74 *Multiple lipomas.*

Clinical features

The individual lesion is a soft, lobulated, subcutaneous mass. Some lesions appear to have a slight increase in surface vascularity. Such lesions are sometimes painful when knocked.

Site(s) of predilection

Lipomas can occur anywhere.

Pathology

Collections of fat cells, sometimes admixed with dilated and aberrant vessels, are seen. The latter appearance is sometimes subcategorized as angiolipoma, and this pathology is thought to correlate with the discomfort that occurs in some lesions when knocked.

Investigation and treatment

Solitary tumours are easily excised. Multiple lesions are best left untouched.

- Chondrodermatitis nodularis is a benign swelling of the ear affecting mainly elderly men; can be confused with dysplastic lesions.
- Keloids and hypertrophic scars are caused by abnormally proliferative scar tissue.
- Lipomas are collections of subcutaneous fat cells that can occur as multiple lesions; extremely common.

chapter 5

Inflammatory Dermatoses

URTICARIA AND ANGIO-OEDEMA

Box 5.1

Urticaria
Raised swellings or wheals caused by leakage of fluid from vascular spaces into the dermis.
Angio-oedema
Deeper diffuse swelling caused by leakage of fluid from vascular spaces into the subcutaneous tissues.

INTRODUCTION

Urticaria is an eruption characterized by the appearance of multiple cutaneous wheals (**Fig. 5.1**). Angio-oedema (**Fig. 5.2**) is the same process, but involving the subcutaneous tissues. Individual wheals, almost by definition, arise and disappear within a short period of time (from about 30 minutes to 3–4 hours) and leave no visible mark. However, during an

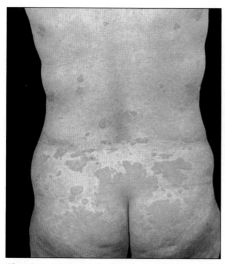

Fig. 5.1 *Urticarial wheals on the buttocks and lower back in a patient with idiopathic urticaria.*

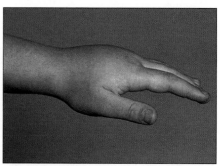

Fig. 5.2 *Swelling of the hand due to angiodema (courtesy of Dr Martin Stern).*

attack of urticaria, crops of wheals continue to appear anywhere on the body surface. In some patients, the whealing tendency lasts for a few days at most. In other patients, the process can continue for months or years, but there may be days free of whealing and others where the problem is much more intense. Rarely, urticaria is part of a more generalized systemic reaction to injected, ingested, or inhaled proteins. This situation — known as anaphylaxis — may be associated with profound lowering of blood pressure and death.

The underlying process in urticaria and angio-oedema is initiated by the release of vasoactive chemicals from mast cells. The most important of these chemicals is histamine, but other compounds are undoubtedly involved in some instances, notably in more severe reactions and in some forms of physical urticaria (*see* below). It is not known what causes the release of these mediators in all cases. In some patients with acute forms of urticaria, the reaction is associated with interactions between antigens and IgE (**Fig. 5.3**) that disrupt the mast-cell membrane. Almost any substance can have antigenic properties, but the most commonly encountered antigens are drugs (e.g. penicillin), foodstuffs, possibly food additives, and some inhaled pollens and moulds. In other patients urticarial lesions may be part of a more generalized 'serum sickness' reaction caused by type-III hypersensitivity. Some chemicals (e.g. aspirin, opiates, and possibly food additives) may trigger mast-cell degranulation directly. In many instances the mechanism remains unclear.

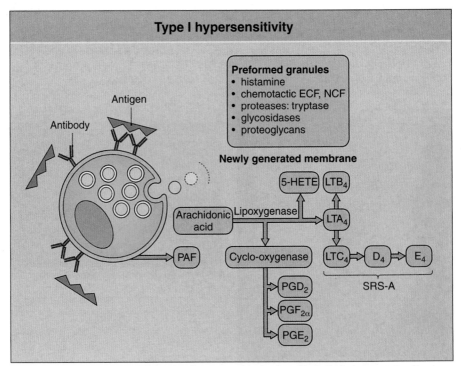

Fig. 5.3 *Type I hypersensitivity leading to urticaria. Specific IgE binds to mast cells; antigen then binds to the free end of IgE leading to release of histamine and other inflammatory mediators.*

CLINICAL FEATURES

A number of clinical patterns and causes of urticaria are recognized (**Figs 5.4–5.8**).

The urticarias - a working classification	
Acute	Attack lasts for a few days and is generally associated with a recognizable trigger, e.g. foods (strawberries, shellfish); drugs (penicillin, aspirin).
Contact	Similar to acute, attacks last for a few hours associated with direct skin contact with offending agent, e.g. grass, animal fur, foods.
Chronic idiopathic *	Attacks last for weeks, months or even years and single aetiological factors are seldom identified, although some authorities believe that food colouring, preservatives and additives may play a role.
Symptomatic dermographism	Wheals appear at the site of scratching (Fig. 5.5); this may occur together with, or independent of, other forms of urticaria.
Cholinergic	Small wheals appear on the upper trunk in young adults in conditions associated with sweating (Fig. 5.6).
The physical urticarias	May be a feature of chronic idiopathic urticaria *
Cold-induced	Wheals appear on exposure to cold: gusts of air, or cold drinks and foods may trigger an attack (Fig 5.7).
Heat-induced	Very rarely, hot substances may set off a whealing tendency; heat is also a non-specific trigger in other forms of urticaria.
Aquagenic	Whealing follows contact with water at any temperature.
Light	Whealing occurs after exposure to light (solar urticaria).
Delayed pressure	Exceptionally in this form, the wheals do not appear for 24 hours; contact with chair-backs and walking may trigger the wheals (Fig 5.8).
Angio-oedema	Deeper, diffuse subcutaneous swellings occur, especially around the eyes and mouth; involvement of the throat can result in airway obstruction; palms and soles may be involved; angio-oedema may be part of a generalized anaphylactic reaction and may accompany urticaria; rarely, angio-oedema is due to an inherited defect of C1-esterase deficiency: **hereditary angio-oedema**.

Fig. 5.4 *The urticarias — a working classification.*

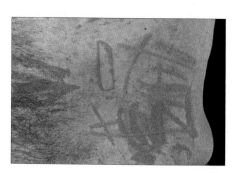

Fig. 5.5 *Symptomatic dermographism; linear wheals at the sites of scratching.*

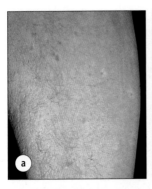

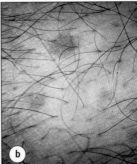

Fig. 5.6 *Cholinergic urticaria: (a) tiny oval urticarial lesions on the forearm induced by exercise; (b) close up.*

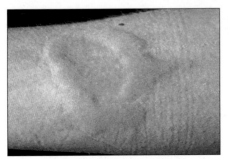

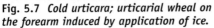

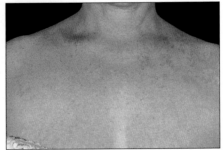

Fig. 5.7 *Cold urticara; urticarial wheal on the forearm induced by application of ice.*

Fig. 5.8 *Delayed pressure urticaria; urticarial wheal induced by weights strapped to the shoulder.*

INVESTIGATION AND TREATMENT

It is important to take a good history, which will help to reveal potential triggers. It is usually prudent to perform simple haematologic and biochemical screening, especially if the condition is associated with any feeling of malaise or there are other general symptoms. Urticarial rashes are sometimes seen with hepatitis and other infections. Some clinical immunologists may wish to follow these tests with a range of IgE-based tests, including skin-prick tests and serum antibody screening (e.g. radioallergosorbent tests, RAST) to pinpoint a specific antigenic trigger. If it is suspected that the urticaria has a physical basis, a challenge test is appropriate: ice applied to the skin for cold urticaria; hot water in a container for heat-induced urticaria; ultraviolet radiation for solar urticaria; water for aquagenic urticaria. To test for delayed-pressure urticaria, a heavy weight should be left in contact with the skin (usually on a strap over the shoulder or thigh); the patient monitors the response over the next 12–24 hours.

The drug treatment of choice for most forms of urticaria begins with the H$_1$ antihistamines. Early H$_1$ antihistamines produced marked sedation in most individuals but there are now a number of agents in which this side-effect is much less troublesome (e.g. fexofenadine, desloratadine, levocetirizine); these would normally be used as first-line therapies. Some authors advocate the addition of H$_2$-receptor antagonists (there are also H$_2$ receptors in the skin) when the urticaria is not easily controlled by monotherapy. Some forms, especially the physical urticarias, are largely unresponsive to antihistamines of either class. A more aggressive approach involving systemic steroids may be required in a few patients, especially those in whom the urticaria is part of a major systemic allergic response.

ANAPHYLAXIS

Very occasionally, the vasoactive mediators released in urticaria may produce a profound vasodilatation, leading to a reduction in blood pressure, lowered cardiac output, and shock. Such reactions may occur with drugs (penicillin is a classical offender, but many other agents may be responsible) or foods (nuts are a common cause). The mechanism involved may either be type I (IgE-mediated hypersensitivity) or the reaction may occur as part of a type-III (immune complex) problem. Unless urgent action is taken, the patient may rapidly succumb to anoxic brain damage and die. The most immediate requirement is adrenaline (epinephrine) to improve circulatory performance. Patients may also need systemic steroids, antihistamines and intensive-care support. It is crucial that potential triggers are identified and avoided as far as possible.

URTICARIAL VASCULITIS (*SEE ALSO* CHAPTER 8)

In some urticarial eruptions, lesions with an otherwise typical morphology last much longer than usual and leave a purpuric stain in the skin (**Fig. 5.9**). Histologic examination of the lesions reveals true, low-grade vasculitis. Such lesions often occur as an isolated phenomenon, but may be part of a more generalized illness such as systemic lupus erythematosus.

- Urticaria is a common eruption of multiple cutaneous wheals caused by fluid leakage from vascular spaces into the dermis; angio-oedema is the same process but involving the subcutaneous tissues.
- Wheals arise and disappear within a short period of time (30 minutes to 3–4 hours).
- Process is initiated by the release of vasoactive chemicals from mast cells.
- Non-sedating antihistamines can be prescribed.
- Urticaria may sometimes be associated with profound vasodilatation, reduced blood pressure, lowered cardiac output, and shock (anaphylaxis); treat with adrenaline (epinephrine).

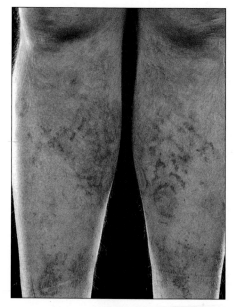

Fig. 5.9 *Purpuric urticarial wheals on the legs in a patient with urticarial vasculitis.*

THE ECZEMA–DERMATITIS GROUP

Box 5.2

Eczema-dermatitis
Term applied to inflammatory skin conditions caused by both exogenous (irritant, allergic infectious) and endogenous (genetic) factors.

INTRODUCTION

Inflammation within the skin is a factor in a number of conditions. This whole chapter is, of course, devoted to 'inflammatory' dermatoses such as psoriasis and lichen planus; skin infections are invariably associated with a degree of inflammation. Indeed, inflammation is one of the most basic and important of all the pathologic processes with which we, as doctors, are required to deal. However, some types of cutaneous inflammation are conventionally grouped together under the working title 'eczema' or 'dermatitis'. This somewhat miscellaneous group of conditions share similar histopathology and an absence of other specific features that would require a reclassification into a group covering of the other disorders dealt with in this section of the book.

It is helpful in studying this group of disorders to produce a sensible working classification (**Fig. 5.10**); a number of recognized complexes of signs provide useful clinical distinctions. We also understand the causes of some forms of eczema and dermatitis; this offers further insights. However, it must be acknowledged that it is impossible (and possibly unhelpful) to ascribe a definitive label to every patient within the working classification.

Eczema-Dermatitis

Exogenous
    Primary irritant
    Contact allergic
    Secondary to pathogens (infective)
Endogenous
    Atopic
    Seborrhoeic
    Discoid
    Hand and foot: hyperkeratotic/fissured vesicular (pompholyx)
    Stasic (varicose)
    Asteatotic
    Superficial scaly dermatosis
    (Xanthoerythrodermia perstans)
    Lichen striatus
    Photo-provoked
    Neurodermatitis (including lichen simplex chronicus and nodular prurigo)

Fig. 5.10 *A classification of eczema-dermatitis.*

It cannot be emphasized enough that nearly all eczema is caused by a combination of both endogenous (i.e. genetic) and exogenous factors. For example, atopic dermatitis clearly has a very significant genetic component (as shown by family involvement and the particularly high degree of concordance for the disease between identical twins). However, it seems highly likely that something in the environment needs to activate this genetic predisposition. The same is certainly true of irritant dermatitis, where the same exposure to irritants such as soaps or detergents will provoke a reaction much sooner in someone with a tendency to eczema than someone without. There may be several overlapping endogenous and exogenous factors at work.

- Eczema-dermatitis describes skin conditions characterized by inflammatory processes.
- Eczema is caused by a combination of both endogenous (i.e. genetic) and exogenous factors (e.g. skin irritants).

CLINICAL FORMS OF ECZEMA–DERMATITIS

Primary irritant dermatitis

The skin is capable of withstanding a significant degree of chemical insult but, if such trauma is excessively prolonged or the materials involved are particularly harsh, an irritant dermatitis may develop (**Fig. 5.11**). As indicated above, this occurs with greater speed in some patients, often because of an endogenous eczematous tendency. For example, irritant dermatitis is very much more troublesome in those with a previous history of atopic dermatitis. Common irritants include soaps and detergents, shampoos (especially in hairdressing), foodstuffs, and cutting oils. Working with the hands in a constant state of wetness may induce the same changes. Thus, certain occupations predispose to the development of condition: hairdressers; cooks and caterers; machine-tool operators; washers-up; nurses; and housewives/homemakers.

It often takes repeated injury over time for the reaction to develop but, once the process has begun, short remissions are followed by rapid deterioration. This is evident in the common experience that industrial hand dermatitis will frequently improve over a weekend away from work, only to return within a few hours of restarting. Longer periods away from the trigger (e.g. summer holidays) may produce longer relief.

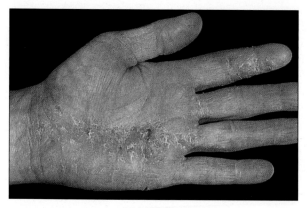

Fig. 5.11 *Irritant contact dermatitis of the hand.*

Investigation and treatment — The only permanent solution to severe irritant dermatitis is the cessation of the provoking activity but, if this is impossible, some relief can sometimes be obtained by the judicious use of topical corticosteroids to suppress inflammation, the liberal use of emollients and non-soap cleansers, and avoidance measures such as gloves and barrier creams.

- Irritant dermatitis results from prolonged or harsh chemical insult (e.g. soaps, foodstuffs, and cutting oils)
- Short remissions are often followed by rapid deterioration.
- Cessation of the provoking activity is the only long-term solution but avoidance means include gloves, barrier creams or topical corticosteroids.

Contact allergic dermatitis

Some people develop type-IV, delayed, cell-mediated hypersensitivity to allergens in their environment. Exposure induces a dermatitis, predominantly at the site of contact. Often, only minute quantities of the offending agent are needed to cause reactions. These reactions begin within the epidermis when antigens, present on the surface of the Langerhans' cells, trigger a T-cell response (**Fig. 5.12**). A large number of agents can induce contact allergic dermatitis (**Figs 5.13–5.17**)

Although dermatitis caused by contact allergy typically occurs at the site of contact, secondary spread onto adjacent or even distant non-contact sites is common and may cause confusion. Certain sites are more often affected than others, especially the eyelids, which are commonly inflamed in sensitivity to epoxy resins, plants, cosmetics and metal, for example.

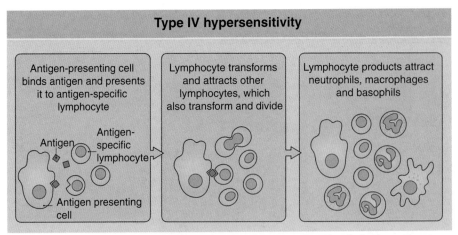

Fig. 5.12 *Type IV reaction — antigen-presenting (i.e. Langerhans') cells in the epidermis bind antigen and present it to T lymphocytes, triggering the release of a variety of cytokines (IL-1, IL-2, IL-4, etc.) which results in an inflammatory response.*

Causes of contact allergic dermatitis

Antigen	Common pattern/sites	Environmental source
Nickel and cobalt (Fig. 5.14)	Eczema under jewellery, watches, fastenings	Non-precious metals
Chromates	Hands; feet; face (due to airborne contact)	Cement; tanned leather; industrial processes
Rubber chemicals (Fig. 5.15)	Hands, forearms, waist, feet	Gloves; shoes; elasticated materials
Colophony	Under sticking plasters	Sticking plasters
Epoxy resins	Face, hands	Domestic and industrial use
Phenylene diamines	Face, especially eyelids, which are often oedematous	Hair dyes
Formaldehyde, the 'parabens', ethylene diamine, and Quaternium 15	Almost anywhere but often eyelids and face; may complicate varicose eczema and otitis externa	Preservatives in medicaments and toiletries - formaldehyde especially in shampoos
Lanolin	Anywhere; may complicate varicose eczema and otitis externa	Medicaments and toiletries
Aminoglycosides (especially neomycin)	Anywhere; may complicate varicose eczema and otitis externa	Medicaments
Corticosteroids	Anywhere	Medicaments
Plant antigens (Fig. 5.17)	Linear streaks at point of contact; face (due to airborne contact)	*Primula obconica*(UK); Rhus (poison ivy) (USA); Parthenium (India); Chrysanthemum and many others
Wood antigens	Hands; forearms; face (due to airborne contact)	Hardwoods, especially mahogany

Fig. 5.13 *Some common causes of contact allergic dermatitis.*

Any material that is volatile, or can be airborne in the form of dust, can give rise to airborne contact dermatitis. The pattern of involvement here is often of a diffuse dermatitis of the face, backs of hands, and other exposed areas, simulating a light-sensitive eczema. However, the classical light-spared areas are usually involved.

Investigation and treatment — Investigation must begin with a careful history of exposure to potential sensitizers. It is important to establish a clear description of possible work and domestic sources. This should include details of all tasks carried out, hobbies and leisure pursuits, and cosmetics, toiletries, and medicaments applied to the skin surface. The key investigative technique is patch testing (**Fig. 5.18**), in which suspected offending agents are applied to the surface of the skin for 48 hours before being removed; the site is then examined for evidence of allergic dermatitis (**Fig. 5.19**). A second examination after 72 or 96 hours is also essential. It has been estimated that up to 30% of positive reactions will be missed if this is not undertaken because some compounds produce later reactions (e.g. lanolin, neomycin). In most instances, a battery of common test allergens is used and these may be modified and adapted for local circumstances or for particular problem areas (e.g. medicaments) or occupations (e.g. hairdressing). It is also often useful to test materials

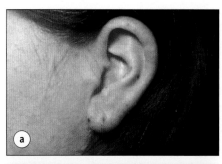

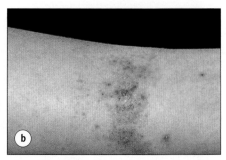

Fig. 5.14 *Common sites of contact allergic dermatitis to nickel* — *(a)* ear lobe (from cheap earrings); *(b)* wrist (from a watch strap); *(c)* back (from metal clasp on a brassiere).

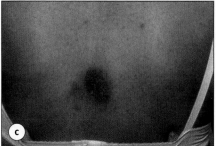

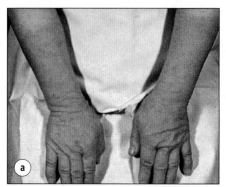

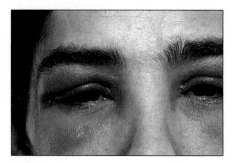

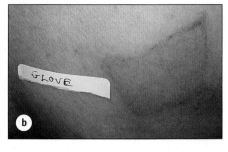

Fig. 5.15 *(a)* Contact allergic dermatitis of the hands and forearms with a sharp cut-off at the mid-forearm due to wearing rubber gloves; *(b)* positive patch test to a piece of rubber.

Fig. 5.16 *Periorbital dermatitis caused by contact sensitivity to preservatives in cosmetics.*

- Contact allergic dermatitis can occur with minute quantities of offending agent at site of contact.
- Secondary spread onto adjacent or even distant non-contact sites is common.
- Investigation involves a careful history and patch testing.
- Treatment with topical corticosteroids may produce symptom relief

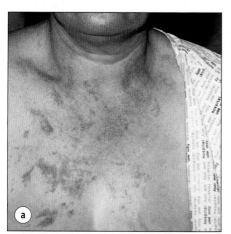
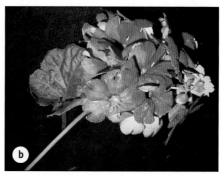

Fig. 5.17 Dermatitis: (a) *linear streaks on the chest caused by* **(b)** *a primula obconica.*

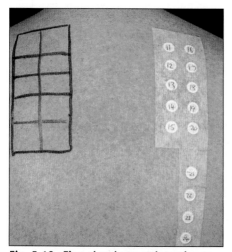
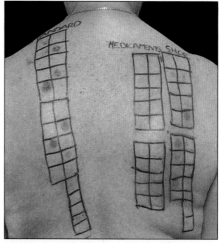

Fig. 5.18 Finn chamber patch testing to the back. *After removal, the site of each patch test is outlined with a marker pen (alternatively, the top of each row of five may be marked).*

Fig. 5.19 Results after 98 hours: several positives in the standard and shoe batteries.

suspected by the patient of being responsible (e.g. make-ups, materials handled at work). However, care must be taken not to place highly irritant chemicals on the skin. If there is any doubt, a specialized test should be used.

It may also be useful to visit the patient's place of work to see precisely what is involved. This may draw attention to tasks and contacts that were not apparent from the history alone.

Treatment of an acute attack with potent topical corticosteroids may produce significant symptom relief; this could perhaps be combined with soaking in potassium permanganate solution if there is a vesicular or bullous component (*see also* Dermatitis of the hands and feet). However, it is essential to remove the causative agent from the environment as far as possible.

Infective eczema

Eczematous changes can be induced by invading organisms. The red, itchy rash that is associated with ringworm (tinea) is nothing more than an inflammatory response to the presence of fungal organisms in the skin (*see* Chapter 3). A bizarre form of this eczematous response to fungal infection is seen with the so-called dermatophytide, in which a widespread eczema and pompholyx of hands and feet develop because of hypersensitivity to a fungal infection, usually of one foot. Typical eczematous dermatitis also occurs commonly around areas of molluscum contagiosum, especially (but not exclusively) in children with an underlying tendency to atopic dermatitis. Bacterial infections may occasionally produce similar changes.

Atopic dermatitis (called also atopic eczema, infantile eczema)

Atopic dermatitis is one of the commonest disorders in the Western world. In the UK at least 15% of children are affected by the age of 4 years. Atopic dermatitis is classically associated with the other common atopic diseases: asthma and allergic rhinitis–conjunctivitis (hay fever). Urticaria and urticarial reactions, especially after contact with foods and animal hair, are also commonly seen in patients with atopic dermatitis.

Definition — One important question that has been addressed recently is the definition of what is and what is not to be considered atopic dermatitis. In many ways, this is one of the easiest skin disorders to diagnose but it can also present real difficulties and, particularly when considering population studies, clinical trials, and pathogenic research, it is essential to have a method of distinguishing atopic dermatitis from other forms of eczematous dermatitis. A set of diagnostic criteria can be derived from work conducted by the UK Atopic Dermatitis Working Party; this is the first properly evaluated diagnostic checklist (**Fig. 5.20**).

Diagnostic criteria for atopic dermatitis

To diagnose atopic dermatitis, the clinician should observe:
- An itchy skin condition (or report of scratching/rubbing in a child)
  plus three or more of the following:
- A history of involvement of the skin creases (folds of elbows; fronts of ankles; around neck; cheeks in children <4 years old).
- Personal history of asthma or hay fever (or of atopic disease in first degree relative in children <4 years old).
- History of generalized dry skin in past year.
- Visible flexural eczema (or eczema of cheeks/forehead and outer limbs in children <4 years old).
- Onset in first 2 years of life (not applicable to children <4 years old).

Fig. 5.20 *Diagnostic criteria for atopic dermatitis (eczema).*

Pathogenesis — It is clear that genetics are fundamentally important in atopic dermatitis. As indicated above, a family history of asthma, rhinitis, atopic dermatitis itself, and other atopic phenomena is common in patients with the condition. Furthermore, a Danish twin study has demonstrated unequivocally that the risk of developing atopic dermatitis is much higher in monozygotic twins than in dizygotic twins or non-twin siblings. It also appears from some studies that there may be a significant degree of specificity in the inheritance of the atopic disorders. However, it is also apparent that this condition, and the other atopic disorders, are complex interactions between this genetic susceptibility and the environment in which the individual lives. Atopic dermatitis is more common in higher socioeconomic groups; in one community-based study in Leicester, we demonstrated that although atopic dermatitis is equally common among children of both (white) European and Asian families, a family history of atopic disease is significantly less frequent among Asians. One interpretation of these findings is that genetic susceptibility exists equally in both groups, but that an element of the Western environment has triggered the development of atopic dermatitis.

It is highly likely that disordered immunologic function is fundamental in this host–environment interaction. It is well known that the majority of patients with atopic dermatitis have high IgE levels and positive prick tests for allergens such as house dust mites, cat and other animal fur, dander, pollens, grasses, moulds, and some foods. However, it is also clear that the immunohistological features of the condition are more in keeping with those of a type-IV hypersensitivity reaction than the type-I reaction classically seen in urticaria. Attempts have been made with some success to reproduce eczematous lesions by the application of airborne allergens and house dust mite, and support for the possible importance of such allergens is beginning to emerge with therapeutic prophylactic and interventional studies.

Two discoveries have been made about the clinically involved skin of patients with atopic dermatitis: epidermal Langerhans' cells bind IgE; IgE was also found to be present on the surface of antigen-presenting cells in the dermal infiltrate. This has led to the hypothesis that antigens absorbed through the skin might bind to allergen-specific IgE on the surface of epidermal Langerhans' cells, thereby inducing T-lymphocyte activation and an eczematous hypersensitivity response.

Further work also appears to indicate that T-cell proliferation in patients with atopic dermatitis results in the preferential expansion of a clone of T cells known as the T-helper 2 subset. This type of work, together with a better understanding of the underlying molecular genetics, will continue to refine our knowledge of the intricacies of the interactions taking place in this disease.

We must not forget, however, that other factors may also play a fundamental or facilitative role in atopic dermatitis. For example, epidermal lipids are qualitatively and quantitatively abnormal. Much interest has in the past focused on cyclic nucleotide metabolism, especially in the leukocytes, and more recently abnormalities in neurotransmitters have attracted attention. There has also been much interest in the role of *Staphylococcus aureus*: nearly all patients with atopic dermatitis are colonized (*see* below). However, immunological dysfunction is clearly important, and further studies may begin to explain how and why atopic dermatitis starts in whom it does and, just as interestingly, why it so often seems to disappear.

Clinical features – Atopic dermatitis usually begins in childhood, often in the first year of life. However, the same skin changes may appear at any age. In its most typical form, beginning in infancy, the face is prominently involved (**Fig. 5.21**) with red, inflamed skin. Similar changes appear over the trunk and limbs (**Fig. 5.22**), often on the extensor surfaces initially. As time passes, there is an increasing tendency for the flexural surfaces to become

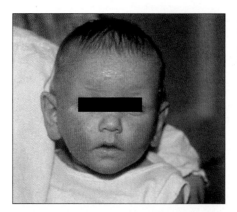

Fig. 5.21 *Atopic dermatitis in childhood typically spares the periorbital and perinasal areas giving a characteristic appearance.*

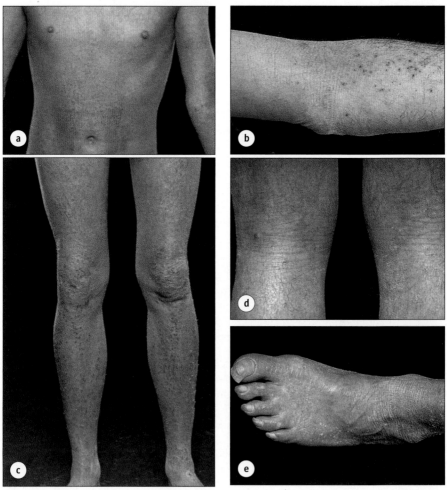

Fig. 5.22 *Atopic dermatitis affecting (a)* the trunk; *(b)* antecubital fossae; *(c)* lower limbs; *(d)* popliteal fossae and *(e)* ankles.

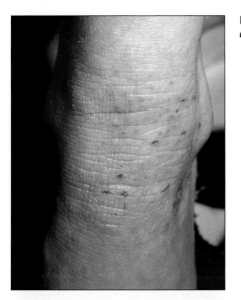

Fig. 5.23 *Lichenification in chronic atopic dermatitis.*

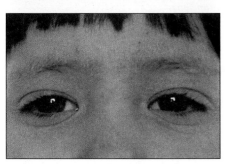

Fig. 5.24 *Arcuate skin creases of both lower eyelids (Dennie–Morgan folds) bilaterally.*

involved (antecubital and popliteal fossae; wrists and ankles) (Fig. 5.22). The skin may also become thickened and rough — a change known as lichenification (**Fig. 5.23**). A similar phenomenon occurs around the eyes, where the 'Dennie–Morgan' infraorbital fold is commonly seen (**Fig. 5.24**). Patients with this disorder often have a generally 'dry' skin. The term xerosis is often used to describe this situation, although a significant number of children have changes amounting to a true ichthyosis (*see* Chapter 11).

There are also, often, multiple scratches and abrasions present because atopic dermatitis is always itchy. The itch is probably the aspect of the disorder that causes the most distress. The symptom seems to become all-pervasive. Patients have feverish bouts of scratching, and some children seem never to stop rubbing and scratching at their skin. They may lie awake at night, keeping other family members from sleeping.

Another frequent finding is weepy, yellow crusts caused by impetiginization (**Fig. 5.25**). However, defining precisely what represents secondary staphylococcal infection in atopic dermatitis is not always straightforward. Most patients with the condition are colonized by *Staphylococcus aureus* all the time, and there seems to be a complex relationship between the skin and the organism: treating the lesions with topical corticosteroids reduces the level of staphylococcal colonization, and the use of antibiotics or antiseptics will frequently bring about an improvement in the skin. It has been suggested that staphylococcal proteins may

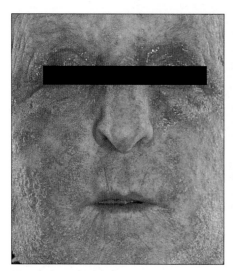 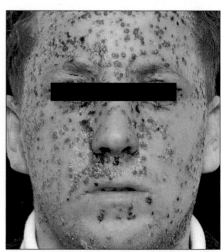

Fig. 5.25 *Impetiginized dermatitis of the face showing yellow-gold crusts indicating infection with* **Staphylococcus aureus.**

Fig. 5.26 *Extensive herpes simplex of the face in a patient with atopic dermatitis (eczema herpeticum/Kaposi's varicelliform eruption).*

be involved in the perpetuation of eczematous changes in atopic dermatitis or the exacerbation of such changes (or possibly both), either directly or by immunological mechanisms.

The natural history of childhood atopic dermatitis is for spontaneous resolution in about 60% of cases. Unfortunately, a significant number of patients continue to have trouble into adolescence and adulthood. Furthermore, a large number of individuals with a past history of the disease develop primary irritant dermatitis from occupational or domestic exposure to chemicals (*see* page 183).

Eczema herpeticum (Kaposi's varicelliform eruption)

It is very important that superinfection with the herpes simplex virus is detected in a patient with atopic dermatitis. Viral lesions spread widely over the skin surface, creating an appearance resembling chicken pox (hence the name originally used by Moritz Kaposi) (**Fig. 5.26**). This may be accompanied by a fever, particularly if the attack is associated with first-time exposure to the virus. This state can be life-threatening for three main reasons.

- The skin may cease to be an effective barrier to the retention of fluid and protein, leading to metabolic disturbances.
- The skin is susceptible to further invasion by bacteria that may cause septicaemia.
- Viraemia and viral encephalitis may occur.

If eczema herpeticum is suspected, and the patient is febrile or unwell, intravenous therapy with aciclovir (acyclovir), or one of the newer alternative drugs, should be started immediately. Topical corticosteroids should also be suspended, and the patient should be kept under close observation.

Investigation and treatment — There are few investigations that assist in the diagnosis or management of atopic dermatitis on a day-to-day basis. Swabs for bacterial culture may be valuable to determine antibiotic sensitivity. Samples for viral culture should be taken before commencing treatment if eczema herpeticum is suspected. Allergy tests (prick tests and serum assays for total IgE and specific IgE) are usually unhelpful, except in confirming the atopic state.

First-line therapies in atopic dermatitis	
Emollients	Liberal use helps to keep the skin comfortable and may reduce the need for corticosteroids; often used in association with bathing, as oils, non-soap cleansers and post-bath applications; in general, the heavier the emollient the better it will work, but cosmetic factors also need to be considered; good emollient bases include white soft paraffin and lanolin.
Corticosteroids	Highly effective in controlling the inflammation; the major concern is with long-term use and the potential for atrophy and, especially in children, systemic absorption; for short bursts, it is reasonable to use stronger steroids but for maintenance, the weakest effective agent should be chosen.
Antihistamines	There is no evidence that histamine is important in atopic dermatitis unless there is a significant element of urticaria; however, older, more sedative agents (trimeprazine, promethazine, hydroxyzine) possess tranquillizing properties and can be very useful if given at night.
Anti-infectives	As indicated, agents that inhibit *Staphylococcus aureus* are useful adjuncts, either in short bursts, or as long-term additions to the regimen; there are several options: antiseptics added to the bath; antiseptic or antibiotic creams, either alone or in combination with corticosteroids; oral antibiotics.
Tar	Tar has been known to soothe itchy skin for many years; the most frequent method of application in atopic dermatitis is probably in the form of impregnated bandages; these are wound around affected limbs and produce both relief and protection from scratching; they are messy and smelly and are not always favourites with children or parents. Two forms are in common use: wood/coal tar and ichthammol.

Fig. 5.27 *First-line therapies in atopic dermatitis.*

Treatment is largely symptomatic. **Figure 5.27** gives a list of first-line agents that most dermatologists would consider using in a patient with atopic dermatitis. **Figure 5.28** records some of the therapies that may need to be considered if symptoms are out of control and the quality of life for patient, family, and friends has reached a critical point.

- Atopic dermatitis is very common and associated with other atopic diseases such as asthma and hay fever.
- Atopic disorders are complex interactions between genetic susceptibility and the environmental factors.
- Begins often in the first year with red inflamed skin, dryness and intense itch.
- Secondary staphylococcal infection is common; superinfection with the herpes simplex virus can be life threatening.
- Treatment is symptomatic and may involve emollients, corticosteroids, antihistamines, anti-infectives, tar.

Second-line therapies in atopic dermatitis

These modalities may need to be considered if measures outlined here fail to produce sufficient control or if, as in the case of topical corticosteroids, they may result in an unacceptable risk of side-effects:

Topical calcineurin inhibitors (tacrolimus, pimecrolimus)	These agents provide an alternative to topical corticosteroids; they do not cause atrophy and are particularly useful for facial and flexural skin, and as an adjunct to conventional therapy: questions have been raised about possible carcinogenicity, but there is no evidence that this is an issue in clinical practice.
Ultraviolet radiation	Both ultraviolet B and PUVA have been shown to be effective in atopic dermatitis (for details, see Psoriasis).
Dietary and other environmental alteration	Anecdotal reports of improvements of atopic dermatitis with diet have led to several studies; a few show benefit, many do not; if all else fails it may be reasonable to try a restricted diet under careful supervision for a few weeks; house dust mite eradication has also been reported to have beneficial effects and may be worth considering.
Evening primrose oil	The evidence for any significant effect is thin.
Immunosuppressives	Systemic steroids and ACTH-like agents may occasionally have a role in producing short-term relief; azathioprine has its advocates and has been shown to be effective in two controlled tests; ciclosporin (cyclosporin) A is highly effective, if rather costly and potentially toxic.
Chinese herbs	There is some evidence that some mixtures of Chinese herbs may be effective in some patients; at this time, these agents have not been licensed.
	There have been reports of toxicity (notably hepatitis) and some creams have been found to be adulterated with steroids.

Fig. 5.28 *Second-line therapies in atopic dermatitis.*

Seborrhoeic eczema/dermatitis

This is a very common clinical pattern of eczema seen in adults. There is a form of eczema known as infantile seborrhoeic dermatitis, which occurs (as the name implies) in infancy. The two are not directly related and must be considered separately. The infantile form is considered below.

Clinical features — There are a number of unmistakeable features seen in classical seborrhoeic dermatitis.

Pathogenesis — Considered to be a purely endogenous disorder for many years, the pathogenesis of seborrhoeic dermatitis has at last begun to be unravelled. Although the precise mechanisms involved have still to be elucidated, it seems clear that the yeast *Malassezia/Pityrosporum orbiculare* (*Malassezia furfur*) plays a major role in inducing and perpetuating the inflammation (*see also* Pityriasis/tinea versicolor and Pityrosporon

- Certain sites are prominently involved:
  - Scalp. Mild scaling (or dandruff) represents one end of the clinical spectrum, with marked scaling and erythema at the other; seborrhoeic dermatitis is also one of the causes of the clinical change known as pityriasis amiantacea (**Fig. 5.29**; *see also* Psoriasis).
  - Nasolabial folds (**Fig. 5.30a**).
  - Upper chest (both front and back) (**Fig. 5.30b**).
  - Behind the ears.
  - Eyebrows (**Fig. 5.30c**).
- On the face the red, scaly, somewhat greasy-looking eruption is characteristic and may spread out on to the cheeks (**Fig. 5.30c**).
- Some patients also suffer from an inflammation of the eyelids (blepharitis).
- Others develop a more flexural (intertriginous) form, with lesions in the axillae, groins, and areas where skin surfaces are apposed; these lesions merge, often indistinguishably, with the clinical appearance of flexural psoriasis (see page 208).
- Flexural seborrhoeic dermatitis may be mild but may also be extremely troublesome.
- Adult seborrhoeic dermatitis usually presents in adolescence or early adulthood and, although the severity may fluctuate, the tendency often persists throughout life.

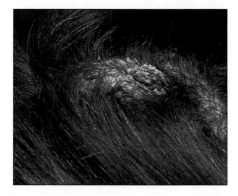

Fig. 5.29 *Pityriasis amiantacea* — *scale enveloping the lower part of hairs in seborrhoeic dermatitis.*

folliculitis, *see* Chapter 3). It is also of considerable interest that seborrhoeic dermatitis is one of the skin signs associated with HIV infection, particularly at the point at which CD4 counts begin to fall.

Investigation and treatment — There are no useful tests to aid diagnosis, but HIV infection must always be considered in any case where the condition appears to be particularly severe or resistant to treatment. Patients will often benefit from either a topical corticosteroid cream or a topical antifungal agent such as miconazole, clotrimazole, or ketoconazole. (Ketoconazole was the first agent to be investigated and the one that, in part, resulted in the re-evaluation of the role of yeasts in this condition.) Sometimes a combination of corticosteroid cream and antifungal agent is helpful. Occasionally, severe seborrhoeic dermatitis requires oral treatment with an agent such as itraconazole.

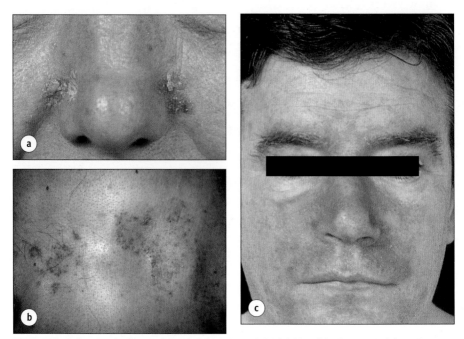

Fig. 5.30 *Seborrhoeic dermatitis of (a)* the nasolabial folds; *(b)* chest and *(c)* eyebrows, cheeks and perioral areas.

Infantile seborrhoeic dermatitis and napkin (diaper) dermatitis

Some children develop a widespread eruption involving the napkin (diaper) area, flexures, and scalp (**Fig. 5.31**). This state, known as infantile seborrhoeic dermatitis, generally appears in the first 3 months of life. The rash appears to cause no symptoms, although the napkin area may be rather sore and weepy. Certainly, itching is not a prominent feature (as judged by a lack of scratching and rubbing), which helps distinguish the rash from atopic dermatitis. However, perhaps 25% or more of children develop typical atopic dermatitis later. The skin lesions respond well to mild topical corticosteroids (often combined with an antifungal agent because of a fear of superadded candidal infection). The scalp changes

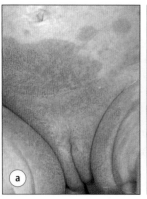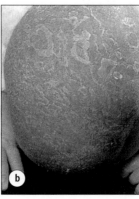

Fig. 5.31 *Seborrhoeic dermatitis in an infant, affecting (a)* the nappy area and *(b)* the scalp.

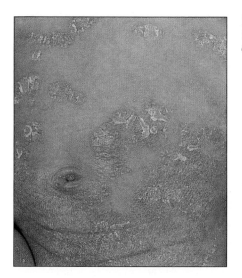

Fig. 5.32 *Psoriasis of the nappy area with typical silver scaled plaques extending onto the abdomen.*

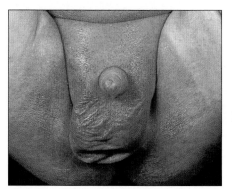

Fig. 5.33 *Irritant contact dermatitis of the nappy area. Note the sharp demarcation on the upper thighs.*

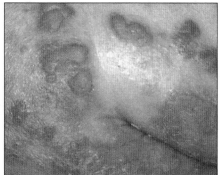

Fig. 5.34 *Herpetiform vesicles in acute primary irritant dermatitis of the nappy area.*

(known as cradle cap) often respond to the application of oils and gentle shampooing but may require more aggressive therapy with salicylic acid.

Occasionally the skin lesions resemble psoriasis (*see* below), and the term napkin psoriasis may be applied (**Fig. 5.32**).

There are also a number of other causes of inflammation in the napkin (diaper) area.

- Primary irritant dermatitis (**Fig. 5.33**). This is generally thought to be caused by faecal enzymes. The skin becomes sore and macerated. Exposure is curative but impractical in most instances. Treatment usually involves attempts to keep the area as dry as possible and the use of emollients and barrier creams. At its most extreme, blisters may occur that resemble herpes (**Fig. 5.34**).
- Jacquet's erythema. This is seen in the older child, who may be somewhat neglected. A strong smell of ammonia is usually present in napkins and over-clothing. Areas of erythema are accompanied, in severe forms, by punched-out ulcers (**Fig. 5.35**).

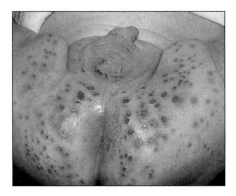

Fig. 5.35 *Punched-out ulcers in severe irritant dermatitis (Jacquet's dermatitis).*

- Candidal infection. *Candida albicans* is usually a secondary invader of other napkin rashes, but may need specific antifungal therapy. Small pustules around the edge of an eruption are highly suggestive of this condition.
- Langerhans' cell histiocytosis (histiocytosis X). (*See* Chapter 6.)
- Zinc deficiency. A napkin rash is part of the complex known as acrodermatitis enteropathica.

Discoid eczema (called also nummular eczema)

Some patients (both children and adults) present with round or oval patches of eczema (**Fig. 5.36**). These are exquisitely itchy and may arise almost anywhere (they are fortunately rare on the face). Lesions, if left untreated, settle over a few days or may grumble on, sometimes merging with adjacent patches. The cause is unknown, although some older patients appear to have a tendency to excessive alcohol consumption.

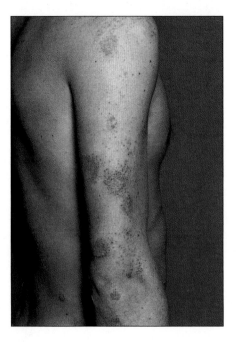

Fig. 5.36 *Discoid eczema — nummular or coin-shaped lesions on the forearm.*

Exudative discoid and lichenoid dermatiosis (the sort of title much-beloved of an earlier generation of dermatologists) is a form of discoid eczema in which the lesions resemble those occurring with lichen and in which, for unknown reasons, the penis is often involved (called also Sulzberger–Garbe syndrome).

The treatment of discoid eczema relies on the use of topical corticosteroids, early enough to prevent lesions from developing into large plaques, but the condition often continues to erupt, causing trouble over many months or years. The lesions in some patients are secondarily infected with *S. aureus*, and oral antibiotics may be helpful.

Varicose eczema (called also stasis dermatitis, gravitational eczema)

In addition to the other changes associated with venous incompetence and hypertension (*see* Chapter 11), patients frequently develop eczematous areas on the lower legs. These may be diffuse, involving the whole gaiter area (**Fig. 5.37**), or more localized. Occasionally, the changes appear directly over varicose veins. Secondary spread to more distant sites is common and may indicate the development of an allergic contact dermatitis to some of the topical medication, a situation which is particularly common in varicose eczema (*see* above). The lesions may also be purpuric, especially around the ankles and on the foot, resulting in an appearance closely resembling one of the pigmented purpuric eruptions described in Chapter 11.

Symptomatic relief can be obtained with topical corticosteroids, but sensitivity to constituents of the base or the steroid molecule itself can be a problem over the longer term. A more radical approach involves active treatment of the underlying venous condition. Support stockings may help but surgery is the ultimate solution. This is not always possible or appropriate, but the advice of a surgeon with an interest in the problem is essential.

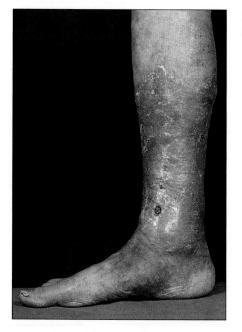

Fig. 5.37 *Varicose eczema affecting the gaiter area.*

Dermatitis of the hands and feet

Hand and foot dermatitis is one of the commonest patterns of eczematous inflammation encountered in clinical practice. It is also a major health problem in industry. Either hands or feet may be involved alone but it is common to see both affected simultaneously. Hand and foot dermatitis may be part of a more generalized eczema (e.g. atopic dermatitis) or may occur as an apparently isolated phenomenon. As indicated above, the hands are frequently involved in primary irritant dermatitis, and both hands and feet may be affected by contact allergic dermatitis. It is very important to ensure that any external contact factor present can be eliminated. Patch testing is therefore a normal part of the investigation of any patient with hand or foot dermatitis. However, common as these problems are, many patients present with dermatitis of the hands and feet for which no obvious external cause can be found, or in whom exogenous factors are only part of the picture. It is a simple, but reasonably useful, rule of thumb that exogenous dermatitis involves the dorsa of the hands and feet, and the finger and toe web-spaces. However, if the changes occur predominantly on the palmar and plantar surfaces, the dermatitis is more likely to have at least a major endogenous component. There are several clinical patterns in which dermatitis appears on the hands and feet. These are, it should be emphasized, not mutually exclusive.

Pompholyx — This term derives from the Greek for blistering, and that is the predominant feature. Most commonly, deep-seated vesicles appear in crops on the palms and soles or along the sides of the digits. These are said to resemble sago grains. Occasionally the lesions may become very large and frankly bullous. The combined symptoms of the disease are very variable, but patients often use words such as 'pricking' and 'tingling' to describe the early phases. There is no doubt that pompholyx lesions itch, but most patients complain that their hands (or feet, or both) are extremely uncomfortable or even painful. As the lesions progress, the skin may become more inflamed (it should be noted that erythema is not commonly seen in early pompholyx), and some splitting and fissuring may follow.

Treatment with potent topical corticosteroids may help to some degree, but the most effective remedy for an acute attack of pompholyx is potassium permanganate, diluted 1:10 000 and used as a soak. Tar is often helpful later in the course of an attack, and oral antibiotics may be required if secondary infection supervenes. Some patients have such severe pompholyx that the use of systemic steroids may be justified, at least in short bursts.

Hyperkeratosis and fissuring — In some patients, the changes are more chronic and result in a degree of hyperkeratosis (Fig. 5.38). The area affected is extremely variable: there may only be one or two plaques present, or the whole palmar and plantar surfaces may be involved. The lesions may be localized to specific sites, such as the finger tips and the base of two adjacent fingers and part of the palm (the so-called apron pattern). The hyperkeratosis may be so marked that it is indistinguishable from palmar or plantar psoriasis. The main symptoms arise from the cracking and splitting that occurs in this form of dermatitis (Fig. 5.38). The tenderness that results can be so severe as to render the

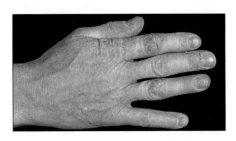

Fig. 5.38 *Chronic dermatitis of the hands with hyperkeratosis and painful fissuring.*

patient nearly completely disabled. The physical stiffness, too, can be a nuisance, especially if the patient has a job which involves fine manual manipulation.

Treatment is difficult. Avoiding external irritants and the use of emollients and potent topical steroids (under occlusion if necessary) may keep some patients comfortable. Others require more aggressive treatment: PUVA (psoralen plus ultraviolet A), particularly using local soaks with psoralen solutions, may be helpful. In the past, low-dose radiation therapy was used by some dermatologists but this seems to have lost favour recently. A few patients need systemic treatment with low-dose systemic steroids and immunosuppressants simply to be able to lead a normal life.

Asteatotic eczema (called also eczema craquelé, xerotic eczema)

This term is applied to skin changes generally attributed to defatting of the skin. An appearance resembling 'crazy paving' is seen (**Fig. 5.39**), often on the lower legs in elderly patients. It may occur more readily in the winter, but is most often seen in patients admitted to care facilities and in whom washing arrangements are radically altered. Rarely, similar changes appear over a wide area. In such patients, an underlying lymphoid malignancy may be present. The treatment of choice is the liberal use of emollients.

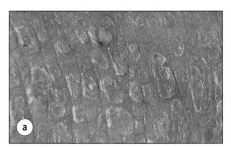 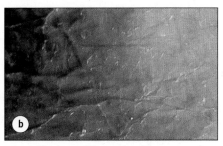

Fig. 5.39 *(a)* and *(b)* *Crazy-paving pattern in asteatotic dermatitis on the shin.*

Chronic superficial scaly dermatosis (called also xanthoerythrodermia perstans, digitate dermatosis)

This is a highly characteristic eruption. It is most commonly seen in older males. Lesions appear on the trunk and limbs. They tend to be round, oval, or elongated, giving a finger-like appearance (**Fig. 5.40**). The surface is slightly scaly and the plaques have a very particular yellowish tinge when present on white skin. Itching is seldom significant. The lesions tend to persist and increase in number over years. Phototherapy can be helpful. The most important point to note about this disorder is that very similar changes are seen in the very early stages of cutaneous T-cell lymphoma (mycosis fungoides). In older literature the term parapsoriasis-en-plaques was used to describe the situation. It is therefore sensible to obtain some histology and, perhaps, to keep an eye on these patients.

Eczema/dermatitis of special sites

There are a number of sites on the body where eczematous inflammation presents particular problems and for which a few additional notes are worthwhile.

Otitis externa — Eczema of the outer ear is common and extremely annoying. There is often no obvious cause and no other history of eczema elsewhere, although there may be subtle features of seborrhoeic eczema (*see* above). Contact allergic dermatitis, especially that which is caused by medicaments, is also a very common complicating feature and all patients with otitis externa should undergo patch testing.

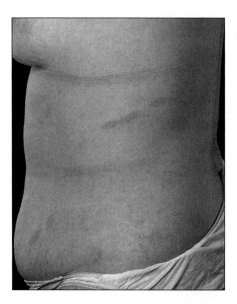

Fig. 5.40 *Finger-shaped lesions on the abdomen in chronic superficial scaly (digitate) dermatosis.*

Eyelid dermatitis — Again, eyelids may be involved as a primary dermatitis, as part of a more generalized endogenous eczema (e.g. atopic dermatitis, seborrhoeic dermatitis) or be caused by contact allergy (**Fig. 5.41**), especially to hair dyes, nail varnish and medicaments. Contact eyelid allergy is often accompanied by oedema.

Paronychial dermatitis — When eczema involves the dorsa of the tips of the fingers and toes, a marked nail dystrophy is commonly seen (**Fig. 5.42**).

Perineal and genital dermatitis — The skin of the vulva, penis, and anus are frequently involved in eczematous dermatitis of various kinds. For example, the intertriginous groin folds may be affected by seborrhoeic dermatitis and the vulva and perianal skin are common sites for lichen simplex chronicus.

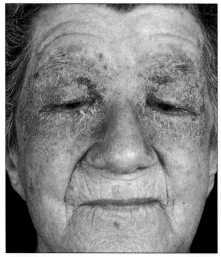

Fig. 5.41 *Eyelid dermatitis due to contact sensitivity to neomycin in eye drops.*

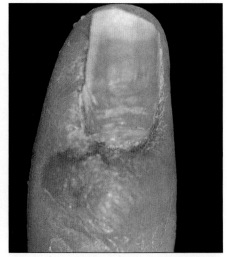

Fig. 5.42 *Nail dystrophy secondary to paronychial dermatitis.*

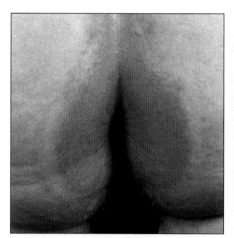

Fig. 5.43 *Perianal dermatitis due to ethylene diamine in triadcortyl cream.*

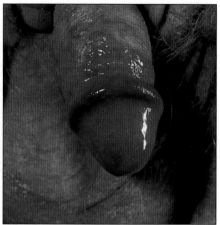

Fig. 5.44 *Well-defined dark red ulcerated lesion extending onto the shaft of the penis in Zoon's plasma cell balanitis.*

The anal skin is subject to irritation for obvious reasons and this may be exacerbated by haemorrhoids or other anal conditions. Anogenital epithelium seems, like the ears, eyelids, and lower legs to be particularly susceptible to contact allergic sensitization by medicaments (**Fig. 5.43**).

The glans penis may also become inflamed (balanitis). In older, usually uncircumcised males, a non-specific balanitis is common and usually responds to mild topical steroids. More troublesome is the florid inflammatory condition known as Zoon's erythroplasia (also called balanitis circumscripta plasmacellularis), in which moist, shiny, deep-red patches appear on the glans, especially around the sulcus (**Fig. 5.44**). Histology reveals a dramatic infiltrate of plasma cells. The condition responds only partially to topical corticosteroids but circumcision is often curative.

Lichen striatus

Lichen striatus is the term used to describe a curious condition in which linear streaks of eczematous skin appear, usually on a limb, often in a child or adolescent (**Fig. 5.45**). Histologically, there is little to be seen, apart from a mild, subacute dermatitis. The streaks last for a variable period of time before disappearing. The main diagnostic differential is that of a linear epidermal naevus (*see* Chapter 4).

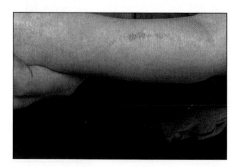

Fig. 5.45 *Linear eczematous lesion on forearm in lichen striatus.*

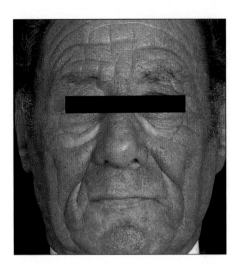

Fig. 5.46 *Photosensitive dermatitis of the face sparing the eyelids, perioral region, and under the chin in chronic actinic dermatitis.*

Chronic actinic dermatitis (called also actinic reticuloid)

The primary photodermatoses are covered later in this chapter, but it should be noted here that some unfortunate patients develop dermatitis in response to light of various wavelengths. Eczematous changes appear on light-exposed sites (**Fig. 5.46**), with characteristic sparing of shaded areas such as the eyelids and under the chin. Occasionally the skin of the face, scalp, and neck become grossly thickened, and the histological appearances also become much more extreme and can be confused with a cutaneous lymphoma by the unwary doctor. Affected patients have a miserable life. Sunscreens do not work well enough and active treatment is required. Patch testing should always be considered because some of these patients have complex photoallergies, particularly to sesquiterpene lactones, a common constituent of flowers of the *Chrysanthemum* genus family. Systemic azathioprine has been found to be helpful, as has ciclosporin (cyclosporin) A.

Neurodermatitis (including lichen simplex chronicus and nodular prurigo)

Some patients develop eczematous changes, either over widespread areas of the body or in localized patches, a significant component in the initiation and perpetuation of the lesions appearing to be the development of an 'itch–scratch' cycle. The lesions are very excoriated (scratched and abraded) and may become heavily thickened (or lichenified — a term used to describe the rather flat-topped nature of the lesions, which therefore begin to resemble those seen particularly in hypertrophic lichen planus — *see* below). Classical sites for the localized plaque form of this disorder (lichen simplex chronicus) (**Fig. 5.47**) include the shins, forearms, palms, perianal and vulval skin (*see* below), and the back of the neck (where it is sometimes called lichen nuchae). Other variants include an otherwise nondescript eczematous eruption with no known exogenous trigger, and the remarkable condition called nodular prurigo.

Nodular prurigo presents a striking clinical picture. Dome-shaped lesions develop almost anywhere on the body surface. These vary in size from a few millimetres to one or two centimetres in diameter (**Fig. 5.48**). There are usually only a few lesions initially, but

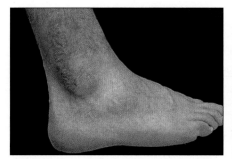

Fig. 5.47 *Lichenified plaque of dermatitis on the lateral aspect of the ankle in lichen simplex chronicus (neurodermatitis).*

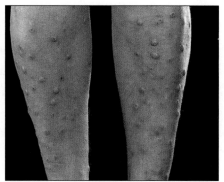

Fig. 5.48 *Intensely itchy nodules on the legs in nodular prurigo.*

gradually more develop until there are often many such lesions. Patients complain of an insatiable and uncontrollable desire to scratch, often coming in intense bursts. Many are atopics, as shown by a history of hay fever, asthma, or eczema.

Treating these forms of skin inflammation, where itching is the major problem, and scratching probably part of the pathogenesis of individual lesions, is extremely challenging. Simple topical therapy with corticosteroids, together with occlusion under medicated bandages impregnated with tar, ichthammol, or zinc paste is the usual starting point, but is often ineffective in the long-term, especially with nodular prurigo. Some authorities recommend the use of tranquillizers and other psychotropic agents. Ultraviolet B phototherapy and PUVA may help some patients, and there are reports of success with powerful immunosuppressive drugs.

- Seborrhoeic eczema commonly affects the scalp and face and responds to topical antifungal/corticosteroid treatment.
- Infantile seborrhoeic dermatitis presents as a non-itchy rash in the napkin (diaper) area and flexures and scalp; responds well to mild topical corticosteroids.
- Discoid eczema presents with round/oval, itchy skin lesions; early treatment with topical corticosteroids is recommended.
- Varicose eczema is associated with venous incompetence and hypertension with eczematous areas on the lower legs; topical corticosteroids and active treatment of underlying condition are advised.
- Hand and foot dermatitis commonly of multiple/mixed aetiology; patch testing alone may fail to establish cause.
- Asteatotic eczema is attributed to defatting in elderly skin; treat with liberal use of emollients.
- Lichen simplex chronicus and nodular prurigo are both characterized by intense itching.

PSORIASIS

Box 5.3

Psoriasis
Common, non-infectious inflammatory skin disorder presenting with erythematous plaques topped with silvery scales.

INTRODUCTION

Psoriasis is a common disorder: in most ethnic groups the incidence is estimated at 1.5–3.0%. There is a strong genetic component, especially in those patients whose disease begins before the age of forty, where there is also a significant association with HLA-Cw6. However, environmental factors are also important. For example, an attack of guttate psoriasis (*see* below) often follows a streptococcal sore throat and patches of psoriasis frequently appear in areas of trauma (the Koebner phenomenon). Some drugs (e.g. lithium, antimalarial drugs) can induce psoriasis and there has been a long-standing belief that stress may be a factor in induction or exacerbation of attacks.

Psoriasis has a highly characteristic histopathology, in which marked acanthosis is accompanied by loss of the granular cell layer, retention of nuclei in the hyperkeratotic horny layer (parakeratosis), and accumulation of polymorphonuclear leukocytes in micro-abscesses. It is now thought that the primary stimulus may be cells of the T-lymphocyte series and that psoriasis may be, in part, an autoimmune disorder.

PATHOGENESIS

There has been a considerable increase in the level of interest in the pathogenesis of psoriasis since the demonstration that ciclosporin (cyclosporin) A, a drug that has very potent effects on T-cell function (and on the T-helper CD4+ subset in particular), is extremely effective in psoriasis. It has been known for many years that the epidermal transit time (the time it takes for a basal cell to mature and differentiate into a corneocyte) is much reduced in psoriasis — from an average of 28 days to 7–8 days. It has also been demonstrated that there is a veritable soup of inflammatory mediators in the epidermis, and that there are abnormalities in the vasculature in psoriatic plaques (especially at the expanding edge of plaques). However, it is now generally believed that these changes are the consequence of some form of immune dysfunction, involving CD4+ T cells, perhaps responding in a genetically predetermined way to environmental stimuli such as streptococcal antigens, trauma, and even stress. Just how these immunoinflammatory processes develop and produce the full-blown picture of psoriasis described above awaits elucidation.

CLINICAL FEATURES

- Most frequently encountered as plaques.
- Size of the plaques and the extent of involvement vary widely: plaques may be a few millimetres or several centimetres in diameter; there may be one plaque or thousands.
- So-called classical sites (**Fig. 5.49**) are the scalp, knees, elbows, base of spine, and umbilicus, but lesions of psoriasis can appear anywhere on the body surface.
- Each plaque shares a number of common signs.
- Plaques are pink or red, scaly, and well demarcated (**Fig. 5.50**).
- Surface scale is said to be silvery (**Fig. 5.50**) — this is best appreciated after gentle rubbing.
- More vigorous rubbing leads to obvious pinpoint bleeding.

These clinical features are all explained by the histopathology of psoriasis.

CLINICAL VARIANTS

In addition to the standard 'plaque' form of psoriasis, several additional presentations are worth noting separately. Localized disease can usually be managed by local means,

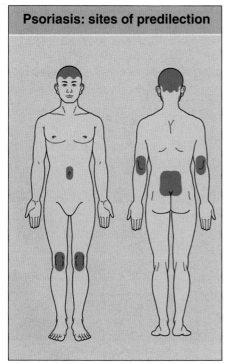

Psoriasis: sites of predilection

Fig. 5.49 *Typical distribution of psoriasis.*

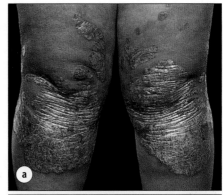

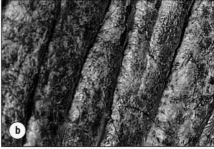

Fig. 5.50 *Well-demarcated plaques on the knees — (a) with a silvery scale; (b) in psoriasis.*

although plantar pustulosis in particular can be so troublesome that systemic treatment may be justified. Local PUVA is often used. Acrodermatitis continua may respond to corticosteroids under polythene occlusion. Widespread forms of pustular psoriasis should be managed in an in-patient setting. Good nursing care is critical. Systemic drugs such as methotrexate and ciclosporin (cyclosporin) A are often needed to bring the condition under control.

Guttate psoriasis

Showers of small plaques develop over the trunk and limbs and lesions may appear on the face and on the scalp (**Fig. 5.51**). This often follows a streptococcal sore throat and may be the first attack the patient has had, or may represent an exacerbation of pre-existing psoriasis. The lesions may resolve spontaneously, but more frequently require some intervention. Ultraviolet B phototherapy is particularly helpful.

Flexural psoriasis

Either accompanied by plaques elsewhere or alone, psoriasis may affect the axillae, perineal creases and inframammary folds. There is some clinical overlap with seborrhoeic dermatitis (*see* page 196), and some dermatologists favour the concept of 'sebo-psoriasis'. Treatment can be difficult because dithranol (anthralin) may burn and corticosteroids are prone to cause atrophy. Tar and vitamin-D analogues are probably the agents of first choice, if mild topical steroids fail. Topical tacrolimus may also be useful.

Nail psoriasis

Psoriatic nail changes (**Fig. 5.52**) are extremely common, and often provide helpful information if the skin lesions are atypical. Most common are irregular pits, onycholysis, or both. Occasionally grosser changes are seen, with severe subungual hyperkeratosis. In

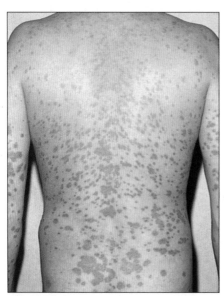

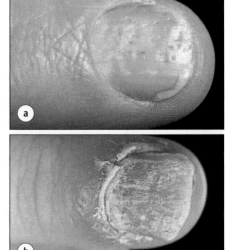

Fig. 5.51 *Oval lesions 1–2 cm in diameter on the trunk in guttate psoriasis.*

Fig. 5.52 *Psoriatic nail dystrophy — (a)* pitting and *(b)* thickening of the nails.

acrodermatitis continua (a form of localized pustular psoriasis) the nails may be destroyed (*see* below). The nail changes typical of psoriasis may occur in isolation and nail changes are almost universal in some forms of psoriatic arthropathy (*see* below).

Confluent or brittle psoriasis

If plaques become very active and merge over widespread areas, psoriasis can be said to have become confluent or brittle (**Fig. 5.53**). This state is highly unstable, the skin ceases to perform its natural functions adequately, and an exfoliative dermatitis may develop (*see* exfoliative erythroderma (dermatitis) page 230). Generalized pustular psoriasis sometimes begins in this way. This state may emerge *de novo*, or arise as a complication of previously entirely stable disease. Sometimes pustular psoriasis is precipitated by treatment with irritant creams, or the cessation of a course of systemic steroids. Patients with this disorder need to be nursed carefully and treated with bland creams topically. Systemic treatment is usually indicated unless there are compelling complicating factors which dictate otherwise. However, once the situation has stabilized it is often possible to withdraw the oral medication and control the psoriasis by other means.

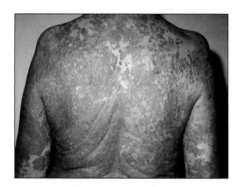

Fig. 5.53 *Extensive unstable psoriasis.*

Pustular psoriasis

Pustule formation in psoriasis can occur either as part of a chronic, indolent form of psoriasis on the palms and soles (**Fig. 5.54**), or as a more explosive, widespread condition. In the most severe form – acute pustular psoriasis (von Zumbusch's psoriasis) — erythematous, oedematous areas are studded with pustules (**Fig. 5.55**). There is usually a pyrexia and the patient looks and feels unwell. Among other abnormalities on investigation, the white count is almost invariably raised. Less severe forms of this state may be seen, notably the curious Lapière form, in which striking rings of pustules appear,

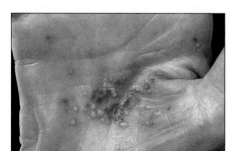

Fig. 5.54 *Characteristic 1–2 mm diameter yellow-white pustules and resolving brown pustules in pustular psoriasis on the palm (palmo-plantar pustulosis).*

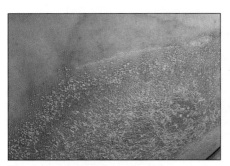

Fig. 5.55 *Sheets of pustules in generalized pustular psoriasis (von Zumbusch's psoriasis).*

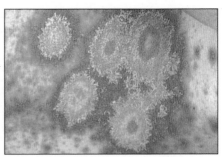

Fig. 5.56 *Striking annular pustular psoriatic lesion in childhood (Lapiere).*

often in an otherwise completely healthy child (**Fig. 5.56**). When severe pustulation occurs on the tips of one or more fingers and toes, the term acrodermatitis continua is often applied. This is generally a chronic state and can result in destruction of the nail apparatus. Occasionally it is seen as part of, or progresses to, generalized pustular psoriasis.

The treatment of psoriasis — It is often said that, if there are several treatments available for a condition, none of them can be very effective. There is certainly a wide range of agents and therapeutic modalities that are used in the treatment of a patient with psoriasis. The choice of which to use depends on many factors.

- The clinical pattern of the psoriasis.
- The site(s) involved.
- The extent.
- The physical health of the patient (both generally and as a result of the psoriasis).
- The age of the patient.
- The psychological impact of the psoriasis.
- The effect of the disease on the patient's ability to carry out normal daily tasks.

Some of the factors to be considered have been mentioned under each clinical variant, but **Figure 5.57** contains some general principles which may be helpful.

PSORIATIC ARTHROPATHY

About 5–10% of patients affected by psoriasis develop arthritis; the authors of a US series found that up to 40% of patients complained of joint pain.

There are a number of specific patterns that can clearly be demarcated.

- Predominantly peripheral monoarthritis or oligoarthritis.
- Distal interphalangeal joint involvement (so-called 'classical').
- Symmetrical rheumatoid-like (but seronegative).
- Arthritis mutilans.
- Spondylitis and sacroiliitis (with or without peripheral arthropathy).

Nail changes are seen in over two-thirds of patients with psoriatic arthritis, and these may be very severe, especially in patients with distal interphalangeal joint involvement and in arthritis mutilans.

The treatment of psoriatic arthritis should be undertaken by a rheumatologist, but will often involve the use of a combination of drugs including non-steroidal anti-inflammatory agents, sulfasalazine, and methotrexate.

Agents/modalities used in psoriasis

Emollients	Useful for reducing scaling and keeping plaques from cracking and bleeding.
Tar	Time-honoured remedy for plaque and guttate patterns; especially useful in combination with ultraviolet B; also helpful for scalp disease and the flexures.
Salicylic acid	Often added to ointments to reduce scaling.
Dithranol (anthranol)	Highly effective, but time consuming (even with 'short-contact' regimens), and potentially messy (dithranol stains everything it touches); dithranol can also cause burning; it is only appropriate for stable plaque psoriasis.
Topical corticosteroids	Effective short-term in plaque psoriasis; milder agents are the mainstay of the treatment of flexural psoriasis and lesions on the face; also widely used in scalp applications.
Vitamin-D analogues	Newly introduced; effective in suppressing plaques in many patients with plaque psoriasis; may have a significant role in widespread, but stable, disease; also useful in the flexures.
Ultraviolet-B phototherapy	About 70% of psoriatics improve with ultraviolet B, which is usually given two to three times weekly, starting with short exposures and gradually increasing as the skin becomes conditioned; some patients worsen and others find ultraviolet B of no value.
PUVA	Psoralen with ultraviolet A (long-wave ultraviolet); highly effective for widespread psoriasis; can be administered either in tablet or 'bath' form; side-effects include burning and induction (long-term) of skin cancers; local PUVA is helpful for limited disease, especially of the hands and feet.
Retinoids	Derivatives of vitamin A are useful in many disorders where keratinization is abnormal; in psoriasis they are reserved for severe disease; they can cause hyperlipidaemia and are teratogenic.
Methotrexate	This anti-metabolite has been used for many years; it is given as a once-weekly dose (usually between 5 and 30 mg) by mouth; parenteral administration is occasionally useful in acute states such as von Zumbusch's pustular psoriasis; long-term use may cause hepatic fibrosis and careful monitoring (including liver biopsies) is needed.
Ciclosporin (cyclosporin) A	Potent immunosuppressive with dramatic effects in psoriasis; the drug is reserved for severe disease because of its cost and its toxicity profile, which includes renal impairment in particular.
Newer Therapies (largely unlicensed)	Mycophendate mofetil; fumaric acid esters; monoclonal antibodies, topical tacrolimus or pimecrolimus for facial and flexural lesions;

Other agents (e.g. azathioprine, hydroxyurea) are favoured by some authorities. Many treatment regimens for psoriasis involve mixtures and combinations of agents (e.g. tar + salicylic acid; corticosteroid + salicylic acid; PUVA + retinoids).

Fig. 5.57 *Therapeutic modalities commonly used for psoriasis.*

- Psoriasis is common with incidence estimated at 1.5–3.0% (most ethnic groups).
- Strong genetic component (especially with onset before age of forty).
- Most frequently encountered as plaques on scalp, knees, elbows, base of spine, and umbilicus.
- Guttate psoriasis: showers of small plaques often following streptococcal sore throat.
- Flexural psoriasis: affects axillae, perineal creases and inframammary folds.
- Nail psoriasis: irregular pits, onycholysis and occasionally severe subungual hyperkeratosis.
- Confluent or brittle psoriasis: active plaques merging over widespread areas.
- Pustular psoriasis: chronic, indolent form of psoriasis on the palms and soles or widespread condition (severe) with erythematous, oedematous areas studded with pustules.
- Wide range of agents and therapeutic modalities available in treatment of psoriasis.

REITER'S SYNDROME

The complex of urethritis, arthritis and conjunctivitis described by Hans Reiter, initially in postdiarrhoeal states, may also be accompanied by striking skin lesions particularly on the hands and feet, but also on typically psoriatic sites. These are known as keratoderma blenorrhagica (**Fig. 5.58**). The histologic features of this condition are essentially those of psoriasis, and the condition represents a link between psoriasis and some of the other associated features of the seronegative arthropathies. The skin lesions of Reiter's syndrome will often respond to the systemic therapy usually used, but may also require topical treatment with corticosteroids.

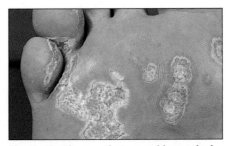

Fig. 5.58 *Plaques that resemble psoriasis on the soles of the feet in Reiter's syndrome.*

LICHEN PLANUS AND OTHER 'INTERFACE DERMATOSES'

LICHEN PLANUS

Box 5.4

Lichen planus
Uncommon inflammatory skin condition presenting with eruptions of violaceous papules of varied morphology and extent.

Introduction

Lichen planus is an uncommon inflammatory skin condition, in which a wide range of clinical features are conventionally accepted as being part of the spectrum. All are characterized, histologically, by the presence of:

- Marked liquefaction degeneration of the basal layer.
- An expansion of the granular cell layer.
- A dense subepidermal infiltrate, predominantly of T lymphocytes.

Clinical features

The signs of the commonest form of lichen planus are instantly recognizable, but there are a number of variants, some of which appear at first sight to bear little or no resemblance to one another. There is also a wide variation in symptoms, even in the so-called classical form (*see* below). Some patients complain of intense itching, others are hardly troubled at all. The time course is also very different between subtypes. The majority of patients with classical exanthematous lichen planus undergo a spontaneous remission within 12 months but, in some (especially in hypertrophic and atrophic forms — *see* below), the disorder pursues a relentless and extremely chronic course, often lasting for the rest of a patient's life.

It is possible to recognize several distinctive clinical patterns and variants (**Figs 5.59–5.67**).

Other clinical features

Because of the marked destruction of basal layer cells in lichen planus, the inflammatory process frequently leaves pigmentary anomalies in its wake. This is particularly prominent, and distressing, in pigmented skins. Furthermore, occasionally patients are seen in whom there appear to be no preceding papules at all, a situation which has been called lichen planus pigmentosus.

It is also worth noting the effects that lichen planus may have in certain specific sites.

- Genitalia. Both male and female genitalia may be affected (**Fig. 5.68**); this is a site where there is a tendency to significant atrophy.
- Nails. These are affected to a mild degree in 10% of patients, but can be severely damaged, or lost completely because of an overgrowth of the nail fold epithelium, a change known as pterygium (**Fig. 5.69**).

The main clinical variants of lichen planus

Classic	An eruption of flat-topped papules appears, often over the course of a few days, affecting especially the wrists, ankles, and the small of the back (Fig. 5.60); the papules are frequently surmounted by whitish dots or lines known as Wickham's striae (Fig. 5.61); the mouth is often affected by a network of lacy white lines (Fig. 5.62); if the palms and soles are affected, the classic violaceous colour is lost, and the papules become translucent (Fig. 5.63); annular lesions may also appear in among the rest of the papules (Fig. 5.64).
Hypertrophi	Lesions become thickened, hyperkeratotic, and form plaques, especially over the shins and forearms (Fig. 5.65); this form of lichen planus is particularly itchy, and rubbing and scratching may play a role in the development and persistence of the lesions; in many instances this form of lichen planus lasts for years.
Atrophic	The pathological process in lichen planus may result in a marked thinning of the epidermis, particularly on the soles of the feet, and in very chronic oral disease (Fig. 5.66); this may severely alter taste and the tolerance of hot or spicy food. (There is an increased risk of oral squamous carcinoma in patients with chronic oral lichen planus.)
Vesiculobullous	Intense sub-epidermal inflammation may lead to separation and bulla formation (Fig. 5.67); in some patients a bullous pemphigoid-like reaction may occur, and bullae may appear without pre-existing lichen planus papules: this is termed lichen planus pemphigoides.
Actinic	The lesions of lichen planus may be induced by exposure to light; the thiazide diuretics may induce a photo-provoked lichen planus-like eruption.

Fig. 5.59 *The main clinical variants of lichen planus.*

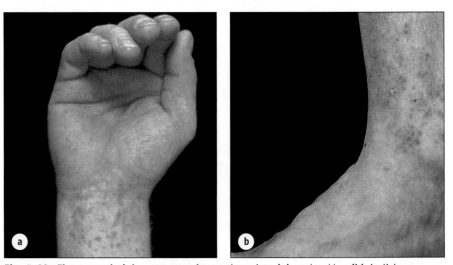

Fig. 5.60 *Flat-topped violaceous papules* at the wrists *(a)* and ankles *(b)* in lichen planus.

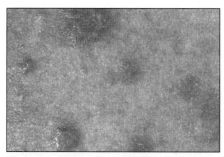

Fig. 5.61 *White lines (Wickham's striae) visible on the surface of lesions.*

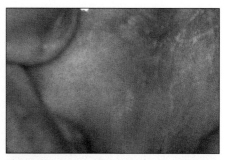

Fig. 5.62 *Lacy white lines in the mouth in lichen planus.*

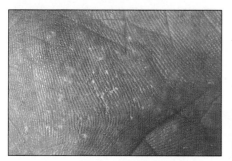

Fig. 5.63 *Translucent papules on the palms in lichen planus.*

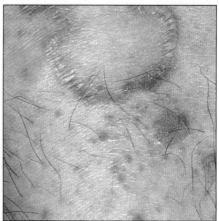

Fig. 5.64 *Annular lichen planus.*

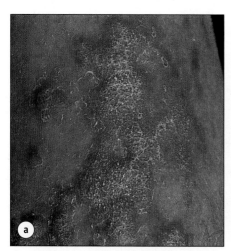

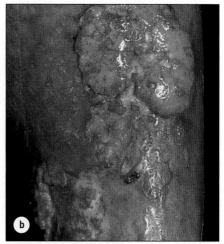

Fig. 5.65 *(a)* Hypertrophic lichen planus on the shins with the development of *(b)* secondary squamous cell carcinoma.

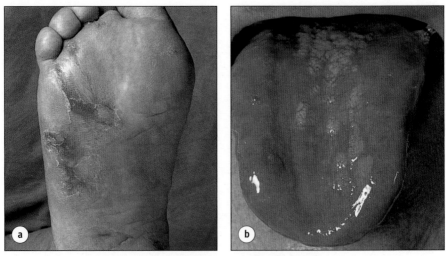

Fig. 5.66 *Atrophic lichen planus of* **(a)** *the soles and* **(b)** *tongue.*

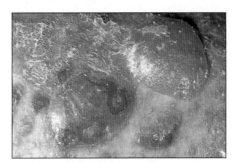

Fig. 5.67 *Bullous lichen planus.*

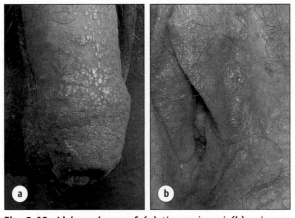

Fig. 5.68 *Lichen planus of* **(a)** *the penis and* **(b)** *vulva.*

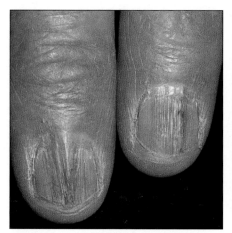

Fig. 5.69 *Nail dystrophy secondary to lichen planus with pterygium formation.*

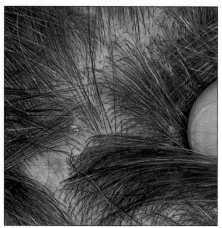

Fig. 5.70 *Scarring alopecia of the scalp secondary to lichen planus.*

- Hair. Follicular involvement by lichen planus (known as lichen planopilaris) may occur anywhere; on the body surface it causes a follicular prominence; in the scalp and other areas of terminal hair, the process may be very destructive and is one of the causes of a cicatricial alopecia (**Fig. 5.70**).

Pathogenesis

When Erasmus Wilson first described lichen planus in 1869, he attributed it unequivocally to stress and this is still offered as an explanation by some today. It seems likely, however, that the reaction in lichen planus is immunologically mediated and, perhaps, represents an assault on the epidermis by T lymphocytes. It further seems plausible that this is triggered by something exogenous that affects epidermal antigenicity (or at least the recognition of the epidermis as antigenic), such as infection or a chemical (it is notable that some drugs can initiate similar changes). There have been suggestions that some chronic erosive oral lichen planus may be associated with hypersensitivity to mercury amalgam in dental fillings.

The treatment of lichen planus

Most patients benefit from the use of topical steroids, at least in reducing the symptom of itching, if prominent. There is some evidence that a short course of oral steroids may shorten the course of the classical, eruptive form of the disease but this hardly seems justified in most instances. However, extensive lichen planus and its atrophic variants often do require a more aggressive approach. Here, oral steroids or other immunosuppressive agents may be helpful. In particular, ciclosporin (cyclosporin) A has been used successfully. Some authorities maintain that oral retinoids are effective in oral disease, but in our experience they are of limited value. Despite a number of reports, there is little to support the use of griseofulvin in clinical use.

Lichen nitidus

Although considered to be a separate entity by some, this disorder, which is characterized by clusters of non-itchy micropapules (**Fig. 5.71**), is probably simply a variant of lichen planus. Lichen nitidus tends to pursue a rather chronic course.

217

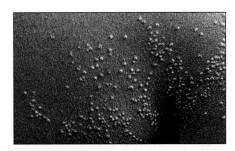

Fig. 5.71 *Lichen niditus.*

Lichenoid drug reactions

As indicated above, lichen planus, or lichen-planus-like changes, may be triggered by some drugs (*see* Chapter 8).

- Lichen planus is an uncommon inflammatory skin condition thought to be immunologically mediated representing an assault on the epidermis by T lymphocytes.
- Presents classically with flat-top papules affecting the wrists, ankles and back.
- Majority of patients undergo spontaneous remission within 12 months; some (especially in hypertrophic and atrophic forms) suffer chronic course.
- Topical/oral steroids or other immunosuppressive agents depending on variant.
- Lichen-planus-like changes may be triggered by some drugs.

CUTANEOUS LUPUS ERYTHEMATOSUS

Skin changes occur commonly in the multisystem disorder systemic lupus erythematosus and these are considered in Chapter 8. However, in some patients skin lesions are the predominant feature, with the systemic manifestations associated with lupus erythematosus being absent or only very mild. Two distinct forms are generally recognized:

Chronic discoid lupus erythematosus (CDLE)

The typical skin lesion of CDLE is an erythematous plaque, usually encountered on the face, neck, ears, or scalp (**Fig. 5.72**), but also occasionally on the arms and hands. Lesions may be photo-provoked or exacerbated. The most important feature of an individual lesion of CDLE that distinguishes it from other inflammatory dermatoses is the presence of follicular plugging (**Fig. 5.72**). This may be seen on the surface of the plaque itself or on the underside of gently lifted surface scale, as the so-called carpet-tack sign. Another important clinical feature is the occurrence of scarring in the plaques. This scarring may be mild but is often quite marked and can give rise to significant distortion of normal tissue anatomy (**Fig. 5.72**). In the scalp, this leads to permanent hair loss (*see* Chapter 9). Lesions of CDLE may also be seen in the mouth, nasal epithelium, and conjunctiva.

Investigations and prognosis — Histologically, in a relatively active lesion, the epidermis and hair follicle epithelium undergo liquefaction degeneration and there is a dense inflammatory cell infiltrate present around dermal vessels and adnexal structures. The follicular plugging seen on inspection is also clearly visible microscopically. Immunofluorescence reveals a linear band of IgG or IgM at the basement membrane.

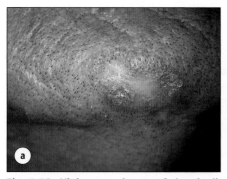
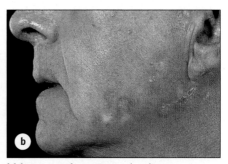

Fig. 5.72 *Violaceous plaques of chronic discoid lupus erythematosus* showing *(a)* *follicular plugging and* *(b)* *secondary scarring.*

Serologically there may be a low titre of antinuclear factor, but there is generally no other evidence of systemic involvement.

A few patients with CDLE progress to develop systemic lupus erythematosus (SLE) (*see* Chapter 8) and some patients with SLE present with lesions of CDLE as well as other features. However, most patients who present with CDLE continue to have skin changes only, often for many years. Active treatment is important for prevention of the scarring that will result from untreated disease.

Treatment — Some patients manage satisfactorily with the intermittent use of topical corticosteroids, although these drugs may have to be at the top end of the potency range to be valuable. Intralesional injections of steroids may also be useful in smallish areas. In some patients, however, lesions continue to spread despite intensive topical therapy and a systemic approach is required. The drugs most commonly used are the antimalarials, of which hydroxychloroquine, at a dose of 200–400 mg daily, seems to provide a reasonable balance of efficacy and side-effects. Chloroquine is also effective but has a higher incidence of ocular toxicity and mepacrine stains the skin yellow. Some authorities find the retinoid acitretin helpful. Occasionally, a short course of systemic steroids may be required. All patients with cutaneous lupus should be advised to use sunscreens and avoid excessive sun exposure. However, some patients actually report benefit from sunlight. Dapsone is also effective in some patients.

Lupus profundus

Deeper extension of the infiltrate in CDLE lesions is found fairly commonly on direct microscopy. However, when the histologic changes associated with CDLE are found deep in the subcutaneous fat without much in the way of overlying change the term lupus profundus is used. This form of the disease which is, in essence, a panniculitis, produces deep nodular swellings which may progress to cause significant hollowing due to fat atrophy.

Subacute cutaneous lupus erythematosus

This is a much rarer entity than CDLE. The patient is usually a middle-aged or elderly woman, in whom a widespread eruption appears, typically over the upper trunk and limbs. The morphology of the eruption is rather variable, but lesions often are annular or have a wavy outline. The individual lesions are not as hyperkeratotic as those seen in CDLE, nor is follicular plugging a prominent feature. Serologically these patients are nearly always ANF

219

(antinuclear factor) positive. There may be mild systemic involvement, and even those that do not are Ro/La positive. This form of lupus erythematosus generally requires systemic treatment, and will respond to some extent to the same range of agents as described above for CDLE. Dapsone has also been used.

Chilblain lupus — One variant of cutaneous lupus erythematosus (LE) produces chilblain-like lesions predominantly on the fingers and toes in cold weather (**Fig. 5.73**). The lesions may accompany cutaneous LE elsewhere, or appear entirely alone. LE serology is positive more often than in other forms of skin change, and full-blown SLE may develop. Therapy is not usually as effective as in other forms of cutaneous lupus.

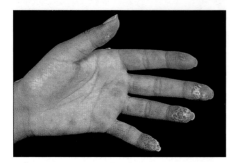

Fig. 5.73 *Chilblain lupus of the hands and fingers.*

- Chronic discoid lupus erythematosus (CDLE) is characterized by an erythematous plaque with follicular plugging and scarring; most patients do not progress to SLE.
- Treat CDLE with topical steroids, sunscreens and sun avoidance.

LICHEN SCLEROSUS
(CALLED ALSO LICHEN SCLEROSUS ET ATROPHICUS)

Box 5.5

Lichen sclerosus
Uncommon disorder characterized by white lichenoid atrophic lesions mainly in the genital region.

Another relatively uncommon condition, characterized by whitish plaques on the skin (hence its older name white spot disease), is lichen sclerosus. Histologically, the epidermis is usually thin. There may be mild liquefaction degeneration of the epidermis and a mononuclear cell infiltrate present in the dermis. The most notable feature, however, is a rather bland band of upper dermal collagen. This disorder presents in a number of ways.

On the genital and perianal skin of adult females — Here, the condition produces white, plaque-like changes (**Fig. 5.74**) in which erosions are common. The changes can give rise to

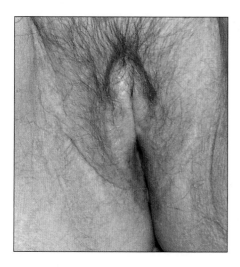

Fig. 5.74 *Ulcerated white plaques in lichen sclerosus of the vulva.*

significant discomfort. Lichen sclerosus sometimes results in loss of tissue and fusion of vulval folds, particularly if lesions are long-standing.

On the genital and perianal skin of prepubertal females — Lichen sclerosus in prepubertal girls is characteristically well circumscribed, often assuming a figure-of-eight distribution around the vulva and anus. Surface areas of purpura are commonly seen, which may break down to leave erosions. The child is often very uncomfortable and may complain of soreness, dysuria, and pain on defecation. Lichen sclerosus is sometimes mistaken for evidence of vulval damage from sexual abuse.

On the male genitalia — In adult males, the equivalent changes caused by this condition are known by a rather quaint but slightly threatening name: balanitis xerotica obliterans. The glans, prepuce, or both, become white and there may be significant fibrosis in longer-standing disease (**Fig. 5.75**). This can lead to occlusion of the meatus, or to phimosis. In young boys, lichen sclerosus probably presents as phimosis but is not even diagnosed in most cases, since the troublesome prepuce is simply removed surgically and discarded.

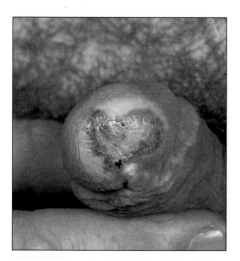

Fig. 5.75 *Lichen sclerosus of the penis (balanitis xerotica obliterans).*

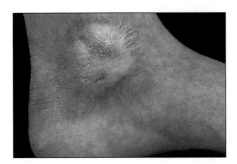

Fig. 5.76 *Lichen sclerosus in a site of trauma at the ankle.*

On non-genital skin — Lichen sclerosus may occur on sites other than the genitalia, either alone, or in combination with genital disease. It has a predilection for the wrists and the flexures, but may arise anywhere (**Fig. 5.76**). Lichen sclerosus has been reported to follow trauma to the skin, including sunburn.

Treatment and prognosis of lichen sclerosus

In prepubertal girls, it is generally accepted that many patients show improvement and resolution of lesions as they enter puberty. Unfortunately, however, this is not true for them all. The judicious use of topical steroids can often provide marked symptomatic relief. In adult women, the disorder appears to respond to potent topical corticosteroids, which are undoubtedly the initial treatment of choice. However, the disorder can be very indolent and chronic. Furthermore, there is a definite risk of vulval malignancy in patients with lichen sclerosus and careful follow-up is essential, with biopsies of any suspect areas. It is important that a good working relationship develops with a gynaecologist with an interest in the subject. Many centres now run joint vulva clinics. The outcome in boys is mentioned above, but lichen sclerosus in adult males can be very troublesome. Lesions often persist for years and may give rise to great anxiety and discomfort. Potent topical steroids are again of value in relieving symptoms. Surgical intervention may be required for phimosis or narrowing of the meatus.

- Lichen sclerosus is a relatively uncommon condition characterized by whitish plaques and bands of upper dermal collagen, most commonly found in genital and perianal skin.
- Topical steroids initial treatment of choice.
- Risk of vulval malignancy and careful follow-up is essential.

GRAFT-VERSUS-HOST DISEASE

The introduction of bone marrow transplantation as a front-line treatment for severe leukaemia and other disorders has brought to the fore a range of problems originally described in the 1950s, usually associated with the administration of blood products. These are collectively known as 'graft-versus-host disease' (GVHD) or 'graft-versus-host reactions'. The general effects of these states is beyond the brief of this book, but the skin changes that may be seen are worth noting.

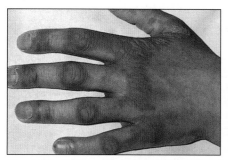

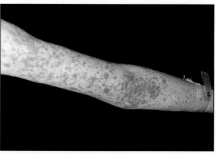

Fig. 5.77 *Erythematous macular lesions of the hands in acute graft-versus-host disease.*

Fig. 5.78 *Lichenoid lesions of the forearm in chronic graft-versus-host disease.*

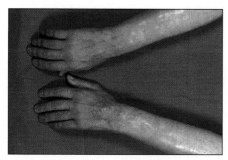

Fig. 5.79 *Sclerodermoid changes of the forearms in chronic graft-versus-host disease.*

There are three main phases to the skin changes of GVHD.
- In the first few weeks after the transplant, an erythematous maculopapular eruption may develop, often exhibiting a predilection for the skin behind the ears and the hands and feet (**Fig. 5.77**); this may resolve (usually following intensive treatment with immunosuppressive agents) or may extend and deteriorate. If left unchecked, widespread blistering may develop, identical to that seen in toxic epidermal necrolysis; such a situation has a very poor prognosis indeed.
- From about 3 months after transplantation, a more lichen planus-like eruption may develop (**Fig. 5.78**); this may be very widespread and often involves the mouth.
- Finally, many months after the transplant, severe sclerodermatous changes may develop; these can cause marked contractures and disability (**Fig. 5.79**).

The histological changes that one would expect to see in cutaneous GVHD will naturally depend on the stage at which it is encountered, and its severity. In brief, however, the changes consist of an invasion of the epidermis by T lymphocytes, which are often found in close apposition to dead or dying keratinocytes (a phenomenon known as satellite-cell necrosis). Liquefaction degeneration of the basal layer and a variable degree of loss of adhesion between the epidermis and dermis occur. In later forms, the changes become those of a more chronic process, with the ultimate sclerodermatous state being reflected in a rather amorphous and featureless dermis composed largely of compacted connective tissue.

PITYRIASIS ROSEA

Pityriasis rosea is one of the most striking eruptions seen in clinical practice. The history and clinical features are almost always the same. An otherwise healthy child or young adult may feel slightly 'under the weather' and develops a scaly red patch somewhere on the trunk, upper thigh, or shoulder. This may be mistaken for a fungal infection or a patch of eczema (**Fig. 5.80**). In fact, this is the so-called herald patch and is followed a few days (or a week or two) later by a florid eruption of pink (hence, rosea), oval patches. These have a highly characteristic distribution, appearing nearly always on the trunk, upper arms, and legs only. It is only rarely that lesions spread to involve the forearms, lower legs, and face. On the trunk, the lesions line up with their longer axis seeming to follow the spinal nerves around the trunk. This is said to produce an appearance resembling an inverted Christmas tree. This can be confusing because the lines appear to sweep downwards from the vertebral column when viewed from behind, but upwards from the centre of the abdomen when viewed from in front (**Fig. 5.81**). Compare this with the perceived, popular appearance of a Christmas tree (as often portrayed on Christmas cards) and the actual architecture and maybe you will see the problem (**Fig. 5.82**). However, there is no doubt

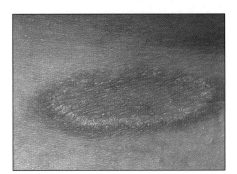

Fig. 5.80 *Herald patch in pityriasis rosea showing characteristic peripheral collarette of scale.*

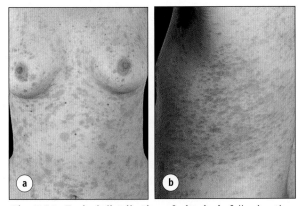

Fig. 5.81 *Typical distribution of pityriasis* following the lines of the ribs — *(a)* chest and abdomen; *(b)* sides of trunk.

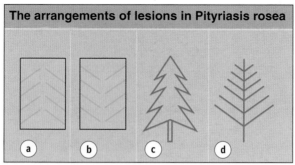

The arrangements of lesions in Pityriasis rosea

Fig. 5.82 *Pityriasis rosea looks like an inverted Christmas tree! (a) on the back and (b) on the front; (c) is a frequent representation of a Christmas tree and (d) real architecture of a Christmas tree.*

that whether the appearance is likened to a Christmas tree, upside down or not, this physical sign is pathognomonic of the disorder. The features of the individual lesions are also very specific. On the surface of each oval patch there is a light, scurfy scale (*see* Gr. pituron bran, dandruff + -iasis). This scale appears centrally and rapidly spreads across the patch to produce the classical peripheral collarette (*see* Fig. 5.80). The eruption lasts for approximately 6–8 weeks before disappearing, usually for ever. Some patients experience significant itching but many have no symptoms. Occasionally, as indicated above, pityriasis rosea may be atypical in distribution and the diagnosis will rest on the individual features of the lesions and the prior appearance of the herald patch. Even more unusually, the lesions themselves may be quite atypical. For example, patches may be surmounted by blisters.

There is some evidence implicating HHV 6 and 7 infection in the pathogenesis of pityriasis rosea.

Investigation and treatment
The only test that is really worth considering is syphilis serology if the appearance of the eruption is somewhat atypical and the patient is in a risk group (*see* Chapter 3). Treatment only needs to be symptomatic as the eruption inevitably settles spontaneously. Mild topical corticosteroids offer relief to some patients. Phototherapy may be useful in slowly resolving cases.

PITYRIASIS LICHENOIDES AND LYMPHOMATOID PAPULOSIS
There are two recognized forms of pityriasis lichenoides: one more acute (pityriasis lichenoides et varioliformis acuta — PLEVA) and one more chronic (pityriasis lichenoides chronica). However, there may be some overlap between the two.

Pityriasis lichenoides et varioliformis acuta (called also Mucha–Habermann disease)
This is the less common of the two variants. Crops of brownish-red papules appear. These evolve over the course of a few days with central vesiculo-pustulation and necrosis developing (**Fig. 5.83**). The lesions dry up to leave small pockmarks and scars. The onset may be accompanied by malaise and even a low-grade fever for the first day or two. Occasionally, there is also joint swelling and, very rarely, more significant systemic

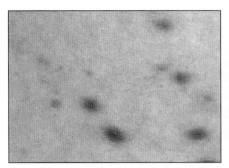

Fig. 5.83 *Lesions in pityriasis lichenoides et varioliformis acuta.*

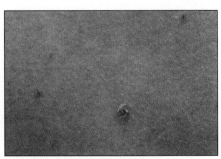

Fig. 5.84 *Scaly papule on the trunk in pityriasis lichenoides chronica showing characteristic 'mica' scale.*

involvement ensues. Attacks usually subside, often after many weeks or months, and seldom recur.

Pityriasis lichenoides chronica

Pityriasis lichenoides chronica is much more frequently encountered in clinical practice than its more acute cousin. The lesions are also papular, but are less florid and last longer. They are surmounted by a small flake or plate of parakeratotic scale (said to resemble mica) (**Fig. 5.84**). Showers of lesions often appear on the trunk, but are less common on sun-exposed sites. In pigmented skins, pityriasis lichenoides chronica may result in a widespread eruption of almost macular hypopigmented lesions. The patients (who are often children or young adults) are invariably fit and well and are really only troubled by the lesions because of their cosmetic appearance.

Occasionally patients are seen in whom a background eruption of apparently typical pityriasis lichenoides chronica is accompanied by some lesions which are more characteristic of PLEVA.

LYMPHOMATOID PAPULOSIS

Lymphomatoid papulosis (**Fig. 5.85**) is the term applied when the lesions are clinically at the more severe end of the pityriasis lichenoides spectrum and when there is significant atypia of the mononuclear cells in the infiltrate. The course of this form of the disease is often more prolonged than that of typical PLEVA and in some circumstances appears to be an overlap state with, or an early phase of, cutaneous T-cell lymphoma (*see* Chapter 4). The presence of the immunocytochemical marker CD30 indicates a more malignant outlook.

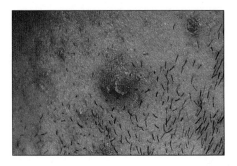

Fig. 5.85 *Papular lesions on the trunk in lymphomatoid papulosis.*

Investigations and treatment

The histology seen in biopsies of lesions of pityriasis will obviously depend on the stage at which the sample is taken, and the intensity of the reaction. However, there is commonly a lymphocytic infiltrate around and in dermal vessels. The vessels themselves show some of the features of a primary vasculitis. The overlying epidermis shows a range of changes from mild acanthosis and parakeratosis at the chronic end of the spectrum, through to complete necrosis at the more severe end. As indicated above, it is important to examine specimens carefully for evidence of cytological atypia and, where necessary, perform extra staining and/or seek the advice of an expert dermatopathologist in interpreting the changes. Treatment is unsatisfactory. Pityriasis lichenoides chronica will often respond to ultraviolet B, and tetracyclines have been used for the more acute forms. However, they are by no means always successful.

PITYRIASIS RUBRA PILARIS

Pityriasis rubra pilaris is rare. There are generally held to be five clinical forms which have, perhaps unsurprisingly, been termed types I to V (**Fig. 5.86**).

The main clinical variants of pityriasis rubra pilaris	
Type I	Adult onset, 'classic'
Type II	Adult onset, 'atypical'
Type III	Juvenile onset, 'classic'
Type IV	Juvenile onset, 'circumscribed'
Type V	Juvenile onset, 'atypical'

Fig. 5.86 *Griffiths classification of pityriasis rubra pilaris.*

Clinical features

As can be seen, the disorder may appear in both children and adults. The term 'classical' refers to the appearance of a widespread eythematous and hyperkeratotic eruption, usually beginning on the head and neck and spreading slowly, inexorably and caudally to involve almost the whole body surface, including the arms, legs, hands, and feet. A particular characteristic is the pronounced tendency for the eruption to surround and involve hair follicles (**Fig. 5.87**). Patches of erythema studded with follicular hyperkeratosis merge to produce a sheeted erythroderma, classically leaving small islands of normal skin (**Fig 5.88**). The face is prominently involved and, if the periorbital skin is affected, eversion of the

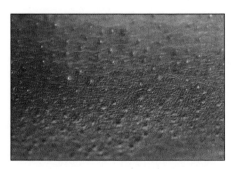

Fig. 5.87 *Follicular scaly lesions on the trunk in classical adult onset (type I) pityriasis rubra pilaris.*

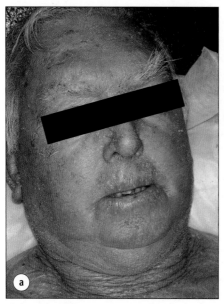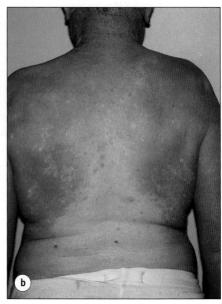

Fig. 5.88 *Widespread erythematous eruption with islands of sparing pityriasis rubra pilaris (a)* on the face and *(b)* on the back.

eyelid (ectropion) may develop. The hands and feet may become severely affected, with marked hyperkeratosis. This may interfere with function to a very significant degree and a particular orange hue is often seen that is quite a useful diagnostic feature. Fingernails and toenails often become markedly dystrophic, but do not show the pits and onycholysis which are so characteristic of psoriasis and are thus quite a useful diagnostic pointer.

Eventually, in most cases, this pattern of pityriasis rubra pilaris (whether in childhood or adulthood — types I and III) resolves spontaneously, although this may take 2 or 3 years. During the interim, however, the patient is often severely compromised by the eruption. A full-blown exfoliative erythroderma may develop, with all the consequences that may ensue (*see* below).

In the atypical adult form (type II) the eruption is usually rather less severe. There is a mixture of scaly erythema and follicular prominence. The disease is usually much more persistent but seldom results in a state of exfoliative erythroderma. It may be extremely difficult to distinguish this form of pityriasis rubra pilaris from other widespread eruptions such as eczema or atypical psoriasis.

The condition that has been termed type IV, circumscribed, juvenile-onset pityriasis rubra pilaris is very different. Here fixed plaques with prominent follicular plugging develop over the knees and elbows (**Fig. 5.89**). There may also be odd lesions scattered elsewhere on the body surface. The lesions are remarkably constant and fixed, but may disappear later in childhood or in early adult life. Some dermatologists have named similar changes as follicular psoriasis, but the classification of such a condition is unclear.

Type V pityriasis rubra pilaris is extremely rare. Cases reported under this heading develop persisting erythema and hyperkeratosis early in life, or even at birth. It is not clear whether all these cases are best considered as variants of pityriasis rubra pilaris or whether some are actually forms of ichthyosiform erythroderma (*see* Chapter 11).

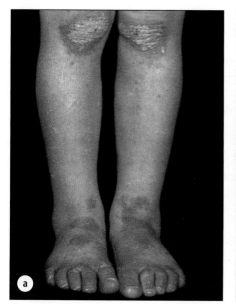 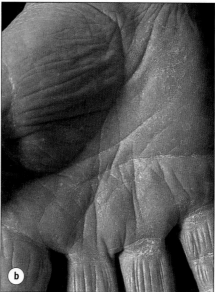

Fig. 5.89 *Well circumscribed psoriasiform lesions* affecting the knees and feet **(a)** and palmar erythema **(b)** in circumscribed juvenile onset (type IV) pityriasis rubra pilaris.

Investigations and treatment

Biopsies may help if there is clinical doubt, because there are differences between pityriasis rubra pilaris and its major diagnostic differential, psoriasis. In particular, epidermal micro-abscesses are not seen, and the degree of acanthosis is much less.

Treatment is generally very unsatisfactory. Topical emollients are helpful in keeping the skin soft in the more extensive forms, but topical corticosteroids are of no value in any of the types described above. Some reports have been made of benefit from the use of retinoids and various cytotoxic drugs, but it is very difficult to assess the real value of these agents in a condition that has such a high rate of spontaneous resolution. For the more localized forms, there is no need for dramatic measures.

- Pityriasis rosea characterized by scaly red ('herald') patch on the trunk, upper thigh, or shoulder of a child or young adult; eruption settles spontaneously (6–8 weeks).
- Pityriasis lichenoides presents (often in chronic form) with papules showing central vesiculo-pustulation and necrosis leaving pockmarks and scars.
- Lymphomatoid papulosis is a severe form of pityriasis lichenoides; important to examine specimens for evidence of cytological atypia.
- Pityriasis rubra pilaris is a rare erythematous and hyperkeratotic local eruption that spreads to cover body surface; high rate of spontaneous resolution.

EXFOLIATIVE ERYTHRODERMA (DERMATITIS)

This is a very important clinical state that can result from a number of different disease processes (**Fig. 5.90**). However, whatever the underlying pathology, there are a number of common features which should be noted. Furthermore, exfoliative erythroderma has significant implications for the patient, however it arises.

Causes of exfoliative erythroderma (dermatitis)	
Dermatitis	Endogenous
	Exogenous
Psoriasis	
Drugs	e.g. sulphonamides, gold.
Cutaneous involvement by	(especially cutaneous T-cell lymphoma and the Sézary
leukaemias and lymphomas	syndrome; *see* Chapter 4)
Pityriasis rubra pilaris	
Pemphigus foliaceus	
Ichthyosiform erythroderma	(*see* Chapter 11)
Miscellaneous causes	e.g. lichen planus, fungal infections, crusted (Norwegian) scabies

Fig. 5.90 *Causes of exfoliative erythroderma (dermatitis).*

Clinical features

The patient's skin becomes red, thickened, and inflamed, and exfoliates continuously. The condition may arise rapidly, or consist of a more chronic and slowly progressive process. Depending where the patient sits on this scale he or she may be acutely unwell. In a rapidly developing erythroderma the patient feels ill, often beginning to shiver from time to time because the skin no longer controls the rate at which heat is radiated into the surrounding environment. This can have dire consequences, especially in the elderly who may suffer from hypothermia as a result. Sudden death from ventricular fibrillation has been described. Whether the situation is acute or longer-standing, several other physical problems may develop.

- High-output cardiac failure may develop as a consequence of the constant perfusion of the skin.
- Insensible water loss from the skin is markedly increased, which can lead to dehydration.
- The high rate of skin loss may lead, ultimately, to protein malnutrition.

On the face, the skin may become so tight that ectropion develops. Similar tightness of the skin of the hands may result in significant impairment of manual dexterity. Patients with exfoliative erythroderma often develop lymphadenopathy. This may be associated with an underlying lymphomatous process, but is more commonly secondary to the cutaneous inflammation (dermatopathic lymphadenopathy).

Investigations and treatment

There are two phases to the management of the patient with exfoliative erythroderma: preventing the secondary effects from leading to significant morbidity or mortality and diagnosing and treating the underlying cause. The two can, of course, proceed simultaneously. Points to consider include the following:

- A full assessment of the general, cardiovascular, metabolic, haematological and biochemical condition of the patient should be undertaken immediately, and any disturbances should be addressed.

- The above assessment should be accompanied by the simple measure of keeping the patient warm.
- Any possible drug triggers should be stopped.
- A skin biopsy should be taken (unless there is a clear and obvious history of a preceding dermatosis).
- A lymph-node biopsy may be indicated.

It is often sensible to initiate treatment with systemic steroids, pending a firm diagnosis. Oral prednisolone in a dose of 30 mg daily is usually adequate. If the cause is known, or proves on investigation, to be psoriasis, the drug of choice is probably methotrexate. This is best administered initially in small doses of say, 5 mg intramuscularly or intravenously. Later, oral therapy, PUVA or other antipsoriatic modalities can be introduced. The treatment of the other major causes will also be that which is appropriate to the condition.

- Exfoliative erythroderma is a potentially fatal condition of sudden onset characterized by red, inflamed exfoliating skin.
- Complications include cardiac failure, hypothermia, lymphadenopathy and infection.
- Full assessment of the general, cardiovascular, metabolic, haematological and biochemical condition of the patient required.
- Initiate treatment with systemic steroids and support therapy.

ACNE AND ERUPTIONS THAT RESEMBLE ACNE

Box 5.6

Acne
Common chronic inflammation of pilosebaceous unit, producing pustules, papules, comedones and scars.

Acne and its variants probably represent the most common of all the cutaneous inflammatory states that are not primarily due to infection. It has been said, for example, that over 80% of people develop some 'spots' at some point in their lives. Perhaps 20–30% of the population seek attention from health professionals for acne. The majority of patients with acne begin to develop lesions at or around puberty and the onset is on average, a year or two earlier, in girls than in boys. The problem usually reaches a peak and subsides over the following 3 to 4 years, but some patients continue to have significant lesions well into their thirties and beyond. Some, particularly women, develop acne for the first time in their late twenties or thirties. Identical changes are also occasionally seen in infants and children (infantile or juvenile acne) (**Fig. 5.91**) and, although this condition usually settles with treatment, it may be followed by a severe recrudescence in adolescence.

A number of clinical entities including acne vulgaris, the severe forms known as acne conglobata and acne fulminans, the phenomenon of secondary acne, the rarer disorders (hidradenitis suppurativa and dissecting cellulitis of the scalp) and, finally, some of the conditions that resemble acne, which can cause diagnostic difficulties will all be expanded in this section:

- Pseudofolliculitis barbae (and acne keloidalis).

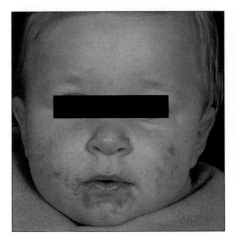

Fig. 5.91 *Infantile acne.*

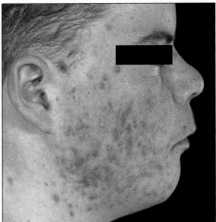

Fig. 5.92 *Erythematous papules on the cheeks of an adolescent male with greasy skin in acne vulgaris.*

- Acne excoriée (des jeunes filles).
- Pityrosporon folliculitis.
- Keratosis pilaris.
- Rosacea, rhinophyma, and perioral dermatitis.

Acne vulgaris: clinical features (Figs 5.92–5.95)

- Acne is a polymorphic eruption arising in skin which is usually visibly greasy (**Fig. 5.92**).
- Lesions characteristically distributed over the face (to which they may be restricted), the back of the neck, the chest, shoulders, back, and upper arms.
- Eruption occasionally more extensive.
- Individual lesions can be classified:
  - Closed comedones or 'whiteheads' — small non-inflamed papules (**Fig. 5.93**).
  - Open comedones or 'blackheads' (**Fig. 5.93**); these may be single or have multiple heads.
  - Papules — small, red, inflamed follicular spots (**Fig. 5.94**).
  - Pustules (**Fig. 5.94**).
  - Scars — these do not occur in all patients, but are the result of the healing process; various types of scar may occur, including atrophic areas, so-called ice-pick scars, which are common on the cheeks, and hypertrophic or keloid scars on the chest and back (**Fig. 5.95**).

Gram-negative folliculitis

Very occasionally, a patient with acne appears to become resistant to antibiotic therapy. The morphology of the eruption may become rather more uniform, with masses of small follicular pustules being seen. Swabs reveal, not the normal skin commensals, but any one of a number of Gram-negative organisms. This condition may be becoming less common as a consequence of earlier retinoid therapy (*see* below).

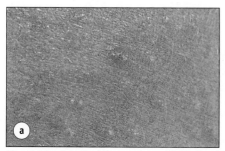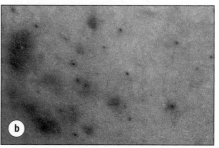

Fig. 5.93 *(a) Closed comedones (whiteheads) and (b) open comedones (blackheads) diagnostic of acne.*

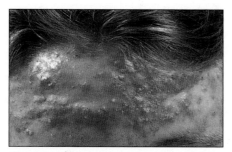

Fig. 5.94 Papules and pustules on the forehead in acne vulgaris.

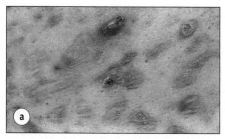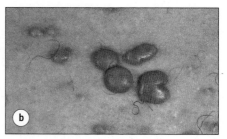

Fig. 5.95 *(a) Atrophic and (b) hypertrophic (keloids) scars in severe acne.*

Nodulocystic acne (acne conglobata)

At the more severe end of the acne spectrum, nodules and cysts may develop (**Fig. 5.96**). The tendency to scarring is increased and the ravages of this severe form of acne may result in a grossly disfiguring appearance.

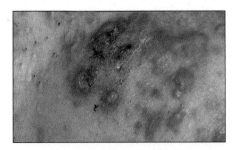

Fig. 5.96 *Nodulocystic acne.*

Acne fulminans

Rarely, a patient presents with severe nodulocystic acne, malaise, fever, and joint pains and/or swelling. Osteolytic lesions may be seen on X-ray. The disease often pursues a stormy course and requires aggressive treatment (*see* below).

Psychological impact of acne

It cannot be stressed enough that, over and above the physical changes in the skin, acne's main effect on the sufferer is on their psychosocial well-being. Personal appearance is central to our feelings of self-worth and acne strikes at an age when the way one looks is particularly critical. We instinctively know that people like us less if we have imperfections, and there is evidence to support this in that employers are inclined to favour those with clear complexions when making job offers. People with facial blemishes are never totally at ease with them and teenagers can become completely obsessed with their acne, even if there are not all that many active lesions. It is all too common to hear that a young person simply will not go out in the evenings but, instead, sits alone in his or her room nurturing feelings of despair and rejection. Suicides have been reported.

Pathogenesis of acne

There appear to be a number of interlocking and interdependent factors involved in the pathogenesis of acne, the interplay of which is illustrated in **Figure 5.97**. In simple terms, there is a marked increase in sebum production at puberty. The rate of excretion of sebum is controlled by tissue androgens which, of course, appear in significantly greater quantities at puberty. However, the levels of circulating androgens are generally normal and are also usually no higher in males or females with acne than in those without. There is a subgroup of girls and women in whom acne presents as only one component of an apparently hyperandrogenized state, some of whom develop mild hirsutism, suffer menstrual irregularities, and have polycystic ovaries, but they probably represent a minority. More common, it is thought, are alterations in the level of the carrier protein sex-hormone binding globulin (SHBG) or tissue androgen metabolism; it may be women affected in this way who have a more prolonged time course, or in whom the acne tends to appear for the first time later than normal.

In addition to the increase in sebum excretion, there is a blockage of the outflow of the hair follicles affected by ductal hyperkeratosis. This leads to the formation of the dilated

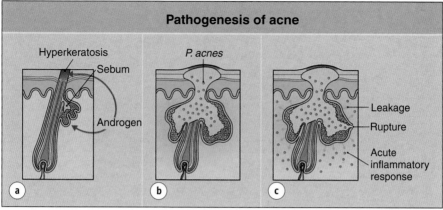

Pathogenesis of acne

Fig. 5.97 *The pathogenesis of acne involves* — *(a)* an increase in sebum production and a blockage of an overflow of the hair follicle; *(b)* an overgrowth of P. acnes and a leakage; *(c)* of inflammatory fatty chemicals into the surrounding dermis, resulting in an inflammatory response.

sac of lipid that is called a comedone. Within the comedone the normal skin commensal *Propionibacterium acnes* multiplies. Numbers of *P. acnes* arise at around the time of adolescence anyway, but the conditions created within the comedone by the pathophysiological changes that take place in acne are perfect for the propagation of this organism. It is thought that this bacterium is, at least in part, responsible for the production of inflammatory mediators which diffuse through the follicle wall and create the dermal inflammation that we call a 'spot', or 'zit'.

Investigations and treatment of acne

Investigations are seldom necessary in acne because the diagnosis is a clinical one and can be made very easily on the basis of the clinical signs described above. However, there are three specific situations in which some further tests may be required:

- If Gram-negative folliculitis is suspected, swabs should be taken.
- If a patient presents with systemic symptoms and acne fulminans is a possibility, a full haematological, biochemical, and immunological screen, and appropriate X-rays, should be performed.
- In the assessments before and during some forms of treatment — especially with the retinoids (*see* below).

The choice of treatment in acne depends on the severity of the condition in terms of:

- Its physical extent and symptoms.
- The degree to which scarring appears to be developing.
- The psychological effects that the condition is having.

Several agents and modalities have been shown to be effective (**Fig. 5.98**).

Most patients will respond to one or other of these modalities, and combinations are also often used (e.g. oral antibiotics with topical benzoyl peroxide). The antibiotics can be very useful in controlling acne but may have to be given for long periods, until the natural peak of severity has passed. Cyproterone acetate is rather slow to take effect but is a very useful adjunct to other treatments in some patients. It may have a role in older women who have completed the rearing of their families but need contraception and anti-acne therapy,

235

Treatments known to be effective in acne

Agent	Mechanism of action	Details of treatment
Benzoyl peroxide	Antibacterial; reduces comedones by keratolytic action?	Topically to whole area daily; begin with weak dose, then increase.
Retinoic acid	Reduces comedones.	Topically to whole area daily.
Antibiotics, especially tetracyclines, erythromycin, clindamycin	Reduces bacteria; inhibits inflammatory processes?	Topically to whole area daily; orally, 1 g daily for 3-6 months initially, for longer if successful.
Cyproterone acetate	Inhibits androgens.	Females only; taken combined with oestrogen as Dianette™.
Isotretinoin	Reduces sebum excretion; inhibits hyperkeratosis; reduces inflammation?	4-month course; dose 0.5-1 mg/kg/day; watch for lipid changes.

Fig. 5.98 *Treatments known to be effective in acne.*

and in younger, sexually active girls who are taking isotretinoin. Isotretinoin is by far the most effective treatment. Over 90% of patients experience complete resolution of lesions and at least 80% remain clear.

However, all of the treatments have some side-effects that patients need to be aware of. The topical agents can be very drying and can make the skin red and sore. Oral antibiotics may give rise to gastrointestinal disturbances, candidal infections, and hypersensitivity rashes and, theoretically at least, can interfere with oral contraceptives. The combined preparation Dianette® containing cyproterone acetate can produce nausea and weight gain, and is contraindicated in patients with a history of thrombosis, epilepsy, or oestrogen-sensitive conditions. Isotretinoin has a number of important side-effects:

- It causes dryness of the skin, lips, nasal mucosa, and conjunctivae.
- It may cause muscle and joint pains.
- Liver function test abnormalities have been reported.
- Fasting triglycerides may rise.
- The drug is teratogenic and all female patients must either refrain from sexual activity or take adequate contraceptive precautions; some dermatologists insist on a pregnancy test before commencement of treatment. A negative pregnancy test is recommended prior to treatment commencing. In the USA, the FDA requires registration of physicians and patients with a central monitoring program (iPLEDGE).
- There is controversy about the effects of isotretinoin on the central nervous system. There are anecdotal reports of episodes of depression and suicide, but adequate controlled data are lacking. Most patients find that their mood improves while on the drug but all patients and their carers should be warned to report any unusual psychological events immediately. Isotretinoin should not be given with tetracyclines because of the theoretical risk of increased intracranial pressure.

Isotretinoin is expensive and is licensed only for use by hospital specialists in the UK, although in other countries it is more freely available. Broadly speaking, the less severe the acne is the more likely it is to respond to less draconian measures. However, in an otherwise uncomplicated world where cost was not a factor and the drug was easily accessible, the retinoid isotretinoin might well be the treatment of choice in far more patients than is currently the case.

In the more extreme forms of acne, where the lesions are highly inflammatory, or in acne fulminans, systemic steroids are required. A short course of oral prednisolone should be administered together with appropriate antibiotics, isotretinoin, or both. Some patients will also need local steroid injections to individual nodules and cysts. This can produce much more rapid resolution. Surgical interventions such as dermabrasion and laser resurfacing may also be helpful in dealing with residual scarring, but this should never be contemplated until after the acne has been brought completely under control. Some patients require psychiatric support.

Secondary acne

Acne may develop alongside several endocrine disorders (*see also* Chapter 8), particularly those in which there are abnormalities of androgens. A rather monomorphic eruption that resembles acne may occur in primary, secondary, and iatrogenic Cushing's syndrome (**Fig. 5.99**). Several drugs can induce or exacerbate acne, e.g. corticosteroids, phenytoin, isoniazid, and lithium. Of greater significance in the modern era than in the past, is the induction of acne by exogenously administered androgens to athletes as part of a performance-enhancing regimen. Topical therapy may also be complicated by the development of comedones and other acne lesions. This is particularly marked with topical corticosteroids but in some patients the use of greasy ointments or pomades is associated with the development of acne, especially across the forehead. Similarly, areas of the skin which are repeatedly soaked in oil may become spotty. Chronic mechanical friction is also reported to cause localized acne under tight-fitting headbands and underwear.

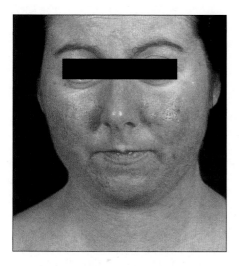

Fig. 5.99 *Monomorphic acne in Cushing's syndrome.*

Comedones are an important feature of chronic sun damage (and are therefore known as solar comedones). They are particularly prominent around the eyes and nose, and on the back of the neck (**Fig. 5.100**). The rest of the skin is generally very wrinkled, and there may be epithelial cysts and other features suggestive of chronic sun exposure. Comedones are also seen in malformations that resemble naevi (*see* Chapter 4).

Comedones are also seen in the rare but important condition, chloracne, which results from the toxic effects of chlorinated hydrocarbon chemicals. Patients may develop a variety of other skin and systemic changes, including hypertrichosis, chronic fatigue, liver function test abnormalities, and neuropathies.

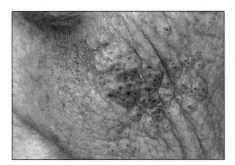

Fig. 5.100 *Senile (solar) comedones on the face.*

- Acne is a polymorphic eruption caused by increased sebum excretion and blockage of outflow of hair follicles affected by ductal hyperkeratosis.
- Presents with comedones, papules, pustules and scars (healing) on face, neck, chest, shoulders, back, and upper arms.
- Can have serious affects on psychosocial well-being.
- Treatment can be topical (e.g. benzoyl peroxide) or oral (e.g. antibiotics and/or isotretinoin).
- Secondary acne may develop with some endocrine disorders (e.g. Cushing's syndrome) or in some drug treatments (e.g. corticosteroids).

Hidradenitis suppurativa

This relatively uncommon condition is a chronic inflammatory process involving skin containing apocrine glands. In mild and early disease, a few comedone-like lesions develop, usually in one or both axillae or in the perineal area, and are accompanied by recurrent swellings, which may give rise to significant discomfort before discharging purulent material and settling down. Later in the course of the disease subcutaneous sinuses develop and whole areas of affected skin may become the subject of permanent and cyclical inflammation and discharge (**Fig. 5.101**). The extent of skin affected varies considerably. The axillae, groins, lower abdomen, and perineum are the most commonly involved sites, but lesions may extend on to the female breast, down the inner thighs, and upwards from the natal cleft. Lesions may also occur on the neck and scalp. Hidradenitis is a difficult condition to treat. Some patients seem to benefit from long courses of erythromycin or tetracyclines in doses of >1 g daily, as for acne. Acute flares may respond to high-dose antibiotics, and a combination of erythromycin and metronidazole (because of the frequent involvement of anaerobes) is well-established. More recently the combination of rifampicin and clindamycin, each at a dose of 300 mg daily has been used with a fair degree of success, and in the authors' experience is the most useful antibiotic regimen. Occasionally, systemic steroids may be helpful. In more extensive disease, success has been reported with both cyproterone acetate (in women only) and retinoids, but others have cast doubt on this. Many patients ultimately require surgical intervention. Plastic surgeons attempt to remove all diseased tissue and, where necessary, perform skin grafts to cover the remaining defects.

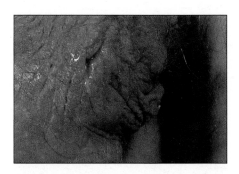

Fig. 5.101 *Hidradenitis suppurativa in the perineum.*

Dissecting cellulitis of the scalp (called also perifolliculitis abscedens et suffodiens)

Even rarer than hidradenitis, dissecting cellulitis of the scalp presents a somewhat similar picture. Initially, chronic sepsis develops in localized areas of the scalp. Papules, nodules, and pustules arise and settle, often discharging pus in the resolving phase. Later, more and more of the scalp becomes affected by a subcutaneous network of sinuses and abscesses. Scalp hair is lost and there is a tendency to scarring. Treatment is similar to that described above for hidradenitis, and with the response to isotretinoin being rather better.

The 'follicular occlusion syndrome'

This term has been used to describe development of a combination of two or more of nodulocystic acne, hidradenitis suppurativa, and dissecting scalp cellulitis. As if this were not enough, some unfortunate individuals appear prone to pilonidal sinuses as well.

Acne excoriée (des jeunes filles)

This disorder is much more common in girls than boys. There are no primary acne lesions, or only very few. The main 'eruption' consists of excoriations and other exogenously induced marks (**Fig. 5.102**). The patients are said to be highly strung and anxious, and the most straightforward therapeutic approach is to initiate treatment with long-term tetracycline or erythromycin and instruct/advise that the picking of spots is to be abandoned. If the problem continues, the addition of a minor tranquillizer may be of benefit.

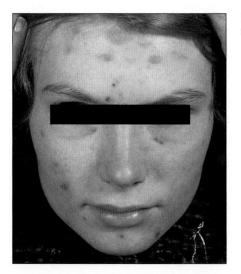

Fig. 5.102 *Excoriated papules on the face in acne excoriée.*

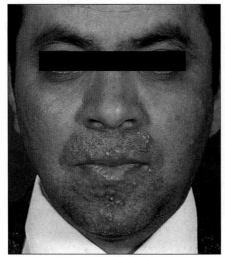

Fig. 5.103 *Pseudofolliculitis barbae.*

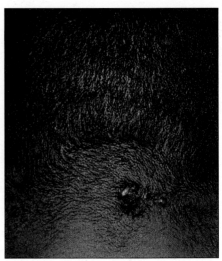

Fig. 5.104 *Keloid on the back of the neck secondary to pseudofolliculitis (acne keloidalis).*

Pseudofolliculitis barbae (and acne keloidalis)

Some men have rather curly beard hairs. Some of these hairs fail to emerge properly from the follicle orifice and continue to grow intradermally. The resulting foreign body reaction produces inflamed spots (Fig. 5.103). This condition is most commonly seen on the neck, but may extend on to the face, particularly around the mouth and chin. The incidence of this disorder is highest in Afro-Caribbeans and it may also be more severe and troublesome, and also more extensive, involving not only the face but the back of the neck as well. The tendency for black skin to form keloid scars may combine with the follicular inflammation to produce multiple scars on the affected area, a situation termed acne keloidalis (Fig. 5.104).

Pityrosporum folliculitis

It has relatively recently been established that the skin commensal *Malassezia* (*Pityrosporum ovale/orbiculare*) can give rise to an eruption of follicular spots, particularly over the upper trunk. This yeast-like fungus is also implicated in seborrhoeic dermatitis (*see* above) and in pityriasis versicolor (*see* Chapter 3). Treatment with one of the azole antifungal agents is usually sufficient.

Rosacea, rhinophyma, and perioral dermatitis

Rosacea is a highly characteristic eruption consisting of erythema, telangiectasia, and recurrent papulopustules. The condition classically affects the forehead, cheeks, nose, and chin (Fig. 5.105), but occasionally similar lesions are seen elsewhere. Patients often complain of facial flushing and may also suffer with migraines. The age of onset is usually over 30 years, although rosacea may occur earlier, but no comedones are present, which helps to distinguish this disorder from a late-onset acne. Patients with rosacea of long standing may also develop facial lymphoedema. Some also develop a specific form of keratitis.

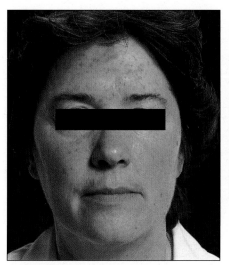

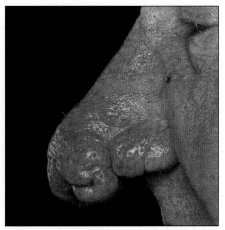

Fig. 5.106 *Bulbous nose in chronic rosacea (rhinophyma).*

Fig. 5.105 *Papules and telangiectasia on the cheeks and forehead in acne rosacea.*

Treatment of rosacea — The condition responds extremely well, in most instances, to treatment with tetracycline antibiotics or erythromycin. A course of 1 g daily for 8 weeks or so will usually result in complete clearance, but the condition often recurs on cessation and maintenance or periodic courses of treatment are thus required. Topical metronidazole has also been shown to be effective. Some patients fail to respond to these drugs and isotretinoin should be tried, but the response in rosacea is not as reliable as it is in acne. There are several associated clinical changes that should be mentioned here.

- Rhinophyma. Significant sebaceous hyperplasia may accompany or follow rosacea of the nose and this may lead to the extraordinary appearance known as rhinophyma (**Fig. 5.106**). This is, of course, highly disfiguring and is one reason for aggressive treatment. Surgical intervention can improve rhinophyma considerably even at a very late stage.
- Perioral dermatitis. Some patients develop a papular, erythematous eruption around the mouth, in the nasolabial folds (**Fig. 5.107**) and, occasionally, further afield. This is not exclusively (but almost always is) associated with topical steroid application, often initially to some other facial dermatosis. The condition responds well to tetracyclines or erythromycin.
- Steroid rosacea. Topical corticosteroids can induce changes identical to those in idiopathic rosacea (**Fig. 5.108**).
- Overlap states. Through experience it is realized that patients with rosacea, perioral dermatitis, or both, may also show some features of seborrhoeic dermatitis.
- Rosaceous 'tuberculide'. Very occasionally, a patient presents with a papular facial eruption, with or without the other features of rosacea. Histology of one of the lesions present reveals granulomatous change indistinguishable from that seen in full-blown tuberculosis, with giant cells and caseation necrosis in evidence. Various names have been applied to such a clinical picture, including granulomatous rosacea and lupus miliaris disseminata faciei. The latter name betrays the fact that such changes were once erroneously considered to be associated with tuberculous infection (for a

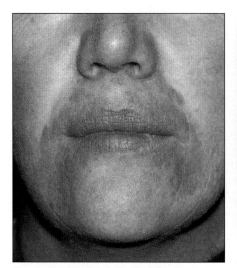

Fig. 5.107 *Perioral dermatitis.*

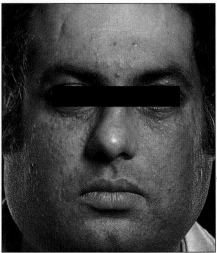

Fig. 5.108 *Rosacea secondary to topical steroids.*

Fig. 5.109 *Granulomatous papules on the eyelids in acne agminata.*

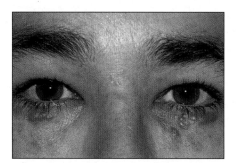

discussion of the true tuberculides *see* Chapter 3). In some patients, granulomatous papules appear around the eyes and nose and are generally grouped in the central area of the face; this pattern is known as acne agminata (**Fig. 5.109**). None of these patients respond well to treatment, but many resolve spontaneously over a period of years.

- Rosacea: highly characteristic eruption consisting of erythema, telangiectasia, and recurrent papulopustules mostly affecting forehead, cheeks, nose, and chin.
- Age of onset is usually over 30 years.
- Treat with tetracycline antibiotics or erythromycin.

LIGHT-INDUCED DISORDERS (ACQUIRED PHOTODERMATOSES)

Many conditions exist in which light plays a role in the induction or exacerbation of skin changes. Some examples are given in **Figure 5.110**.

This section is primarily concerned with those disorders which are generally considered to be true photodermatoses and the reader is referred to the appropriate section of this book for the other conditions mentioned.

Some important conditions in which light plays a role in the induction or exacerbation of skin changes	
Acute photosensitivity	Sunburn, xeroderma pigmentosum (*see* Chapter 11), the porphyrias (see Chapter 11), solar urticaria (*see above*), pellagra.
Primary photosensitivity disorders	Polymorphic light eruption, juvenile spring eruption hydroa vacciniforme, actinic prurigo.
Disorders sometimes exacerbated by sunlight	Drug reactions (*see* Chapter 8), lupus erythematosus (*see above*), rosacea (*see above*), Darier's disease (*see* Chapter 11), eczema including chronic actinic, dermatitis (see above) psoriasis, lichen planus (*see above*).

Fig. 5.110 *Some important conditions in which light plays a role in the induction or exacerbation of skin changes.*

Polymorphic light eruption

Many people develop a rash that they may call 'prickly heat' (discussed briefly below — *see* Miliaria) when they are exposed to bright sunshine. This may occur early in the summer in temperate climates, or only with light of greater intensity than normally encountered at home. The dermatologist may often have to make the diagnosis on history alone because the eruption only appears on holiday and has long since vanished. The most common story is of the onset of a papular eruption on light-exposed surfaces within some hours of exposure to sunlight (**Fig. 5.111**). The rash is erythematous and often intensely itchy. Occasionally, more extensive lesions develop, or the papules merge to form plaques. Blisters can form in very severe reactions. In most patients the reaction subsides with time, and the rest of the summer is trouble-free, suggesting some degree of 'conditioning' of the skin. All patients should be screened for lupus erythematosus (with which polymorphic light eruption shares many histological features). In cases where the history is more vague, porphyrin screens (*see* Chapter 11) should also be undertaken. Photobiology units usually perform sophisticated challenge tests with ultraviolet and visible light, but the results are inconsistent and not generally helpful in most patients. The most successful form of active therapy is probably prophylactic PUVA in a pre-season course, but oral hydroxychloroquine 200 mg twice daily is an alternative and helps many patients to enjoy their holidays without their rash. Some authorities recommend narrow band UVB (TL-01).

Juvenile spring eruption

This name is given to the appearance of blisters on the ears, usually in small boys, typically every spring (**Fig. 5.112**). Some patients also develop polymorphic light eruption, suggesting that the two disorders are closely related.

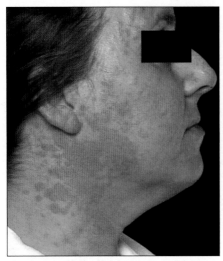

Fig. 5.111 *Urticarial lesions on the face in polymorphic light eruption.*

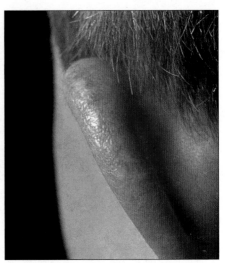

Fig. 5.112 *Papules and vesicles on the ear in juvenile spring eruption.*

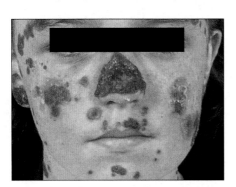

Fig. 5.113 *Facial vesicles and bullae on the face lead to pock-like scars in hydroa vacciniforme (courtesy of Dr D A Burns).*

Hydroa vacciniforme

This is a rare condition seen almost exclusively in childhood. It is characterized by the appearance of multiple vesicles and bullae on light-exposed areas, particularly the face and hands (**Fig. 5.113**). These heal gradually but leave pock-like scars in their wake. Patients should be screened for other causes of photosensitivity including lupus and porphyria. Treatment is largely directed at avoidance of exposure because interventional therapies are largely ineffective. Fortunately the condition tends to subside as adulthood dawns.

Actinic prurigo

This term embraces two distinct clinical presentations. The first, and the most common in Europe, is a sporadic disorder of prepubertal children. The second is a familial disorder, most commonly described in native Americans, in which the condition appears in both children and adults. The appearances of the eruption are, however, very similar: itchy, papulonodular lesions appear on light-exposed surfaces and tend to persist throughout the summer months. As the years pass, the lesions may last longer, into the autumn (fall) and beyond. They may also begin to appear on areas that are mostly covered by clothing. As may be imagined, the condition can be very disabling because of its persistence. Treatment is difficult. Claims have been made for prophylactic ultraviolet B or PUVA and thalidomide has been reported to be very effective. Unfortunately, however, this drug is not only highly teratogenic, but it also causes a neuropathy in a high proportion of patients. Measures are largely aimed at sun avoidance, using barrier sunscreens. In the sporadic form a relatively good prognosis can be anticipated, as the condition often clears at or around puberty.

- Polymorphic light eruption is an erythematous and itchy rash upon exposure to bright sunlight.
- Treatment options include prophylactic PUVA or oral hydroxychloroquine.
- Actinic prurigo presents with itchy, papulonodular lesions on light-exposed surfaces; sun avoidance or barrier creams most effective treatment.

MILIARIA

In hot and humid conditions, some people develop occlusion of sweat ducts for reasons which are not entirely clear. This gives rise to an accumulation of sweat within the skin. This may occur at three distinct levels, giving rise to three entirely different clinical pictures:
- Miliaria crystallina — small non-itchy vesicles appear almost anywhere on the body surface (**Fig. 5.114**); this is most often encountered in patients being nursed in intensive care facilities.
- Miliaria rubra — this is the form known colloquially as 'prickly heat'; itchy papules develop over flexural surfaces and, in infants, in the napkin (diaper) area.
- Miliaria profunda — deep-seated nodules develop as sweat is extruded into the dermis; these lesions are more often symptomatic or painful than itchy.

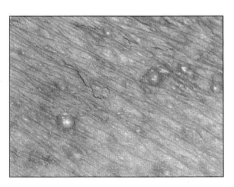

Fig. 5.114 *Tiny pearly superficial vesicles in miliaria crystallina.*

chapter 6

Infiltrative Disorders

INTRODUCTION

A number of disorders exist in which the skin, rather than being involved in a primarily inflammatory or infective process, is infiltrated by cellular and other elements. This chapter will cover the most important of these.

NECROBIOTIC DISORDERS

Box 6.1

Necrobiosis
Term applied to a particular change in the dermal collagen in which there is a loss of the normal pattern, and some swelling, of collagen bundles, thought to be due in part to necrosis. The collagen is also more basophilic in its staining reaction to haematoxylin and eosin (H&E) than normal.

Necrobiosis may be found in several clinical conditions (**Fig. 6.1**). Perhaps not surprisingly, patients have been reported with combinations of two or more of these disorders, the most common being the association of necrobiosis lipoidica and granuloma annulare.

Conditions in which necrobiosis may be a feature	
Necrobiosis lipoidica	'Typical' associated with diabetes 'Typical' without diabetes 'Atypical'
Granuloma annulare	Localized Disseminated
Rheumatoid nodule	
Necrobiotic xanthogranuloma	
Sarcoid	

Fig. 6.1 *Conditions in which necrobiosis may be a feature.*

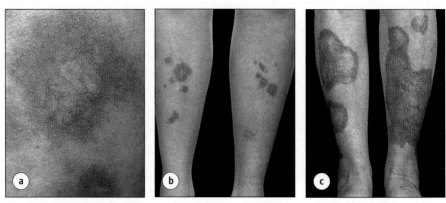

Fig. 6.2 *Necrobiosis lipoidica* — *(a)* *there is a yellowish, waxy, central area with telangiectatic vessels, and a reddish-purple 'active' margin;* *(b)* *several lesions on the shins in the same patient as a);* *(c)* *very extensive lesions.*

NECROBIOSIS LIPOIDICA (DIABETICORUM)

Lesions of necrobiosis lipoidica are atrophic. The skin is waxy and, often, has a yellowish colour, with a raised, purplish margin (**Fig. 6.2a**). Telangiectatic blood vessels are easily seen on the surface. Lesions may be multiple (**Fig. 6.2b**) and may become very extensive (**Fig. 6.2c**). Lesions of necrobiosis may break down and ulcerate. By far the most common site for necrobiosis lipoidica is the shins, lesions occasionally occuring on the arms and trunk.

Much less commonly, a necrobiotic process involves the scalp, causing a cicatricial alopecia (**Fig. 6.3** — *see also* Chapter 9). Similar changes may occur in sarcoidosis (*see* page 255). However, for cases in which sarcoidosis has been excluded and the histology is definitively necrobiotic, the term atypical necrobiosis is used.

Fig. 6.3 *Atypical necrobiosis of the scalp.*

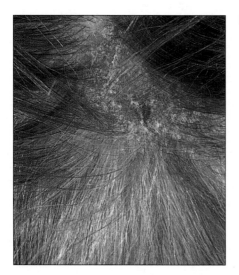

The histological features of necrobiosis lipoidica are somewhat variable. A marked degree of necrobiosis is always present, the lesions mostly being scattered diffusely in the lower dermis. The necrobiosis is accompanied by a rather loose surrounding inflammatory infiltrate, which may be granulomatous with giant cells, but may be more histiocyte-predominant. Thickening of the walls of small dermal vessels is an inconstant feature. Some lesions contain a large number of foam cells.

The most important association with necrobiosis is diabetes mellitus. Although necrobiosis only occurs rarely in patients with diabetes (perhaps in no more than 0.5–1.0%), over two-thirds of patients with necrobiosis lipoidica have diabetes (and the disorder, therefore, sometimes attracts the additional label diabeticorum). A further subdivision of patients are said to have abnormal glucose tolerance, especially when the test is performed under 'stressed' conditions (e.g. steroid-loaded). The microangiopathy of diabetes is thought to be an important aetiological factor.

- Necrobiosis lipoidica is an infiltrative disorder presenting with atrophic ulcerating lesions commonly on the shins.
- Most important association with necrobiosis is diabetes mellitus.
- Difficult to treat; topical steroids or injected corticosteroids, excision and grafting.

The condition is extremely difficult to treat. Topical steroids, with or without polythene occlusion, or injected corticosteroids may help control the spread of lesions, and there are many reports of other drugs and potions that have apparently helped a case or two. Methotrexate has been found to be helpful in atypical necrobiosis of the scalp. Excision and grafting certainly has a place for treating severe, ulcerating, painful lesions.

GRANULOMA ANNULARE

In granuloma annulare (GA), as the all-important second word would suggest, the overall architecture of the lesions is annular and the rings can be seen to be composed of individual round elements (**Fig. 6.4a** and **b**). The most typical sites are the knuckles of the fingers and hands, the dorsum of the feet (**Fig. 6.4c**), and the extensor surfaces of the knees and elbows. Much less commonly, lesions may be scattered diffusely over wide areas of the trunk and limbs (**Fig. 6.4d**). Very occasionally, lesions may be subcutaneous.

Histologically, annular condensations of necrobiosis are found in the mid-dermis, surrounded by a pallisading granuloma. Lesions may occasionally show histological breaching of the necrobiotic centre through the epidermis, a situation known as perforating GA.

There has been some controversy about the association of GA with diabetes mellitus. It seems that this association is mostly found in patients with the widely disseminated form of GA, although there is a (much weaker) association between localized GA and diabetes, too.

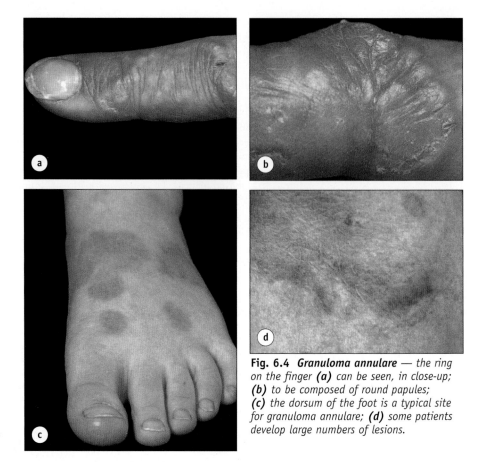

Fig. 6.4 *Granuloma annulare* — *the ring on the finger* **(a)** *can be seen, in close-up;* **(b)** *to be composed of round papules;* **(c)** *the dorsum of the foot is a typical site for granuloma annulare;* **(d)** *some patients develop large numbers of lesions.*

If lesions need treatment, a few respond quite well to potent topical steroids and local injections of triamcinolone. Disseminated GA may be helped by PUVA therapy.

RHEUMATOID NODULE

The occurrence of subcutaneous nodules in seropositive rheumatoid arthritis is well known (*see* Chapter 8). The central area is, histologically, characterized by extensive necrobiosis.

NECROBIOTIC XANTHOGRANULOMA

Necrobiotic xanthogranuloma is an extremely rare condition in which plaques of waxy, yellow, infiltrated skin appear (**Fig. 6.5a**) in association with xanthelasma-like lesions (**Fig. 6.5b**). Affected patients always have a monoclonal gammopathy.

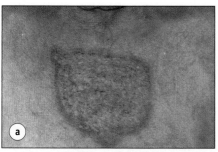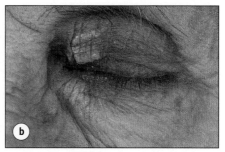

Fig. 6.5 *Necrobiotic xanthogranuloma* — *(a) plaque on the chest; (b) xanthelasma-like lesions around the eyelids.*

SARCOIDOSIS AND OTHER GRANULOMATOUS INFILTRATES

SARCOIDOSIS

The skin is frequently involved in sarcoidosis and there are several recognizable forms (**Fig. 6.6**), although a degree of overlap between them is common (*see* Chapter 8).

Box 6.2
Sarcoidosis Multisystem granulomatous disorder characterized by the development of lymphocyte-poor epithelioid cell granulomas (*see* Chapter 8).

Cutaneous sarcoid
Erythema nodosum (see Chapter 8) Scar sarcoid Papular Lichenoid Nodular Lupus pernio

Fig. 6.6 *Cutaneous sarcoid.*

In the skin, in common with several other disorders, sarcoid has a predilection for scars, and the infiltration of the skin and subcutis around a previously traumatized area is well recognized (**Fig. 6.7a**). Skin involvement may also be diffuse (**Fig. 6.7b**), with the clinical appearances ranging from small erythematous papules to large nodular and ulcerating lesions. The lesions may be flat-topped and may closely resemble lichen planus (*see* Chapter 5) or lichen scrofulosorum (see Chapter 3).

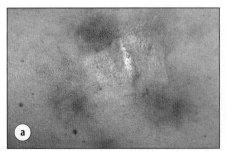

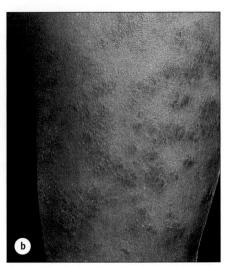

**Fig. 6.7 *Sarcoidosis* — *(a)* deep *granulomas in a previously scarred area — the patient had systemic sarcoidosis; (b) papulonodular lesions of sarcoid.*

One specific form of sarcoidosis deserves special mention: lupus pernio (**Fig. 6.8a**). Here, granulomatous areas appear particularly on the nose and ears, and are virtually always accompanied by chronic changes elsewhere, including pulmonary fibrosis and cystic changes in the bones of the digits. The skin and nails of the fingers may also be involved (**Fig. 6.8b**).

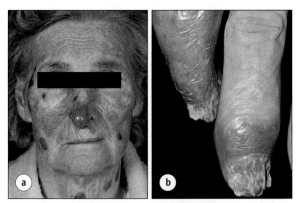

**Fig. 6.8 *Lupus pernio* — *(a)* infiltration of the nose and other facial lesions; *(b)* finger involvement in the same patient.*

OTHER GRANULOMATOUS INFILTRATES

Crohn's disease

Crohn's disease of the lower colon and rectum quite commonly extends to involve the skin, resulting in infiltrated plaques and perianal sinuses (*see* Chapter 8). Very rarely, granulomatous infiltrates appear at distant sites (metastatic Crohn's disease).

Granulomatous cheilitis

In granulomatous cheilitis, the lips become puffy and swollen as a consequence of their infiltration by tuberculoid/sarcoidal granulomas. Initially, there is often a localized area (**Fig. 6.9**), but gradually the process extends to involve the whole lip or lips. Granulomatous swelling of the lips may occur alone, as part of the manifestations of Crohn's disease, or in a condition known as the Melkersson–Rosenthal syndrome, which comprises granulomatous cheilitis, facial nerve palsy, and fissured (or scrotal) tongue.

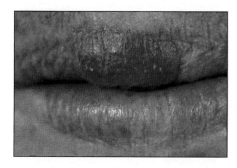

Fig. 6.9 *Granulomatous cheilitis.*

Patients with persistent swelling of the lips should be biopsied. If granulomas are found, a search for Crohn's disease may be justified, although this is probably unnecessary if there are no symptoms. Intralesional steroids will often reduce the swelling significantly. There are many reports of granulomatous cheilitis induced by flavourings and other food additives. In the authors' experience this is uncommon, and such patients will volunteer that they have found certain foods which aggravate their problem.

- Sarcoidosis is characterized by lymphocyte-poor epithelioid cell granulomas with frequent skin involvement.
- Sarcoid has a predilection for scars.
- Diffuse skin involvement ranges from erythematous papules to large nodular, ulcerating lesions.
- Crohn's disease can extend to involve the skin, resulting in infiltrated plaques and perianal sinuses.
- Granulomatous cheilitis is characterized by puffy/swollen lips due to infiltration by tuberculoid/sarcoidal granulomas.

MASTOCYTOSIS

The occurrence of a solitary naevoid infiltrate by mast cells has already been mentioned in Chapter 4 (*see* mast cell naevus). More commonly, cutaneous mastocytosis takes the form of multiple lesions. This is seen in both adults and children, and can lead to several different clinical appearances: notably, diffuse cutaneous mastocytosis, urticaria pigmentosa, and telangiectasia macularis eruptiva perstans. All these forms are characterized by the infiltration of the dermis by an abnormal number of mast cells. This is best demonstrated microscopically by the use of one of the special stains. Mastocytosis may also be systemic, with mast cell infiltration involving internal organs, especially bones, liver, and spleen. Very rarely, patients may present with a mast cell leukaemia.

DIFFUSE CUTANEOUS MASTOCYTOSIS

Diffuse cutaneous mastocytosis is rare and usually occurs in infancy and childhood. The skin is diffusely infiltrated with mast cells and, clinically, is thickened and yellowish. The skin wheals and blisters on the slightest friction. There is no satisfactory treatment except to try to reduce the whealing using antihistamines.

URTICARIA PIGMENTOSA

Urticaria pigmentosa can affect both children and adults. Multiple, pigmented macules, papules, or nodules are present, which, in children, tend to be rather fewer in number and yellowish-brown (**Fig. 6.10a**). On first inspection, they can be difficult to distinguish from juvenile xanthogranuloma (*see* page 255). In adults, especially later in the course of the disease, the lesions are more numerous and have a dusky reddish hue (**Fig. 6.10b**). A classical diagnostic feature is that lesions of urticaria pigmentosa urticate when rubbed ('Darier's sign' — **Fig. 6.10c**).

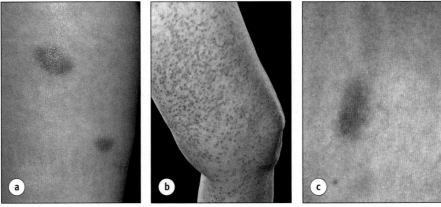

Fig. 6.10 *Urticaria pigmentosa* — *(a)* in a child (compare this with Fig 6.11); *(b)* in an adult; *(c)* 'Darier's' sign — a lesion of urticaria has been rubbed gently and is urticating.

Patients complain of a variable degree of pruritus. Some develop spontaneous whealing and may also exhibit dermatographism. Flushing attacks can occur with extensive skin involvement. The prognosis is generally quite good in children, as the disease improves and clears spontaneously in many patients. Adult disease tends to persist and gradually extend. Treatment with antihistamines may relieve some of the symptomatology. PUVA improves the appearance of extensive urticaria pigmentosa by darkening the surrounding 'normal' skin.

- Cutaneous mastocytosis is characterized by infiltration of the dermis by an abnormal number of mast cells.
- Diffuse cutaneous mastocytosis (rare) occurs mainly in infancy and childhood with skin wheals and blistering; reduce the whealing using antihistamines.
- Urticaria pigmentosa affects both children and adults presenting with pigmented macules, papules, or nodules; lesions of urticate when rubbed.

TELANGIECTASIA MACULARIS ERUPTIVA PERSTANS

Telangiectasia macularis eruptiva perstans presents a rare cutaneous picture, and is almost invariably seen in adults, but rarely in children. Instead of pigmented papules, the skin is covered in a telangiectatic macular eruption. Whealing is not a prominent feature and the diagnosis may be made only on biopsy.

JUVENILE XANTHOGRANULOMA (NAEVOXANTHOENDOTHELIOMA)

Juvenile xanthogranuloma occurs in children, often those aged under 1 year. Typically, a solitary lesion or a crop of yellow–orange papules suddenly appears on the head and neck or on the trunk (**Fig. 6.11**). Occasionally, there are hundreds of lesions present. This is essentially a clinical diagnosis, but, histologically, xanthogranulomas show a mixed dermal infiltrate, with histiocytes and Touton giant cells. In established lesions, the presence of foamy histiocytes is an important diagnostic feature.

Lesions generally disappear spontaneously over the course of a year or so.

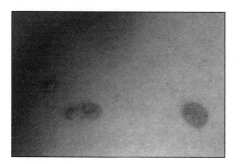

Fig. 6.11 *Juvenile xanthogranuloma.* *Lesions can be difficult to distinguish from urticaria pigmentosa, but are usually rather more orange and do not urticate.*

LANGERHANS'-CELL HISTIOCYTOSIS (HISTIOCYTOSIS X)

The term Langerhans'-cell histiocytosis is preferred to histiocytosis X because it reflects the true nature of this group of conditions and reduces some of the 'mystery' implicit in the older name. However, both are found in common usage. There are also a number of 'older' clinical terms that have been applied to manifestations of Langerhans'-cell histiocytosis: eosinophilic granuloma, Hand–Schüller–Christian disease, Letterer–Siewe disease, and Hashimoto–Pritzker syndrome.

Many systemic features are seen, particularly reflecting infiltration of bones, liver and spleen, lymph nodes, lungs, and pituitary fossa.

Cutaneous involvement is relatively common. The following may occur:

- A rather greasy, seborrhoeic, dermatitis-like eruption of the scalp.
- A rash of brown, scaly, purpuric papules (**Fig. 6.12**).
- A persistent napkin dermatitis.

255

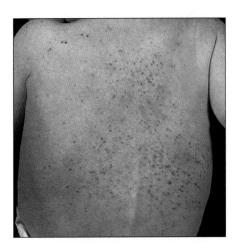

Fig. 6.12 *This child's rash was due to Langerhans'-cell histiocytosis.*

AMYLOIDOSIS

Box 6.3
Amyloidosis Infiltration of the skin and other organs by material with the staining characteristics of starch (amylum).

Amyloidosis has a number of recognizably different forms, in which the deposits of material, although looking identical under light microscopy, derive from different sources (Fig. 6.13).

A classification of amyloidosis	
Primary (immunoglobulin-derived)	Associated with plasma cell dyscrasia.
Secondary	Associated with chronic inflammatory disorders.
Primary cutaneous	Macular (frictional). Papular (lichen amyloidosus) Nodular Atypical
Secondary cutaneous	Amyloid deposits may be seen in association with a number of other skin conditions, e.g. basal cell carcinomas, naevi, seborrhoeic keratoses.

Fig. 6.13 *A classification of amyloidosis.*

Of these forms, only the primary cutaneous types commonly present in the skin clinic. The amyloid deposits found in the dermis in these disorders appear to be derived from the keratin of degenerating epidermal cells in macular and papular amyloidosis.

There is significant racial variation, with the macular and papular forms of primary cutaneous amyloidosis being much more common in Asians than in whites or Afro-Caribbeans.

PRIMARY CUTANEOUS AMYLOIDOSIS

Macular (frictional) amyloidosis

Patients with macular amyloidosis develop macular hyperpigmentation, particularly over the upper back, arms, and legs (**Fig. 6.14**). There is a characteristic 'rippled' effect. Patients often describe the areas affected as being remarkably itchy. Some authors believe the term frictional amyloidosis is more appropriate because of reports of the condition developing after long periods of cutaneous rubbing.

Histologically, there are small deposits of amyloid present in the dermal papillae.

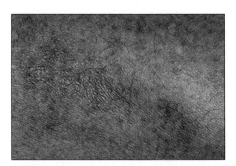

Fig. 6.14 *Macular amyloid. There is pigmentation that has not been preceded by any inflammatory episode. The so-called rippled effect is seen to one side of this plate.*

Papular amyloidosis (lichen amyloidosus)

The changes are more marked in lichen amyloidosus, with the development of (**Fig. 6.15**). Thus, the condition may closely resemble lichen simplex chronicus (with which it may, indeed, be aetiologically linked).

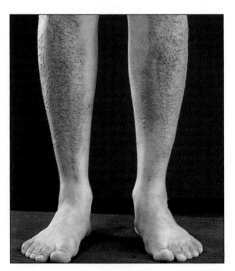

Fig. 6.15 *Lichen amyloidosis.*

Nodular amyloidosis

Nodular amyloidosis is rare. One or more nodules develop more or less anywhere in the skin, but before biopsy they are frequently not recognized as being due to amyloid. The deposits contain light chains, and patients need to be followed up long-term in case they develop a significant plasma cell dyscrasia (*see* primary amyloidosis in Chapter 8).

ATYPICAL PRIMARY CUTANEOUS AMYLOIDOSIS

There have been a number of descriptions of unusual cutaneous eruptions made; on biopsy, these eruptions have been shown to be due to cutaneous amyloid deposition.

PRIMARY AND SECONDARY AMYLOIDOSIS

Primary (immunoglobulin-derived) amyloidosis is covered in Chapter 8. In secondary amyloidosis, amyloid is deposited in various internal organs as a consequence of long-standing, chronic, systemic inflammation (e.g. familial Mediterranean fever, chronic empyema, rheumatoid arthritis). The skin is not generally involved.

- Amyloidosis is characterized by skin infiltration by material with the staining characteristics of starch (amylum).
- Presents with macular ('frictional') hyperpigmentation over upper back, arms, and legs; or sheets of flat-topped papules on the shins ('papular'); or rarely as nodules ('nodular').

LYMPHOCYTIC INFILTRATES

Infiltration of the skin by lymphocytes is a feature of many inflammatory dermatoses. Large collections of lymphocytes are seen in skin lesions caused by lupus erythematosus, light reactions, insect bites, and lymphomas. There are, however, some patients in whom lymphocytic infiltration of the skin cannot be classified as due to any of these pathological states. There are three reasonably distinct clinical presentations that have been described:
- The benign lymphocytic infiltrate of Jessner–Kanof (often simply called 'Jessner's').
- Lymphocytoma cutis.
- Pseudolymphoma.

The most important diagnostic aspect of these conditions is their distinction from cutaneous lymphoma, for which careful study by a histopathologist with an interest in dermatopathology may be required.

JESSNER–KANOF BENIGN LYMPHOCYTIC INFILTRATE

In Jessner's, red or pink, smooth dermal swellings, similar at first sight to wheals (**Fig. 6.16**), are seen on the face or the upper trunk. These fluctuate in severity over time and may disappear completely. Some patients report exacerbation of the condition by light exposure. Histologically, there are areas of dense perivascular aggregations of mature lymphocytes seen in the dermis. The overlying epidermis is normal (and this distinguishes the eruption from lupus erythematosus).

Treatment is very difficult. Some patients find topical steroids helpful and a few have been seen in whom antimalarials appear to have helped.

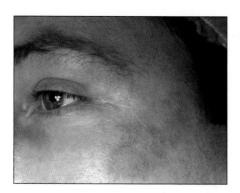

Fig. 6.16 *Jessner–Kanof lymphocytic infiltrate on the face of a young woman.*

LYMPHOCYTOMA CUTIS (SPIEGLER–FENDT SARCOID)

The lesions in lymphocytoma cutis may be very similar to those in Jessner's, but the colour is often rather duskier. The face is by far the most common site for the lesions of lymphocytoma cutis (**Fig. 6.17**). Lesions do not fluctuate to the same degree as those in Jessner's, and the histology is different. In lymphocytoma cutis, there is a striking follicular arrangement of the infiltrate, simulating a lymph node. Intralesional steroids may produce temporary improvement. Solitary lesions can be excised and some authors have recommended radiotherapy.

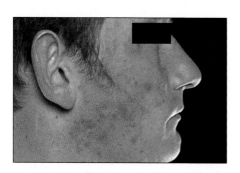

Fig. 6.17 *Lymphocytoma cutis.*

PSEUDOLYMPHOMA

Patients occasionally present with lesions that both clinically and histologically closely resemble a cutaneous lymphoma, but which behave benignly over many years (**Fig. 6.18**). Occasionally these lesions eventually evolve into true lymphomas.

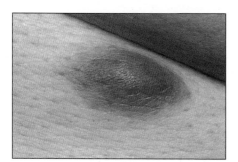

Fig. 6.18 *Pseudolymphoma. This lesion, and three others like it, were initially thought to represent cutaneous B-cell lymphoma, but remained largely unchanged over a decade.*

MUCINOUS INFILTRATES

Several conditions exist in which the skin is infiltrated by mucin (**Fig. 6.19**).

Cutaneous mucinoses
Myxoedema (see Chapter 8) Pretibial myxoedema Lichen myxoedematosus (papular mucinosis; scleromyxoedema) Reticulate erythematous mucinosis (REM) syndrome Scleroedema (adultorum of Buschke) Mucopolysaccharidoses Follicular mucinosis (alopecia mucinosa)

Fig. 6.19 *Cutaneous mucinoses.*

PRETIBIAL MYXOEDEMA

The skin in pretibial myxoedema is infiltrated by acid mucopolysaccharides, with affected areas being overwhelmingly localized to the fronts of the shins and the feet. The lesions may be circumscribed (**Fig. 6.20a**) or there may be diffuse infiltration (**Fig. 6.20b**). Hypertrichosis may occur over the affected areas (*see* Fig. 6.20a). There is a generalized increase in mucinous material in much of the skin, but this is rarely evident clinically. Patients have autoimmune thyroid disease and are usually thyrotoxic (*see* Chapter 8).

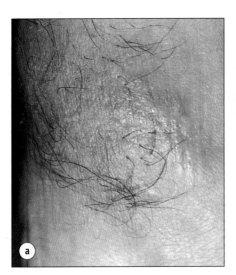

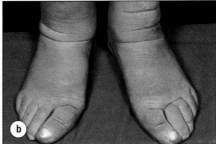

Fig. 6.20 *Pretibial myxoedema —*
(a) localized area with hypertrichosis;
(b) more diffuse infiltration affecting the lower legs and feet.

LICHEN MYXOEDEMATOSUS (PAPULAR MUCINOSIS, SCLEROMYXOEDEMA)

Lichen myxoedematosus is rare. Papules develop almost anywhere on the skin surface (**Fig. 6.21**). These may continue to extend and become aggregated into confluent sheets. In the early stages, the term papular mucinosis seems the most appropriate. Later, lichen myxoedematosus is highly descriptive. In some patients, the pseudo-sclerodermatous changes that may occur on the hands result in the term scleromyxoedema being applied.

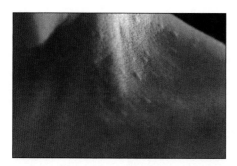

Fig. 6.21 *Papular mucinosis.*

These terms however, indicate a single condition. The dermis is extensively infiltrated by mucinous material. A circulating paraprotein can be found in most patients.

It is claimed that some patients improve with melphalan.

RETICULATE ERYTHEMATOUS MUCINOSIS (REM) SYNDROME

There is some doubt as to the nosological position of REM syndrome, but the patients who have been given this diagnostic label have had a reddish, reticulate eruption on the upper trunk, often in an apparently photosensitive distribution. The skin contains an increase in mucin, but also a perivascular lymphocytic infiltrate. It may be a variant of cutaneous lupus erythematosus.

SCLERODEMA (ADULTORUM OF BUSCHKE)

Sclerodema is another rare dermatosis characterized by mucinous infiltration of the skin. Despite the tag 'adultorum' that is occasionally appended, the disease may affect any age group. The typical history is of a sudden onset of stiffening and induration of the skin of the upper trunk. This gradually extends and can involve the face, lower trunk, and limbs. In most instances, the changes subside and clear after a period of some months to several years. There may have been an infectious illness at the onset and some patients are diabetics.

FOLLICULAR MUCINOSIS (ALOPECIA MUCINOSA)

Follicular mucinosis is a rare condition in which there is inflammation and an extensive mucinous degeneration of hair follicles. Lesions present as plaques of infiltrated skin with follicular prominence (**Fig. 6.22**). When the plaques involve terminal hairs, alopecia may be evident. In most patients, there are only one or a few plaques and these usually settle spontaneously with time. In others, multiple lesions develop and these can be very disfiguring, particularly on the head and neck.

The aetiology of follicular mucinosis is unknown, but the mucinous deposition change appears to follow, rather than precede, the inflammation. In a few cases, the cutaneous

- Mucin can infiltrate skin causing a range of conditions.
- Lichen and pretibial myxoedema are skin manifestations associated with autoimmune thyroid disease.
- Sclerodema is characterized by sudden onset of stiffening/induration of the skin of the upper trunk; subsides over months to several years.
- Follicular mucinosis is a rare condition with inflammation and mucinous degeneration of hair follicles.

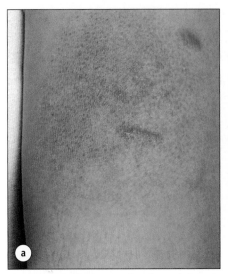 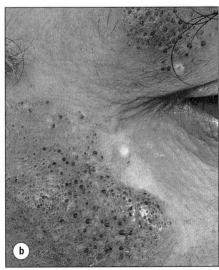

Fig. 6.22 *Follicular mucinosis* — *(a)* a plaque on the upper arm of a young woman; *(b)* this man presented with numerous lesions — he was later diagnosed as having cutaneous T-cell lymphoma.

cellular infiltrate is lymphomatous, and follicular mucinosis may be the presenting feature of a cutaneous T-cell lymphoma (mycosis fungoides) — *see* Chapter 4.

EOSINOPHILIC CELLULITIS

Eosinophilic cellulitis is a rare condition in which raised, itchy, erythematous areas develop, evolve into flatter plaques with a greenish hue (**Fig. 6.23**), and then subside. A mixed dermal infiltrate of eosinophils and polymorphs, and, classically, eosinophilic 'flame figures', are present.

EOSINOPHILIC FASCIITIS (SCHULMAN'S SYNDROME)

Eosinophilic fasciitis is characterised by rapid-onset, generalized cutaneous induration, particularly of the limbs, associated with a high ESR, eosinophilia and fascial inflammation and fibrosis on biopsy. It may be associated with systemic features (arthritis, pulmonary fibrosis, pericarditis) or haematological disease.

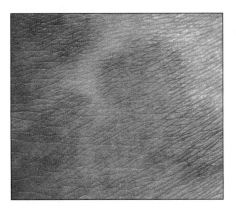

Fig. 6.23 *An area of eosinophilic cellulitis.*

chapter 7

Bullous Diseases

INTRODUCTION

Blistering, or bulla formation, is one of the more dramatic ways in which the skin can respond to insult, injury, or inflammation. There are a large number of unrelated pathological processes that can result in blister formation (**Fig. 7.1**). Blistering is essentially due to splitting in the skin. This may occur within the upper dermis beneath the basement membrane, within the basement membrane zone itself, or at various levels within the epidermis.

The pathological processes involved in blistering also vary considerably, but the most important can broadly be considered under a number of headings (*see* Fig. 7.1):

- Congenital faults in skin adhesion.
- Physical — the skin splits because of damage caused by mechanical or other injury to the tissues.
- Infections — various infections disrupt the skin, usually within the epidermis, and cause blistering.
- Inflammation — blistering occurs as a secondary phenomenon in many inflammatory skin diseases.
- Immunobullous — immunologically mediated damage results in cleavage within the epidermis or between the epidermis and the dermis.

- Blistering or bulla formation is a skin response to insult, injury, or inflammation.
- Due to splitting in the skin by congenital, physical, infectious, inflammatory or immunological processes.

CONGENITAL/INHERITED CAUSES OF BLISTERING

Blistering due to congenital disease usually presents very early in life. However, it should be noted that the rare event of blistering presenting in a neonate may be due to pathological processes other than truly congenital or inherited diseases — especially infections with staphylococci and viruses. These will be considered briefly here, but discussed more fully in Chapter 3.

Some inherited causes of blistering do not result in any clinical problem until much later in life.

The causes of blistering		
Congenital/inherited	Epidermolysis bullosa	Simplex, Junctional, Dystrophic
	Incontinentia pigmenti* Porphyria cutanea tarda (some)† Benign familial pemphigus (Hailey–Hailey disease)	
Acquired	Physical injury	Thermal (burns), Chemicals, Mechanobullous/ friction, Radiation-induced (including Ultraviolet radiation)
	Infections	Staphylococci‡, Viruses, e.g. herpes‡, Fungal infections‡
	Secondary to inflammation	Eczema/dermatitis (including pompholyx)§, Lichen planus§, Insect-bite reactions‡, Bullous erythema multiforme§, Toxic epidermal necrolysis, Pityriasis lichenoides et varioliformis acuta§, Drug Reactions†
	Immuno-bullous	Bullous pemphigoid, Cicatricial pemphigoid, Herpes (pemphigoid) gestationis, Pemphigus, Dermatitis herpetiformis, Linear IgA disease and Chronic bullous disease of childhood, Epidermolysis bullosa acquisita, Bullous SLE, Lichen planus pemphigoides
	Metabolic, miscellaneous/unknown	Porphyria cutanea tarda (most)†, Diabetes mellitus, Renal failure, Subcorneal pustular dermatosis

see also Chapter 11   †*see also* Chapter 8   ‡*see also* Chapter 3   §*see also* Chapter 5

Fig. 7.1 *The causes of blistering.*

THE EPIDERMOLYSIS BULLOSA GROUP OF DISORDERS

There are various ways of classifying EB, based on clinical appearances, the mode of inheritance, and the level at which cleavage takes place within the skin. Using the last of these, there are three main 'types':

- EB simplex — the cleavage lies within the basal cells of the epidermis.
- Junctional EB — the cleavage lies within the structures of the basement membrane.
- Dystrophic EB — the cleavage is subepidermal.

Box 7.1

Epidermolysis bullosa (EB)
Term that is used to describe a group of genetically determined conditions in which the adhesive mechanisms within the skin are defective causing cleavage with the formation of bullae.

Epidermolysis bullosa simplex

There are several different clinical patterns that share the same or similar pathological defect (**Fig. 7.2**) and are hence considered to be forms of EB simplex. Some of these are rare. Most are inherited as autosomal dominant traits. The most common and important patterns are:

Generalized EB simplex
- Tense bullae appear on areas of friction and trauma, often beginning in infancy around the napkin (diaper) area and other points where clothing rubs.
- Blisters begin to occur on the hands and feet (**Fig. 7.3a**) as the child grows and becomes more mobile, and this continues into adult life.
- Blisters heal without scarring but the intensity and severity of the blistering may be extremely incapacitating.
- Disorder is inherited in an autosomal dominant manner in most families.

EB simplex of the hands and feet (Weber–Cockayne)
- Bullae (identical to those seen in generalized EB simplex) appear exclusively on the hands and feet (**Fig. 7.3b**).
- Problem may appear in childhood, the onset is often delayed until adolescence or early adult life.
- Degree of trauma required to induce blistering is variable.
- Inheritance of this condition is also autosomal dominant.

Herpetiform EB simplex (Dowling–Meara)
- Most severe form of EB simplex but rare.
- Severity and intensity of the blistering is such that the clinical picture may closely resemble junctional or dystrophic EB.
- Bullae are much more extensive than in other forms of EB simplex and may involve the mouth and other 'mucous membranes'.
- Condition usually subsides after a year or so, but blistering on the hands and feet continues, together with intermittent crops of 'herpetiform' blisters on the trunk and limbs.

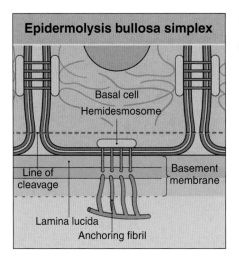

Epidermolysis bullosa simplex

Basal cell
Hemidesmosome
Line of cleavage
Basement membrane
Lamina lucida
Anchoring fibril

Fig. 7.2 *Epidermolysis bullosa simplex.* *The line of cleavage is intraepidermal, through the base of the basal cell.*

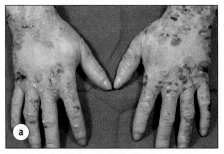
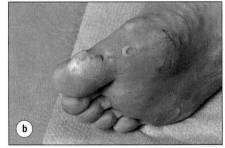

Fig. 7.3 *Epidermolysis bullosa simplex* — *(a)* blistering on the hands; *(b)* blistering on the feet in the Weber-Cockayne type.

Junctional epidermolysis bullosa

The term junctional EB is applied to a group of very rare inherited blistering disorders in which the line of cleavage is within the lamina lucida of the basement membrane zone (**Fig. 7.4**). They are all also characterized by an autosomal recessive mode of inheritance. Mutations in the genes encoding Laminin 5, BP180 (type XVII collagen) and alpha 6 beta 4 integrins have been reported.

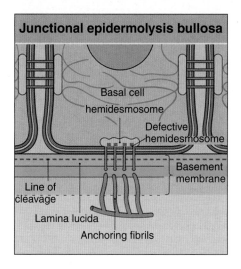

Fig. 7.4 *Junctional epidermolysis bullosa.* *The hemidesmosomes are hypoplastic and the line of cleavage is through the lamina lucida of the basement membrane.*

- Blistering usually appears early in the neonatal period, may be very widespread, and may involve the mouth and pharynx.
- Areas become eroded and heal slowly, if at all.
- Child often becomes extremely unwell because of the loss of skin integrity; some children die in this neonatal phase; the diagnostic label EB letalis (Herlitz) is often applied here.
- Other children survive with appropriate support and intensive care, but continue to develop blisters and erosions: some authorities recognize this as the 'mitis' form of junctional EB.
- Children are sickly and anaemic, and may die at any time from sepsis.
- There are also other, still rarer, subtypes of junctional EB in which lesions may be localized to the extremities or to the flexures.

Dystrophic epidermolysis bullosa

In the dystrophic type of EB, the cleavage is subepidermal (**Figs 7.5 and 7.6**), due to loss of anchoring fibrils. It is caused by mutations in the gene coding for type VII collagen (COL7A1). This may be the result of excessive collagenase activity. The healing phase is characterized by scarring and milia formation. There are two important presentations, one due to a recessive gene, the other being inherited as an autosomal dominant disorder.
Autosomal recessive dystrophic epidermolysis bullosa — Autosomal recessive dystrophic EB, without doubt, can be one of the nastiest skin diseases of all. Patients with recessive dystrophic EB have a miserable existence, in and out of hospital, requiring constant attention to dressings and their general health and nutrition.

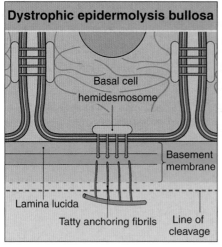

Dystrophic epidermolysis bullosa

Basal cell
hemidesmosome
Basement membrane
Lamina lucida
Tatty anchoring fibrils
Line of cleavage

Fig. 7.5 *Dystrophic epidermolysis bullosa.* *The anchoring fibrils are largely missing and the line of cleavage is through the upper dermis.*

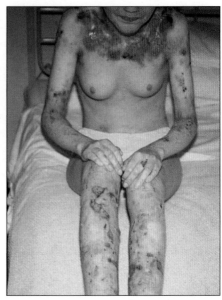

Fig. 7.6 *Autosomal recessive dystrophic epidermolysis bullosa.* *Severe blistering with scarring continues throughout life.*

- Blistering develops soon after birth and is initiated by friction or trauma, but may also appear spontaneously.
- Areas often become secondarily infected and heal to leave atrophic scars in a process that continues throughout life (**Fig. 7.6**).
- More severely affected patients develop 'psuedo-webbing' of the fingers and toes and scarring of the mouth and oropharynx, leading to difficulty with eating and swallowing.
- Ocular scarring may result in blindness.
- Nails are lost and dentition abnormal.
- Degree of scarring is not as marked in other, less severely affected patients, but the chronic blistering continues.
- Squamous cell carcinomas may develop in atrophic areas.

Autosomal dominant dystrophic epidermolysis bullosa — Autosomal dominant dystrophic EB is a less serious problem, but can still result in significant disability. Small blisters develop, particularly on the limbs and at sites of trauma. These heal to leave scars and milia (**Fig. 7.7**) that may occasionally be very marked. The blistering tendency continues throughout life.

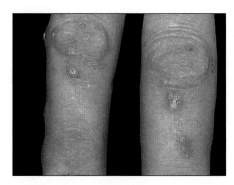

Fig. 7.7 *Autosomal dominant EB.*
Blistering leads to scarring and milia
formation.

Investigation and treatment of epidermolysis bullosa

Although EB may present fairly late, this is a feature of the milder forms and the accurate diagnosis of these disorders is most critical in a neonate with extensive blistering. The same diagnostic principles apply whatever the age of onset. Once other causes of blistering have been considered and excluded as necessary (especially staphylococcal or herpetic infection, or incontinentia pigmenti — *see* Chapter 11), the most important information is obtained from a biopsy for electron microscopy. This will demonstrate the level at which the split is occurring and, therefore, place the process within one of the three categories described above. More recent work has focused on the use of antibodies to various components of the basement membrane zone, and these, or modifications of them, may form the investigations of choice in due course.

The treatment of EB is not easy. There are four areas that need special mention:

- General measures — good nursing care is required in all types of EB, but is absolutely fundamental for the most severely affected patients.
- Specific measures — sadly, there are few.
- Counselling and information.
- Genetic advice.

General and specific measures — The application of simple measures can significantly improve the situation in all forms of the EB simplex group. In EB simplex, the blistering generally heals without scarring, and the main thrust of treatment is to prevent secondary infection and wait for each area to heal, as it will in time. The use of astringent solutions such as potassium permanganate or Burow's solution can be helpful. The patients are often also hyperhidrotic, therefore measures to reduce sweating, especially topical aluminium chloride hexahydrate, may also be valuable.

A similar approach to the individual blisters is appropriate in autosomal dominant dystrophic EB, but in the recessive forms treatment needs to be rather more pro-active. It is essential that all areas are dressed carefully and that secondary infections are minimized. Patients are often unwell and may require attention to systemic problems, such as nutritional deficits and blood-borne infections. As the disease process advances, surgical interventions may be required to try to reduce the damage that will inevitably occur, especially to the hands and feet. Some authorities recommend the addition of drugs that inhibit collagenase, notably phenytoin, but there is no very good evidence of benefit.

Patients with junctional EB need a high level of nursing care and anti-infective measures. There are no known specific treatments available.

Counselling and information — Probably the most important aspect of managing EB is the need to provide information and support to the patients and their families throughout what is often a most distressing time. It is, of course, essential that an accurate diagnosis is made as soon as possible because this will enable at least some form of prognosis to be offered. In the dominant forms, the family will often already have some experience of the condition; however, for the severe recessive forms, this is often not the case (unless there is a previously affected sibling).

Genetic advice — Families will often wish to discuss particularly the genetic aspects of the problem and the implications for their child and for any future children. In this, the assistance of a trained clinical geneticist is invaluable. Prenatal diagnosis is now available using tissue obtained through a fetal biopsy.

- Epidermolysis bullosa (EB) is used to describe genetically determined skin conditions characterized by defective adhesive mechanisms.
- EB simplex shows cleavage within the basal cells of the epidermis and presents with several clinical variants; inheritance is autosomal dominant.
- Junctional EB represents a rare group of inherited blistering disorders with line of cleavage within the lamina lucida of the basement membrane; presents in neonatal period with serious, extensive blistering.
- Dystrophic EB shows subepidermal cleavage with the healing phase characterized by scarring and milia formation.
- Electron microscopy can determine level of split and treatment approach.

BENIGN FAMILIAL PEMPHIGUS (HAILEY–HAILEY DISEASE)

Box 7.2

Benign familial pemphigus
Rare genodermatosis characterized by recurrent blistering and erosions, particularly of flexural areas but also on other parts of the body.

Benign familial pemphigus (**Fig. 7.8**) is inherited as an autosomal dominant condition and is due to mutations in the ATP2C1 gene, which encodes for the calcium transporting ATPase type 2c. This is a magnesium-dependent membrane integrated enzyme which catalyses the hydrolysis of ATP coupled with the transfer of Ca ions.

Histologically, the changes are virtually indistinguishable from pemphigus vulgaris (*see* below), with a suprabasal split within the epidermis and marked loss of adhesion of epidermal cells (acantholysis).

Treatment is difficult. The use of steroid–antiseptic combinations may help and there are reports of improvement following ablation by surgery, lasers, or low-dose superficial X-rays.

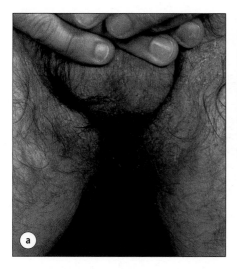

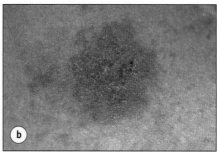

Fig. 7.8 *Hailey–Hailey disease* — *(a) erosions, inflammation and maceration in the groins are a common feature; similar changes are often seen in the axillae; (b) blistering may also occur elsewhere.*

OTHER CONGENITAL/INHERITED CAUSES OF BLISTERING

- Porphyria cutanea tarda — there have been a few families recorded in whom the biochemical and clinical changes of porphyria cutanea tarda appear much earlier in life than usual (see Chapter 8).
- Incontinentia pigmenti — a rare, X-linked dominant disorder that is characterized by a period, usually shortly after birth, when the skin produces crops of vesicles and bullae (see Chapter 11).

ACQUIRED CAUSES OF BLISTERING

PHYSICAL CAUSES

The skin may respond to a number of insults by blistering. Among the most commonly encountered are:

- Thermal injuries — contact with heat or cold beyond 'normal' temperature differentials and for long enough causes the skin to blister. This is due to death of the epidermal keratinocytes. The management of severe burns is beyond the scope of this book, but extensive skin loss from thermal burns is potentially fatal.
- Chemicals — many chemicals, such as acids, alkalis, and petrochemicals, are highly injurious to the skin and may, on contact, cause acute blistering. Occasionally, this may result in widespread skin loss (see toxic epidermal necrolysis below).
- Mechanobullous/friction — the degree of injury required to induce blistering is quite variable, with some people seeming to be much more prone than others. The mechanisms involved are similar to those seen in EB simplex (see page 265). Blisters generally appear at sites of obvious trauma or friction, including the mouth; oral blisters are relatively common and may be haemorrhagic.
- Radiation-induced — by far the most common, harmful ionizing radiation that causes blistering in human (and animal) skin is ultraviolet light. Many of us will have experienced the results of excessive sun exposure; blistering is but an extreme

reaction to such exposure and is caused by inflammatory oedema and cell death in the epidermis.

INFECTIONS

Blistering is a common feature of several important skin infections (for a fuller account, *see* Chapter 3):

- Staphylococcal infection — superficial infection of the skin by *S. aureus* classically causes fragile blisters that progress to honey-coloured crusts. The split is in the subcorneal region of the epidermis. When this occurs in neonates, the term pemphigus neonatorum is classically used (a good example of the clinical basis of the diagnostic terminology in use in dermatology). True pemphigus is, of course, an entirely different pathological process, but the clinical features may be very similar (see page 278).
- Viral infection — blistering is a feature of a number of cutaneous viral infections: for example, herpes simplex, herpes varicella-zoster, vaccinia, smallpox (now 'extinct'), and hand-foot-and-mouth disease. In most instances, the blistering is due to virus-induced cell destruction within the epidermis.
- Fungal infection — as discussed in Chapter 3, blistering is common in tinea pedis. Rarely, too, an allergic or 'side' reaction to fungal infection may cause pompholyx on uninfected hands.

BLISTERING SECONDARY TO CUTANEOUS INFLAMMATION

If cutaneous inflammation is sufficiently intense, blistering may occur irrespective of the primary cause. This is most common in the eczema/dermatitis group, especially on the hands and feet. Some people are prone to develop large, tense blisters at the site of insect-bite reactions. The primary aetiology may not always be obvious on first presentation if the urticarial wheal and evidence of a punctum are obscured by the blister.

Special mention must also be made here of four other important causes in this category:

- Bullous erythema multiforme — the inflammation in erythema multiforme may become so intense that epidermal death may occur. If this happens, the centre of the classical 'target' lesion may be bullous (**Fig. 7.9a**). Involvement of the eyes (**Fig. 7.9b**), mouth (**Fig. 7.9c**), genitourinary tract (**Fig. 7.9d and e**), and bronchial tree may also occur — the Stevens–Johnson syndrome — and the patient may be extremely unwell. The pulmonary involvement or secondary renal failure may be fatal.
- Toxic epidermal necrolysis (TEN) — full-thickness damage to the epidermis may result in sheets of skin separating and leaving raw, oozing dermis. Such a picture may be due to contact with chemicals and drug reactions (see Chapter 8) and may also occur in the Stevens–Johnson syndrome and in severe graft-versus-host disease. The clinical picture may closely resemble staphylococcal scalded-skin syndrome (see Chapter 3), but the level of split is deeper in true TEN, and Staphylococci are not responsible.
- Pityriasis lichenoides — as mentioned in Chapter 5, pityriasis lichenoides et varioliformis acuta may occasionally present with vesiculobullous lesions, which heal to leave pock-like scars.
- Bullous drug reactions — bullae may occur as a consequence of several types of drug reaction. Some are of a 'general' kind: severe, acute eczematous reactions; fixed drug eruptions (**Fig. 7.10**); drug-induced immunobullous disease. Some are more specific to a particular agent: photo-induced blistering of the legs with nalidixic acid; barbiturate-induced or coma-related bullae.

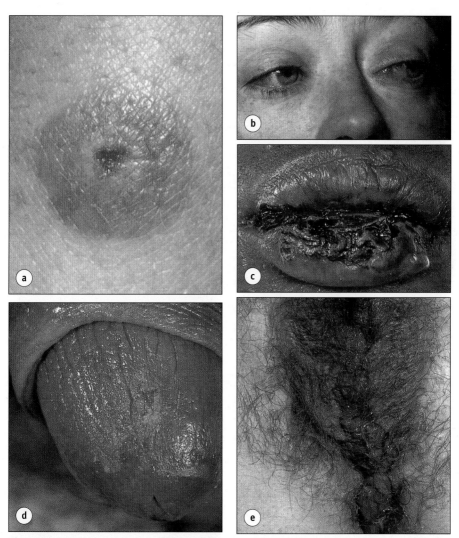

Fig. 7.9 Bullous erythema multiforme (Stevens–Johnson syndrome) — *blisters arise on the surface of the target lesions (a) inflammation and erosions may occur in the conjunctivae (b) in the mouth (c) in the genitalia (d and e) and elsewhere.*

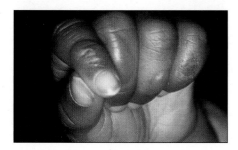

Fig. 7.10 Bulla due to a fixed drug eruption (in this case, carbamazepine was the offending agent, but several drugs may have the same effect).

THE IMMUNOBULLOUS DISORDERS

Immunological reactions of various kinds are a very important cause of blistering. The resulting clinical disorders are all relatively uncommon (apart, perhaps, from bullous pemphigoid), but they require careful assessment and investigation. They also provide some difficult therapeutic challenges.

PEMPHIGOID

Bullous pemphigoid

Box 7.3

Bullous pemphigoid
Most common of the immunobullous disorders due to a subepidermal split, induced by the presence of an antibody directed against part of the basement membrane complex (probably in the hemidesmosomes).

The disorder is usually seen in patients over the age of 65 years, but may occur in younger individuals. Most of the classical clinical appearances are illustrated in **Figure 7.11**. Notable features are:

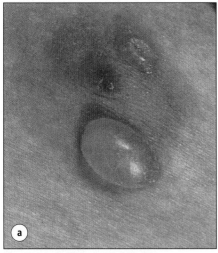

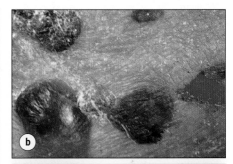

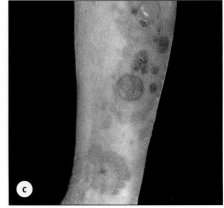

Fig. 7.11 *Bullous pemphigoid —*
(a) tense blisters on an erythematous background; (b) the bullae may be haemorrhagic; (c) the limbs are sites of predilection.

- Irritation.
- 'Background' erythematous eruption with an urticarial or eczematous appearance.
- Tense blisters that may be haemorrhagic.
- Predilection for the arms and legs.
- Oral involvement may occur, but is relatively uncommon.
- Nikolsky sign is negative.

Rarely, bullous pemphigoid may be localized to a single area for long periods of time. There are also reports of the immunological findings associated with bullous pemphigoid in patients with nodular prurigo and a pompholyx-like eruption of the hands and feet. *Investigation and treatment* — The essential investigations in bullous pemphigoid are histology and direct immunofluorescence. A skin biopsy for histology should be taken from the edge of a new blister. This will reveal a subepidermal split, with an inflammatory infiltrate often containing eosinophils. Occasionally, eosinophilic spongiosis is seen. If an older blister is biopsied, the process of re-epithelialization may begin along the floor of the blister. This can, on superficial inspection, cause difficulty in distinguishing the lesion from pemphigus. However, acantholysis does not occur in bullous pemphgoid. Direct immunofluorescence is best performed on skin adjacent to the blister, or on the erythematous background rash. There is a linear band of immunoglobulin (almost always IgG) and C3 at the basement membrane. Indirect immunofluorescence is positive for the same finding in about 70% of patients. Split skin immunofluoresecence increases the yield (to about 80%).

The treatment of bullous pemphigoid is similar to that for pemphigus except that it is seldom necessary to use such high doses of steroids. A common combination is prednisolone and azathioprine, with which many patients can be controlled on very small doses. As affected patients are often very old, and therefore at risk of diabetes, osteoporosis, and other complications, this is clearly an advantage. Many patients' disease 'burns out' after a year or so.

- Bullous pemphigoid is a common immunobullous disorder due to subepidermal split.
- Presents mainly in patients over age 65 but may occur in younger individuals.
- Tense blisters that may be haemorrhagic against 'background' erythematous eruption.
- Treatment with low-dose steroids often effective.

Cicatricial ('benign' mucous membrane) pemphigoid

The term cicatricial is used to describe a form of subepidermal immunobullous disease in which there is a marked tendency for the lesions to heal leaving scarring (it is not in the least 'benign' and we prefer the first name above, to that in parentheses). This is much rarer than bullous pemphigoid. It is characterized by identical tense blisters, although the erythema in the background is generally less pronounced. There is also prominent involvement of the mouth, genital epithelium, and conjunctivae. The lesions heal to leave

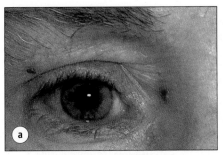

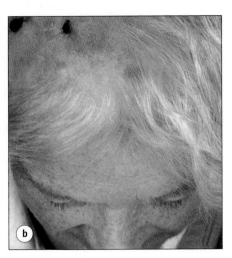

Fig. 7.12 *Cicatricial pemphigoid —*
(a) conjunctival involvement has led to fusion of the eyelids (symblepharon); (b) cicatricial alopecia in the Brunsting–Perry form of the disease.

atrophic areas and, sometimes, milia. In the conjunctival sac, this can cause severe damage (**Fig. 7.12a**). In one form of the disease (eponymously named Brunsting–Perry), the scalp is involved, leading to a cicatricial alopecia (**Fig. 7.12b**).

The histology and the findings on direct immunofluorescence are identical to those seen in bullous pemphigoid. Indirect immunofluorescence may be negative or show a similar pattern to bullous pemphigoid. Immunoblotting may reveal binding to Laminin 5 (epiligrin) or beta 4 integrin.

Treatment is difficult. Patients are much less responsive to steroids and immunosuppressive agents than 'ordinary' bullous pemphigoid, and the disease may pursue a relentlessly destructive course. Dapsone, tetracyclines and nicotinamide may be helpful, and cyclophosphamide is worth considering in resistant cases. Ophthalmological advice may be valuable in reducing damage to the conjunctival sac.

Herpes (pemphigoid) gestationis
A bullous eruption with histological findings identical to those seen in bullous pemphigoid occasionally accompanies pregnancy. It, too, appears to be mediated by an igg class of antibody directed against elements of the basement membrane zone. In contrast to the other pregnancy-related dermatoses (*see* Chapter 8), it occurs in only a tiny minority of patients.

DERMATITIS HERPETIFORMIS
Another rare dermatosis in which bullae are an important feature is dermatitis herpetiformis (DH). However, the most characteristic presenting feature of this disease is irritation. Patients describe the occurrence of waves of severe itching on the sites of predilection: the elbows and forearms (**Fig. 7.13a**), knees and shins (**Fig. 7.13b**), buttocks (**Fig. 7.13c**), shoulders, and scalp. Inspection of the affected areas often reveals a rather non-specific papular and excoriated eruption, but small vesicles do occur (*see* **Fig. 7.13a**), which patients will usually have noticed if questioned directly.

The disease is notable for one important association: gluten sensitivity. Most patients have some demonstrable abnormality of the gut. In some this is mild and consists of an increase in the jejunal intraepithelial lymphocyte count. In others it is more marked, with partial villous atrophy. In a few, a full-blown symptomatic or asymptomatic coeliac disease is present.

276

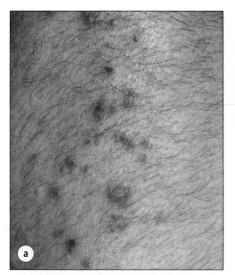

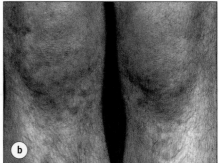

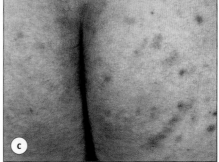

Fig. 7.13 *Dermatitis herpetiformis* —
(a) typical excoriated papules on the extensor surface of the forearm — a few early vesicles can be seen among the lesions; (b) on the knees and shins; (c) on the buttocks.

Histology of the skin shows a polymorphonuclear infiltrate in the papillary tips (microabscesses) in the very earliest papular lesions, and a subepidermal bulla in later lesions. Direct immunofluorescence of normal (not perilesional) skin reveals granular deposits of IgA in the dermal papillary tips. There is no circulating antibody present.
Investigation and treatment — Biopsies should be taken from:
- A very early lesion — to show papillary tip microabscesses.
- Normal skin — for direct immunofluorescence.
- Jejunum.

The disease responds almost immediately to dapsone in a dose of 100 mg daily or less. Itching vanishes and lesions cease forming in most patients. The condition may also be controlled by strict observance of a gluten-free diet alone. Such a diet is certainly recommended, especially for younger patients, not only because it may achieve control but also because there is an increased rate of intestinal lymphoma in DH patients and this might help to prevent this complication.

LINEAR IgA DISEASE AND CHRONIC BULLOUS DERMATOSIS OF CHILDHOOD
Linear IgA disease (predominantly a disorder of adults) and chronic bullous dermatosis of childhood are considered by some to be one and the same disorder, but having two distinct age peaks. Others feel that they should be classified separately, particularly as the childhood version appears to be self-limiting in the majority of cases.

Linear IgA disease
So-called linear IgA disease was at one time confused with DH in the classification of bullous disease; however, it is now apparent that linear IgA disease is a separate disorder in

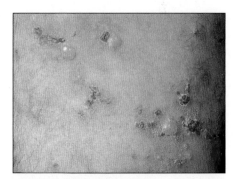

Fig. 7.14 *Linear IgA disease* — *tense blisters.*

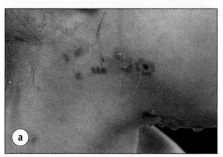

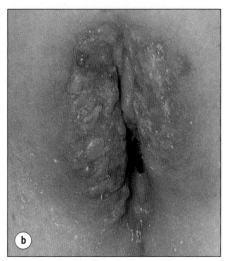

Fig. 7.15 *Chronic bullous dermatosis of childhood* — *(a) tense blisters around the neck in a young child; (b) vulval involvement.*

which subepidermal blistering occurs accompanied by a linear basement membrane band of IgA (**Fig. 7.14**). The clinical appearances may resemble those of DH or bullous pemphigoid. The disease is not associated with gluten-sensitive enteropathy (unlike DH, but like bullous pemphigoid), but responds to sulphones (like DH) better than to corticosteroids (unlike pemphigoid).

Chronic bullous dermatosis of childhood

Identical findings to those found in linear IgA disease in adults are also seen in children.

Clinically, the childhood form of the disease is characterized by tense blisters, often in a rather centripetal distribution (**Fig. 7.15a**). Involvement of the genital region is very common (**Fig. 7.15b**). The disease generally responds well to sulphones and is not associated with coeliac abnormalities of the gut.

PEMPHIGUS

In pemphigus the epidermis contains an antibody directed against the intracellular proteins. This antibody (which is also complement-fixing) leads to the breakdown of epidermal cell adhesion, a change known as acantholysis.

The pemphigus diseases appear to have an immunogenetic component, at least in some patients, but they may also be induced by drugs (e.g. penicillamine, rifampicin).

> **Box 7.4**
>
> **Pemphigus**
> Uncommon though severe acquired bullous disorder, the main feature of which is an immunologically mediated dissolution of the adhesion of the intracellular cement of the epidermal keratinocytes.

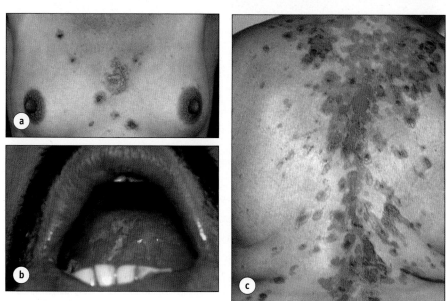

Fig. 7.16 *Pemphigus vulgaris — (a) flaccid blisters and erosions surrounded by new blisters are seen on the chest of this young woman; (b) the mouth is often involved, with severe erosions and inflammation; (c) blisters and erosions may become very extensive.*

The subclassification of the pemphigus group of disorders depends largely on the level at which the split occurs, and on accompanying clinical features.

Pemphigus vulgaris

In pemphigus vulgaris, the split occurs immediately above the basal layer (suprabasal). The skin lesions begin as small, flaccid blisters, but usually break down to become erosions (**Fig. 7.16a**). These areas are extremely slow to heal spontaneously and, indeed, often extend rapidly to cover large areas (**Fig. 7.16b**). If the edge of the erosions is pressed gently or picked up in a pair of tweezers, the epidermis can easily be slid or stripped away from the lesion — a clinical sign of great importance known as the Nikolsky sign. This is only seen in pemphigus, staphylococcal infections, and toxic epidermal necrolysis. The mouth (**Fig. 7.16c**) and other mucosal surfaces are commonly involved early in the disease.

Unless these changes are halted by treatment, the patient gradually becomes more and more unwell, with a greatly increased loss of fluid and protein from the skin surface and a tendency to develop secondary infections.

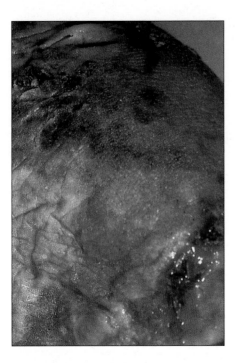

Fig. 7.17 *Pemphigus vegetans.* There is thickening and vegetation at the edge of the erosions on this patient's inner thigh.

Pemphigus vulgaris is more common in some ethnic groups — Ashkenazy Jews and Indians.

Pemphigus vegetans

'Pemphigus vegetans' is used to describe the appearances that can develop as a consequence of the same level of epidermal split as that seen in pemphigus vulgaris, but in which there is a marked tendency for the skin to produce epidermal hyperplasia and 'vegetations' as a response to the immune damage. The thickening begins at the edge of the eroded areas (**Fig. 7.17**), but, later in the course of the disease, there may be little or no obvious blistering or erosion.

Pemphigus foliaceus

In pemphigus foliaceus, the epidermal split is higher in the epidermis — within the granular layer, or even subcorneal. The roof of the lesions is, accordingly, even more fragile than in pemphigus vulgaris, and true blisters may never be seen (**Fig. 7.18**). The Nikolsky sign may be positive, and very severe erosions, similar to those seen in pemphigus vulgaris, may occur.

A form of pemphigus foliaceus, known as fogo selvagem, is endemic in parts of Brazil.

Pemphigus erythematosus

The term pemphigus erythematosus is applied when a patient has the clinical and histological features of pemphigus foliaceus with a tendency for lesions resembling lupus erythematosus (LE) to appear on the face; serological evidence of LE is also present. This situation may represent the concurrence of the two conditions.

Investigation and treatment of pemphigus — The processes involved in establishing the diagnosis in the various types of pemphigus are essentially the same, regardless of the clinical variant, and include the following elements:
- A biopsy for histopathology — best taken from the edge of a fresh lesion.

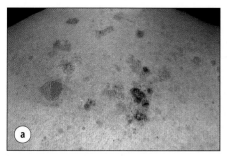

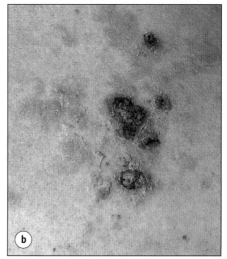

Fig. 7.18 *Pemphigus foliaceus —
(a) there is one eroded area present, but
many of the lesions are very non-specific,
crusted lesions; (b) lesions are seen here
more clearly in close-up.*

- A sample of skin for immunofluorescence — this may be cut from the piece obtained for histopathology, as long as enough is removed for proper interpretation.
- A serum sample for indirect immunofluorescence.
- Serology for LE, if pemphigus erythematosus is suspected.

The findings expected in the various types of pemphigus are summarized in **Figure 7.19**.

The cardinal feature of all forms of pemphigus is acantholysis. In most cases, acute inflammatory cells are present. Although these are usually predominantly neutrophil polymorphs, eosinophils may be very numerous.

The pathological findings in pemphigus				
	Vulgaris	**Vegetans**	**Foliaceus**	**Erythematosus**
Level of epidermal split	suprabasal	suprabasal	high*	high*
Acantholysis	+ve	+ve	+ve	+ve
Direct immunofluorescence	+ve	+ve	+ve	+ve
Indirect immunofluorescence	+ve†	+ve†	+ve†	+ve†
Lupus erythematosus serology	–ve	–ve	–ve	+ve

* within the granular layer or subcorneal
† the titre of indirect immunofluorescence is related, to some extent, to the severity of the disease process

Fig. 7.19 *The pathological findings in pemphigus.*

Occasionally, particularly in pemphigus foliaceus, the histological changes may be more subtle. It may be hard to spot acantholytic cells, and the appearance may be difficult to distinguish from that of simple epidermal oedema (spongiosis). Eosinophils are often present in large numbers in the presenting lesions — a situation known as eosinophilic spongiosis. Immunofluorescence is required to make the definitive diagnosis, as the histological changes can also occur in bullous pemphigoid (*see* below) and in some eczemas.

The treatment of all forms of pemphigus relies on immunosuppression. The most important single agents are systemic corticosteroids, which, particularly in pemphigus vulgaris and vegetans, often have to be given in very high doses initially. The use of additional agents, such as azathioprine, alkylating agents, gold, and ciclosporin (cyclosporin), can help to reduce the daily steroid requirement. Cyclophosphamide and intravenous immunoglobulin (IVIG) may be useful in resistant disease. A careful watch must be kept for secondary infections, which need to be treated quickly and effectively to avoid septicaemia. There is also a need for good nursing care to the cutaneous erosions and to the mouth. Fluid balance and metabolic management are also important.

In some patients, the disease appears to go into a degree of remission and may even remit completely, although usually this only occurs, if at all, after a number of years.

Pemphigus foliaceus does not always require such aggressive treatment. Some patients can be managed by a judicious mix of topical steroids and oral immunosuppressive drugs.

- Pemphigus is an acquired disorder with immunologically mediated dissolution of intracellular cement in epidermal keratinocytes.
- Pemphigus vulgaris presents with small, flaccid blisters that usually break down to become erosions.
- Diagnosis of pemphigus involves biopsy, immunofluorescence (skin sample and serum) and serology.
- Treatment of all forms of pemphigus relies on immunosuppression.

Epidermolysis bullosa acquisita (EBA)

This term is applied to a bullous disorder in which changes apparently identical to those of bullous pemphigoid can be shown to be due to a different level of split in the basement membrane zone, the details of which are summarized in **Figure 7.20**. Clinically EBA is very variable. It may resemble bullous pemphigoid or linear IgA disease, with quite large blisters, or it may be very difficult to distinguish from porphyria cutanea tarda (*see* page 283; Chapter 8). It is generally resistant to the treatments conventionally used in bullous disorders.

Bullous systemic lupus erythematosus

Although rare, bullae are a very striking feature in some patients with systemic lupus erythematosus (**Fig. 7.21**). Dapsone usually produces a dramatic resolution of the blisters.

Lichen planus pemphigoides

Lichen planus is another inflammatory disease in which blistering is a very distinctive, if rather rare, feature (*see* Fig. 5.67). It would appear that a bullous-pemphigoid-like reaction may occasionally be triggered by the immunologically driven damage seen in lichen planus.

Differentiating findings in bullous pemphigoid (BP) and epidermolysis acquisita (EBA)		
	BP	**EBA**
Direct immunofluorescence	IgG + C3 (IgA/IgM rare)	IgG (IgA/IgM more common)
Indirect immunofluorescence	IgG in 75%	IgG in 50%
NaCl split-skin immunofluorescence	Roof of split or both roof and floor of split	Floor of split
Electron microscopy	Blister within lamina lucida	Blister below the basal lamina
Antigen	Hemidesmosome	Type VII collagen and localized to anchoring fibrils

Fig. 7.20 *Differentiating findings in bullous pemphigoid (BP) and epidermolysis bullosa acquisita (EBA).*

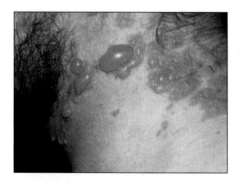

Fig. 7.21 *Bullae in a young man with SLE.*

METABOLIC, MISCELLANEOUS, AND UNKNOWN CAUSES OF BLISTERING

Porphyria cutanea tarda

In porphyria cutanea tarda, small vesicles, which heal with scarring and milia formation, are seen on exposed sites and areas subject to trauma (e.g. the knees and elbows). Hypertrichosis is also commonly seen (*see* Chapter 8). Patients have a genetic abnormality of uroporphyrinogen decarboxylase. The disease is precipitated by many different factors, in particular liver disease from alcohol abuse or hepatitis, but also from iron overload (haemochromatosis) and oestrogen therapy.

Diabetes mellitus

A small minority of patients with diabetes develop blisters of unknown aetiology.

Bullae of renal failure

Some patients on haemodialysis, or receiving high-dose furosemide (frusemide), develop large bullae of unknown cause.

Subcorneal pustular dermatosis (Sneddon–Wilkinson disease)

Sneddon–Wilkinson disease is one of the rarest dermatoses and is properly a pustular dermatosis rather than truly characterized by blisters — however, it finds a place here for convenience. The patients are usually middle-aged to elderly and often female. The lesions are flaccid pustules, often on a serpiginous erythematous background (**Fig. 7.22**). The main differential diagnoses are bullous impetigo (but the lesions are sterile) and pustular psoriasis (of which some authorities believe this to be a form). True subcorneal pustular dermatosis responds to dapsone.

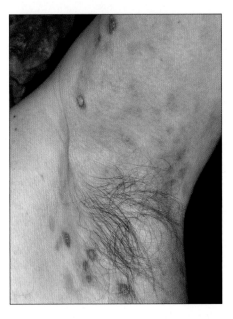

Fig. 7.22 *Subcorneal pustular dermatosis.* *There remains debate as to the proper classification of this very rare dermatosis.*

chapter 8

Systemic Disease and the Skin

INTRODUCTION

Clinical and pathological changes in the skin may be due to the skin's secondary involvement in disease processes affecting one or more other organs. There is no room in this book to discuss all such associations, nor to describe the details of the systemic disorders themselves. This chapter, however, will cover a number of conditions that the dermatologist will encounter with reasonable frequency or in which the implications of recognizing the association of cutaneous symptoms and signs with systemic diseases are especially important.

Although it may seem slightly artificial, these clinical conditions are dealt with in the following sections:

- Skin changes that are frequently signals of other organ disease and which may reflect multiple pathologies.
- Skin changes that are associated with disease in a specific organ or system.
- Skin changes that are due to a pathophysiological process: the skin signs of internal malignancy, the connective tissue diseases, some 'multisystem' disorders, pregnancy (noting that pregnancy is NOT a pathological state).
- Skin changes caused by drugs given for systemic or cutaneous disease.
- The cutaneous effects of psychological disturbances.

SKIN CHANGES ASSOCIATED WITH MULTIPLE PATHOLOGIES

Figure 8.1 gives a list of the most important skin signs in which systemic associations are particularly significant and which may involve several different organs.

Cutaneous symptoms and signs frequently associated with systemic disease
Pruritus
Erythema nodosum
Pyoderma gangrenosum
Necrotizing vasculitis
Acanthosis nigricans

Fig. 8.1 *Cutaneous symptoms and signs frequently associated with systemic disease.*

PRURITUS

Box 8.1

Pruritus
Generalized itching.

Generalized itching is a most distressing symptom. It may, of course, be caused by many skin diseases, and the discussion here is relevant only to those patients in whom the pruritus is not due to a primary skin disorder. This does not mean that skin changes are not found in such patients. Itching results in scratching, and scratching may cause significant secondary damage to the skin (**Fig. 8.2**). It is therefore very important, before proceeding to look for systemic causes for generalized itching, that a careful examination of the skin is conducted to exclude primary skin disorders in which the skin changes can be subtle, such as scabies or dermatitis herpetiformis.

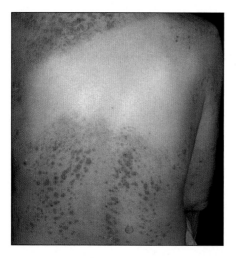

Fig 8.2 *Generalized pruritis.* *It is important to exclude a primary skin disorders. This elderly man with chronic renal failure only had skin lesions on areas that he could reach to scratch.*

Figure 8.3 lists a number of important systemic conditions in which itching may be a prominent feature.

Cholestasis is usually accompanied by some itching and may be due to bile-duct obstruction or damage, or to semi-physiological changes associated with swelling of the liver cells (e.g. in hepatitis). Some patients also develop cholestasis during pregnancy. It is important to recognize that hepatobiliary cholestasis may occur without obvious icterus, at least for a while. Patients with primary biliary cirrhosis in particular may present with

Systemic causes of pruritus
Cholestasis (including pruritus of pregnancy)
Renal failure
Iron deficiency
Polycythaemia vera (aquagenic)
Thyroid disease
Cancers (especially lymphomas)
Psychological states
Old age (senile pruritus)

Fig. 8.3 *Systemic causes of pruritis.*

itching some months or even years before jaundice appears. Cholestasis is a feature of the early, oedematous phases of hepatitis.

The itching of chronic renal failure is not related to levels of creatinine or urea and therefore persists despite dialysis.

The itching associated with iron deficiency is said to occur whether the haemoglobin is low or not, although it must be extremely uncommon not to find some alteration of routine haematology. More typically, the patient has a chronic iron-deficiency state, with a lowish haemoglobin and other indices. The patient is often a woman, and dietary factors, perhaps combined with menorrhagia, are usually relevant. The itching in polycythaemia vera is characteristically triggered by contact with water ('aquagenic').

Patients with either hyperthyroidism or hypothyroidism present with itching. The typical signs of thyroid dysfunction are usually also present, but may be subtle.

The association of itching with cancers is relatively uncommon, except in the case of Hodgkin's disease, where pruritus is important enough to be one of the symptoms that is used in classification of the disease. Cancers of the pancreas or secondaries in the porta hepatis may, of course, give rise to itching, due to cholestasis. Occasionally, however, a patient with another cancer may present with generalized pruritus.

In a number of patients, there is no demonstrable physical cause for their chronic, generalized itching. Some have features of psychological morbidity: 'stress', anxiety states, neuroses. However, attributing generalized itching to psychological factors alone is a process of exclusion and should, we believe, also involve appropriate opinions from a psychologist, or a psychiatrist, or both.

Although not strictly a 'disease', cutaneous senescence is a very important cause of generalized pruritus. The reason is unknown, but the problem is real. Some elderly people are plagued by interminable, intolerable itching. Once again, this diagnosis — labelled senile pruritus — should be made after excluding physical causes.

Investigation and treatment

Patients with pruritus must be examined carefully: for signs of primary skin disease and for evidence of systemic disorders. The appropriate blood tests should be performed for each of the major causes outlined in Figure 8.3. A chest X-ray is prudent. If nothing is found on this initial screen and the itching persists, there is a strong case for a whole-body scan to search for evidence of lymphoma.

The itching associated with iron deficiency, polycythaemia, thyroid disease, and lymphoma responds to treatment for the underlying condition. Psychologically based itching may respond to interventions directed at the root cause.

Treating the itching of chronic cholestasis is more difficult. If the underlying cause cannot be tackled effectively, resins designed to reduce the concentration of bile salts may help, and there are some patients who benefit from phototherapy. The same is true for the itch of chronic renal failure, where phototherapy has its advocates. Naltrexone may be useful in the itch of renal failure.

Patients with senile pruritus also usually continue to suffer to a greater or lesser degree, despite attempts to help. In these last three groups, the patient may have to make the best use they can of topical and systemic antipruritic agents: emollients and topical steroids; old-fashioned remedies such as menthol and calamine; mild oral sedatives (unless contraindicated by other general health factors).

- Careful examination is important to exclude primary skin disorders in generalized itching before seeking systemic causes.
- Cholestasis is usually accompanied by some itching as are iron deficiency and renal failure.
- Pruritis associated with Hodgkin's disease is important enough to be used in classification of the disease.
- Senile pruritus is characterized by interminable, intolerable itching in some elderly patients.
- Treatment for the underlying condition can stop associated itching but some patients may need topical and systemic antipruritic agents.

ERYTHEMA NODOSUM

Box 8.2

Erythema nodosum
Term applied to repeated occurrence of tender, deep-seated lumps, predominantly on the shins (**Fig. 8.4**) but occasionally elsewhere.

The lesions are red initially, and the skin over the surface is often rather shiny. Over the course of the succeeding days, the colour becomes duskier and eventually fades through the same range as might be seen in a bruise. The lesions are initially tender to contact and the legs may be generally sore.

There are a number of causes (**Fig. 8.5**), all of which need to be considered. A careful history and examination must be carried out, seeking, among other things, the symptoms of gastrointestinal disease. It is also important to perform the relevant screening investigations:

- Full haematology and biochemistry.
- Antistreptolysin-A titre.
- Chest X-ray.
- Faecal occult blood.
- Mantoux test and search for active tuberculous infection.
- Appropriate bacteriological screens.

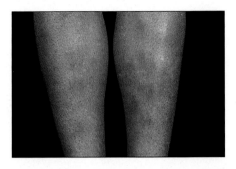

Fig. 8.4 *Typical lesions of erythema nodosum in a young woman.*

Causes of erythema nodosum

Sarcoidosis ('acute' with bilateral hilar lymphadenopathy)
Tuberculosis
Post-streptococcal infection
Inflammatory bowel disease
Infections
• histoplasmosis
• coccidioidomycosis
• yersinia
Drugs
Idiopathic

Fig. 8.5 *Causes of erythema nodosum.*

If a cause is found, appropriate treatment is necessary. If no cause is found, empirical management must follow. Bed rest with or without use of non-steroidal anti-inflammatory drugs is usually very helpful in alleviating the symptoms, and the condition usually subsides on its own in time. However, more specific drug therapy may be needed. Oral dapsone may prevent lesions developing, but the most effective drugs are oral corticosteroid

PYODERMA GANGRENOSUM

Box 8.3

Pyoderma gangrenosum
Term applied to acute painful ulcers with a purple edge that are histologically characterized by a dense neutrophilic infiltrate and ulceration.

Clinically, the lesions often begin suddenly with induration and redness (**Fig. 8.6a**). There is rapid expansion and the centre breaks down, leaving an ulcer with a purplish margin and an overhanging and undermined edge (**Fig. 8.6b**). When pyoderma gangrenosum heals (as it may, both spontaneously and with treatment), it often does so from the centre. It can be very difficult to distinguish pyoderma gangrenosum from severe infective ulceration due to synergistic bacterial gangrene (*see* Chapter 3).

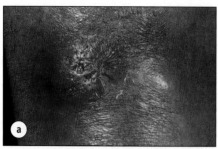 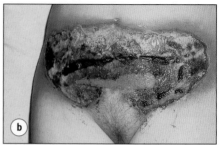

Fig. 8.6 Pyoderma gangrenosum — *(a)* *a small area of lesions — there is induration, redness, and early ulceration present; **(b)** the typically undermined, purplish edge.*

Causes of pyoderma gangrenosum
Rheumatoid arthritis Inflammatory bowel disease Paraproteinaemia Chronic active hepatitis Idiopathic

Fig. 8.7 *Causes of pyoderma gangrenosum.*

There are a number of important causes that need to be considered in any patient with this condition (**Fig. 8.7**).

Investigation and treatment

It is probably good practice to perform a skin biopsy to help confirm the diagnosis and it may be necessary to send away bacteriological samples (including biopsy material) to exclude synergistic gangrene. It is also important to perform the appropriate tests and investigations for the disorders listed in Figure 8.7 and to treat any cause so identified. However, pyoderma gangrenosum may require specific therapy in its own right. If there is any diagnostic doubt, full antibiotic cover should be instituted. Very potent topical steroids may help, particularly for small areas, but most patients need systemic treatment, for which there are a number of active drugs to choose from: minocycline, oral corticosteroids, clofazimine, and ciclosporin (cyclosporin). Each of these has a role to play in some patients because none works in everyone and some patients may not tolerate the side effects of any one agent.

VASCULITIS

Box 8.4

Vasculitis
Term applied when superficial blood vessels become inflamed and damaged, allowing red cells and other blood constituents to leak into surrounding dermis.

Cutaneous blood vessels are prominently involved in many disorders (*see* urticaria in Chapter 5, and urticarial vasculitis and erythema multiforme on page 292). When the superficial vessels are inflamed and damaged, they become leaky and allow red cells (and other blood constituents) into the surrounding dermis. This is known as vasculitis, frequently augmented by adjectives such as 'allergic' (because the cause is sometimes immunological) or 'necrotizing' (because, although there is no serious damage in mild cases, more severe inflammation generally leads to some tissue necrosis). This type of vascular inflammation is usually triggered by the presence in the circulation of immune complexes that adhere to, and damage, the vessel walls. Similar damage may occur in the renal vasculature and in other internal organs. The combined occurrence of this type of cutaneous vasculitis, joint pains, fever, abdominal discomfort, and renal damage is known as the Henoch–Schönlein syndrome. Histologically, the main inflammatory cells are polymorphonuclear neutrophils, which are often fragmented (leucocytoclasis).

Clinically, there is purpura present, predominantly on the lower legs (**Fig. 8.8a**). The purpuric areas are usually palpable, at least after a few hours have elapsed, and may blister (**Fig. 8.8b**), break down, and ulcerate as the damage progresses.

The causes associated with these changes are listed in **Figure 8.9**.

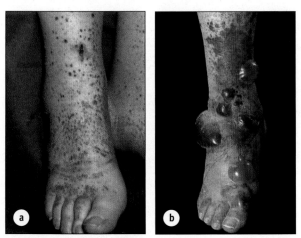

Fig. 8.8 *Vasculitis* — *(a) typical purpuric lesions; **(b)** the inflammation and damage are severe, leading to haemorrhagic blisters.*

Causes of vasculitis
Drug reactions
Infections
Autoimmune diseases
• systemic lupus erythematosus (often 'urticarial' vasculitis) rheumatoid arthritis
Paraprotein-associated
• benign
• malignant

Fig. 8.9 *Causes of vasculitis.*

Urticarial vasculititis

A particular clinical pattern is sometimes seen in which urticarial lesions last much longer than normal and fade to leave purplish staining. This is known as urticarial vasculitis and is seen in a number of systemic disorders, including systemic lupus erythematosus.

Erythema multiforme

The term erythema multiforme is given to a highly characteristic disorder in which vasculitis is a fundamental component. The lesions are round and are therefore called 'iris' or 'target' lesions (**Fig. 8.10a**). They can appear anywhere, but involvement of the extensor surfaces of the limbs, and of the palms and soles, is often prominent. If the vasculitis results in significant ischaemia, the epidermis may become separated from the underlying dermis, and bullae may form (**Fig. 8.10b**). This is known as the Stevens–Johnson syndrome (*see also* Chapter 7). As with other types of vasculitis, erythema multiforme is essentially a reaction state, and there are a very large number of well-documented causes (**Fig. 8.11**) and many other reports where the link is less clear.

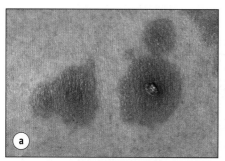

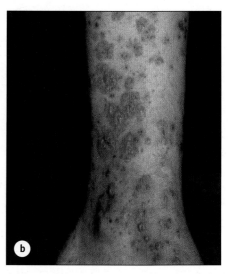

**Fig. 8.10 *Erythema mutliforme —
(a)* target/iris lesions; *(b)* multiple lesions with superficial blistering in severe disease.**

Investigation and treatment of vasculitis

When investigating vasculitis, a good history, focusing on possible drug or infective triggers, should be followed by screening for evidence of the diseases listed in Figures 8.9 and 8.11. Infection (streptococcal or viral) is the most common trigger of the Henoch–Schönlein syndrome, and herpes simplex infection is the most common trigger of erythema multiforme. It is particularly important to keep a close watch on renal function: regular urinalysis and biochemistry are mandatory while the process is active.

In leucocytoclastic vasculitis, strict bed rest is usually followed by complete clearance, but, as with erythema nodosum, the lesions often recur on remobilization. Drug treatment may be necessary and dapsone (or as an alternative, sulphone) or a systemic corticosteroid is the agent of choice. Urticarial vasculitis may be suppressed by dapsone, but systemic corticosteroids are more effective. Erythema multiforme seldom needs specific treatment because the reaction settles over 10–21 days. Occasionally, in the more severe forms with

Some important causes of erythema multiforme
Drugs   barbiturates, sulphonamides phenytoin, thiazides various NSAIDs, phenylbutazone, rifampicin, phenothiazines, sulphones
Infections   herpes simplex, orf, mycoplasma, psittacosis, AIDS, mumps, poliomyelitis, lymphogranuloma inguinale, hepatitis B, histoplasmosis
Sarcoidosis   Lupus erythematosus   Wegener's granulomatosis   Pregnancy   Radiotherapy

Fig. 8.11 *Some important causes of erythema multiforme.*

blistering, patients need extra nursing and medical support. There is controversy over the role of systemic corticosteroids.

ACANTHOSIS NIGRICANS

One of the more peculiar skin changes that the dermatologist encounters is acanthosis nigricans. Clinically, a rather velvety, brown change occurs, which may involve:

- The skin of the flexures (especially the axillae — **Fig. 8.12**).
- The sides of the neck.
- The angles of the mouth.
- The umbilicus.
- The hands ('tripe palms').

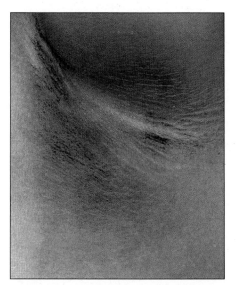

Fig. 8.12 *The velvety, brown appearance of acanthosis nigricans in the axilla.*

Mild versions (sometimes called 'pseudo-acanthosis nigricans') accompany simple obesity in individuals with dark or auburn hair, but more extreme examples are seen in association with cancers, usually of the foregut, and syndromes characterized by insulin resistance (Fig. 8.13).

Conditions associated with acanthosis nigricans	
Malignancy	Especially adenocarcinoma of the stomach
Insulin-resistance	Obesity
	Acromegaly
	With hyperandrogenism — + insulin receptor defects
	— + insulin receptor antibodies
	Lipodystrophies
	Drugs (e.g. sc-thyroxine, testosterone)

Fig. 8.13 *Conditions associated with acanthosis nigricans.*

- Erythema nodosum presents with tender, deep-seated lumps often in response to infection, drugs or internal disease.
- Pyoderma gangrenosum is characterized by indolent areas with dense neutrophilic infiltrate and ulceration associated with a variety of disorders including rheumatoid arthritis.
- Vasculitis causes damage and dermal leakage from cutaneous blood vessels, sometimes with internal organ involvement; underlying causes include drug reactions, infection and autoimmune disease.
- Acanthosis nigricans is characterized by a velvety brown colour change in skin and can be associated with GI cancers.

SKIN CHANGES ASSOCIATED WITH DISEASE IN A SPECIFIC ORGAN OR SYSTEM

Skin changes may accompany disease in almost any organ of the body. However, some associations are more common or more important, and these will be the areas of focus in this section.

VASCULAR DISORDERS

Diseases of arteries, veins, capillaries, and lymphatics may all present with skin changes. Arterial insufficiency leads to the so-called trophic changes of rather tight, shiny skin with little or no hair. The skin is generally cold, and ulceration or gangrene may supervene (Fig. 8.14). Arterial insufficiency is common in atherosclerosis, where the arteries may be narrowed generally or may become embolized from plaques on the vessel wall. Similar changes are seen in Buerger's disease and some forms of arteritis. In Raynaud's phenomenon, the digital arteries go into sudden spasms on exposure to cold. The fingers (or toes) whiten and feel stiff and numb. There are numerous causes, including many of the 'connective tissue' diseases, cryoglobulinaemia, cervical ribs, and the long-term use of vibrating machinery.

Skin signs commonly associated with vascular disease

Arterial

Insufficiency

Loss of hair, cold extremities, ulceration, gangrene

Spasm

Raynaud's phenomenon

Venous

Incompetence

Dermatoliposclerosis, pigmentation, dermatitis, atrophie blanche, varicose veins, ulceration

Lymphatic

Obstruction

Lymphoedema, Stewart–Treves lymphangiosarcoma (*see* Chapter 4), elephantiasis

Hypoplasia

Lymphoedema, recurrent cellulitis

Capillaries

Inflammation

Pigmented purpuric eruptions

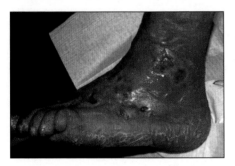

Fig. 8.14 *Multiple ulcers in a patient with arterial insufficiency due to atherosclerosis.*

Venous disease has more protean manifestations. External varicosities (either large bunches of tortuous veins or finer, 'star-burst' or 'thread' veins may be in evidence), but there may be none present. The skin gradually may become more sclerotic, around the ankles and over the lower third of the leg — a change known as dermatoliposclerosis (**Fig. 8.15a**). Pigmentation and eczema are also common and the skin is liable to ulcerate after minor trauma (**Fig. 8.15b**). Another characteristic change seen in venous disease is atrophie blanche (**Fig. 8.15c**). Once established, venous leg ulcers are very slow to heal and treatment entails rest, elevation of the leg(s), and compression bandaging.

Chronic lymphatic obstruction leads to lymphoedema, sometimes of astronomical proportion — elephantiasis, which is particularly troublesome in tropical infections with filarial parasites. Congenital hypoplasia of the lymphatics also leads to swelling of the affected limb, and recurrent streptococcal cellulitis may complicate the situation. Affected patients may have to stay on low-dose penicillin for life.

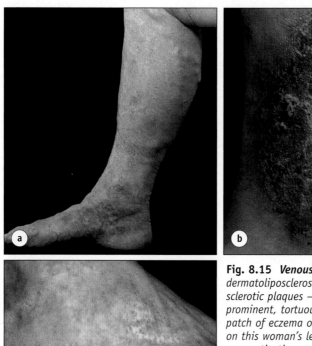

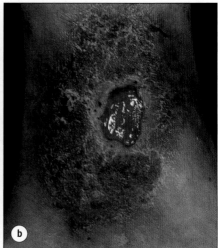

Fig. 8.15 *Venous disease — (a) early dermatoliposclerosis, showing reddened, sclerotic plaques — note also the prominent, tortuous veins and the small patch of eczema over the medial malleolus on this woman's leg; (b) pigmentation and eczematization around a typical venous leg ulcer; (c) atrophie blanche — note the ivory white areas in which dilated capillaries are visible as small pink dots.*

Inflammation of the capillaries, or capillaritis, occurs in a number of relatively uncommon conditions, some of which have extraordinary and/or eponymous names (e.g. purpura annularis telangiectoides — Majocchi's disease; pigmented purpuric lichenoid dermatosis of Gougerot and Blum). The vessels are leaky and, clinically, capillaritis leads to a characteristic combination of pigmentation and purpura. When the patch is solitary, the lesion is termed lichen aureus (**Fig. 8.16**). There are no systemic implications.

- Arterial insufficiency leads to 'trophic' skin changes that may lead to ulceration or gangrene.
- Venous disease manifestations include external varicosities, dermatoliposclerosis, ulceration and atrophie blanche.
- Lymphatic obstruction can lead to lymphoedema with complicating infections.

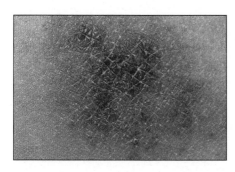

Fig. 8.16 *Capillaritis. A solitary localized patch like the one shown here is known as lichen aureus. The changes can be very widespread and may be given a number of other names.*

HEPATOBILIARY DISORDERS

The skin is an important marker of liver disease, especially chronic forms.

Skin signs commonly associated with liver disease

- Jaundice
- Pruritus
- Palmar erythema
- Spider telangiectases
- Caput medusae (umbilical varicosities)
- Hyperpigmentation
- 'Paper-money' skin
- Xanthelasmas
- Urticarial rashes
- Vasculitis
- Pyoderma gangrenosum (*see page* 289 and Fig. 8.7)
- Pale nails
- Lichen planus (?)

Jaundice, or icterus, is due to the accumulation of bilirubin in the skin and occurs in both parenchymal and obstructive liver disease. Its association with pruritus is discussed on page 286. There are a number of vascular changes associated with liver disease, of which multiple spider telangiectases (**Fig. 8.17**) and palmar erythema are the most common. Portal

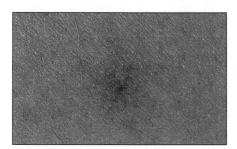

Fig. 8.17 *A typical spider telangiectasis. Small numbers of telangiectases are very common, but larger numbers (the oft-quoted figure of >6 is arbitrary and misleading) may occur in pregnancy or reflect underlying liver disease.*

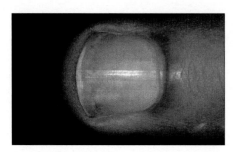

Fig. 8.18 *The pale nail of hypoalbuminaemia in a patient with severe liver disease.*

hypertension may lead to the formation of varicosities in the umbilical area (caput medusae). Pigmentation may be profound in primary biliary cirrhosis. Xanthelasmas may also be seen (*see* page 306). Various forms of vasculitis are seen in liver diseases, especially in those with an autoimmune or viral aetiology. There is some controversy about the relationship between lichen planus (LP) and the liver. Although there are several reports of LP occurring in primary biliary cirrhosis and chronic active hepatitis, there is some disagreement as to whether liver disease is significantly associated with otherwise uncomplicated LP. Recent reports have suggested that hepatitis C may be associated with LP, especially in some countries, but the precise relationship remains to be clarified.

The pale nails of hypoalbuminaemia may occur in liver as well as renal disease (**Fig. 8.18**).

RENAL DISEASE

The skin signs associated with renal disease are listed below.

Skin signs associated with renal disease

- Pruritus
- Vasculitis
- Pale nails
- Hyperpigmentation
- Keratoses and cancers (post-transplant)
- Bullae

Pruritus is probably one of the most troublesome consequences of chronic renal failure (*see* page 287). Many renal disorders are associated with vasculitis and this may be reflected in cutaneous lesions. Renal disease is a feature of many connective tissue disorders and these have cutaneous manifestations. The occurrence of pale nails (*see* Fig. 8.18) has already been mentioned. One significant recent problem has been the tendency for post-transplant patients on immunosuppressive drugs to develop keratoses and skin cancers. Patients on dialysis sometimes develop porphyria cutanea tarda and pseudoporphyria, which can be particularly difficult to treat.

GASTROINTESTINAL DISEASE

The skin signs associated with gastrointestinal disease are listed below.

Skin signs associated with gastrointestinal disease

Erythema nodosum
Crohn's disease
Pyoderma gangrenosum
Crohn's disease
Ulcerative colitis
Cutaneous infiltration
Crohn's disease
Dermatitis herpetiformis
Coeliac disease (*see* Chapter 7)
Panniculitis
Pancreatitis and carcinoma of the pancreas
Thrombophlebitis migrans
Bruising and haemorrhage (Grey–Turner's sign)

The association of inflammatory bowel disease with erythema nodosum and with pyoderma gangrenosum have been discussed earlier.

Other important cutaneous markers of gastrointestinal disease include:

- Cutaneous infiltration and sinus formation in Crohn's disease (**Fig. 8.19**) — as mentioned in Chapter 6, Crohn's disease is also very occasionally accompanied by metastatic infiltrated lesions.
- The association of dermatitis herpetiformis (*see* Chapter 7) with coeliac-type changes in the gut — this is only rarely symptomatic.
- Cutaneous signs of pancreatic disease, including thrombophlebitis, bruising, and panniculitis (**Fig. 8.20**), which may accompany either benign or malignant disease.

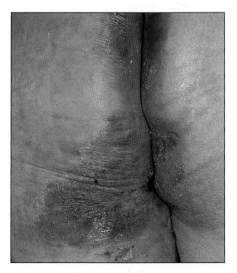

Fig. 8.19 Cutaneous signs of Crohn's disease. *Cutaneous involvement of the perineum is quite common in Crohn's disease of the lower colon and rectum.*

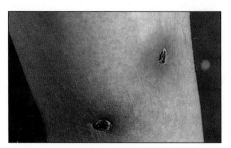

Fig. 8.20 *Cutaneous signs of pancreatic disease. Deep-seated inflammation in the fat (panniculitis) results in the formation of nodular lesions. These may form spontaneously, or may be a sign of pancreatic disease.*

ENDOCRINE DISEASE

There are numerous cutaneous markers of endocrine disease. Some of the more important are listed below.

Skin signs associated with endocrine disease

Hyperthyroidism
Pruritus, palmar erythema, telangiectasia, pretibial myxoedema (*see* Chapter 6), onycholysis (Baker's nails), hair loss (*see* Chapter 9), excessive sweating

Hypothyroidism
Pruritus, dryness, loss of outer third of eyebrows, yellow skin (carotenaemia)

Hyperadrenalism
Striae, hirsuties

Hypoadrenalism
Hyperpigmentation

Acromegaly
Thickened acral skin, acanthosis nigricans

Ovarian
Acne, hirsuties, acanthosis nigricans

Pituitary deficiency
Fine hair

Carcinoid syndrome
Cutaneous telangiectases

Thyroid disease may present with itching or other cutaneous signs, most of which are covered elsewhere in this book. Loss of the outer third of the eyebrows is characteristic of myxoedema, as is the faint yellowish tinge of carotenaemia.

Patients with hyperadrenalism (either primary or secondary) often develop secondary acne, hirsuties, and striae. Hypoadrenalism (Addison's disease) characteristically results in hyperpigmentation — especially of the gums (**Fig. 8.21**), skin creases, and scratch marks.

Patients with acromegaly have thickened skin and may develop acanthosis nigricans. Those with polycystic ovarian disease may be hirsute, and may develop acne and, rarely, acanthosis nigricans; such patients may be extremely resistant to insulin and have a defect of the insulin receptor (*see* acanthosis nigricans).

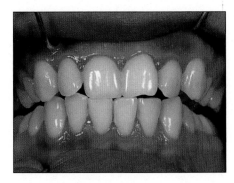

Fig. 8.21 *Hyperpigmentation of the gums in a young Asian woman with Addison's disease.*

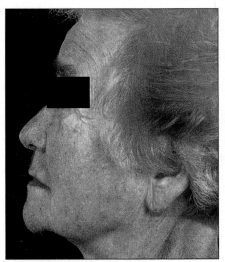

Fig. 8.22 Carcinoid syndrome. *This woman presented with flushing, ascites, and tricuspid regurgitation.*

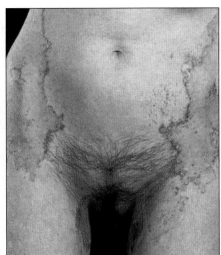

8.23 *Necrolytic migratory erythema.*

Patients with carcinoid syndrome develop flushing attacks and persistent, widespread telangiectases (**Fig. 8.22**). A very striking eruption known as necrolytic migratory erythema is a characteristic sign of a glucagonoma (**Fig. 8.23**).

HAEMATOLOGICAL DISEASE

There are an enormous number of ways in which haematological disease may manifest itself in cutaneous symptoms and signs.

301

Skin signs associated with haematological disease

Red cell

Iron deficiency (+/– anaemia)
Koilonychia (*see* Chapter 9), hair loss (*see* Chapter 9), pruritus

Pernicious anaemia
Yellow skin (carotenaemia), premature grey hair

Polycythaemia vera
Aquagenic pruritus, brick-red colour, erythromelalgia

Haemolysis
Jaundice

Haemoglobinopathies
Leg ulcers

White cell
Leukaemias
Purpura and ecchymoses, infiltration, Sweet's syndrome

Plasma cell
Lymphomas
Infiltration, vasculitis, erythroderma, pruritus

Myeloma and gammopathy
Pyoderma gangrenosum, vasculitis, Sweet's syndrome, amyloidosis

Platelet
Thrombocytopenia
Purpura and ecchymoses

Thrombocythaemia
Infarcts/thromboses, erythromelalgia

Pruritus has been mentioned on page 286. Erythromelalgia is the name given to the occurrence of spasmodic reddening, swelling, and pain, particularly of the feet. It is usually a sporadic, spontaneous phenomenon, but may be associated with polycythaemia vera (**Fig. 8.24**) or thrombocythaemia. Leg ulcers are quite common in sickle cell disease and

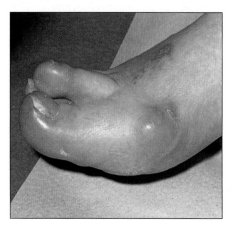

Fig. 8.24 *Erythromelalgia in a woman with polycythaemia vera.*

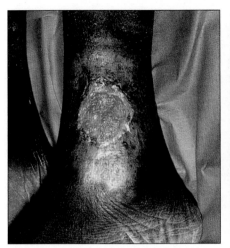

Fig. 8.25 *Chronic leg ulceration in a Nigerian girl with sickle cell disease.*

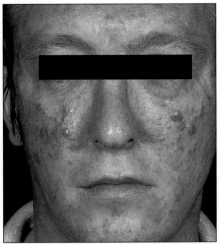

Fig. 8.26 *Infiltration of the skin by a B-cell lymphoma.*

thalassaemia (**Fig. 8.25**). The skin is quite frequently infiltrated by leukaemias or lymphomas, and the resulting eruptions may be very striking (**Fig. 8.26**). Two other associated cutaneous disorders deserve special mention: primary (myeloma-associated) amyloidosis and Sweet's syndrome.

Primary (myeloma-associated) amyloidosis

The accumulation of immunoglobulin-derived light chains in the skin as a consequence of plasma cell malignancy is very rare, but leads to a highly characteristic eruption. The lesions are yellowish, waxy, and purpuric (**Fig. 8.27a**). The tongue is often infiltrated (**Fig. 8.27b**), as are other organs. Histology reveals amyloid deposits which can be distinguished from benign amyloidosis (*see* Chapter 6) by electron microscopy.

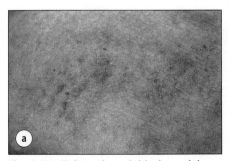
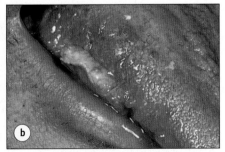

Fig. 8.27 *'Primary' amyloidosis* — *(a)* waxy, purpuric lesions; *(b)* tongue involvement.

Sweet's syndrome

Acute febrile neutrophilic dermatosis of Sweet is also uncommon. However, most dermatologists will see a case from time to time. Patients present with juicy, purplish plaques (**Fig. 8.28**). There may be a fever, although this is not a constant feature. The histological appearances are characteristic and include dense neutrophilic infiltration and eosinophilic 'flame' figures. Patients should be screened for evidence of white-cell malignancy. Treatment with oral steroids is usually effective.

- Jaundice is due to accumulation of bilirubin in skin and occurs in liver disease with associated pruritus and vascular changes including spider telangiectases and palmar erythema.
- Skin signs associated with renal disease include pruritis, vasculitis, keratoses and cancers.
- Gastrointestinal disorders with important skin manifestations include Crohn's disease, ulcerative colitis and pancreatic cancer.
- Skin changes are often associated with thyroid and adrenal disease. Cutaneous manifestations are common in haematological disease.

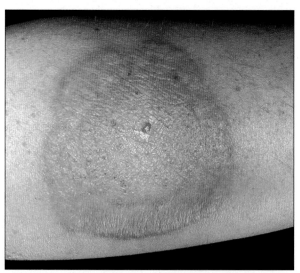

Fig. 8.28 *Painful erythematous plaque in Sweet's syndrome.*

DIABETES MELLITUS

Skin changes in diabetes are common, particularly neuropathic ulceration and the effects of secondary arterial disease.

Skin signs associated with diabetes mellitus

- Neuropathic ulcers
- Atherosclerotic arterial insufficiency
- Necrobiosis lipoidica (*see* Chapter 6)
- Granuloma annulare (*see* Chapter 6)
- Scleroedema of Buschke (*see* Chapter 6)
- Diabetic sclerosis (cheiroarthropathy)
- Bullae

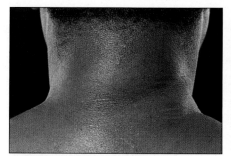

Fig. 8.29 *Scleroedema of Buschke.*
Thickening and induration over the neck and upper back in a patient with insulin-dependent diabetes.

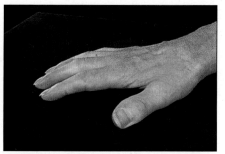

Fig. 8.30 *Diabetic sclerosis.* *This man cannot flatten his hand fully because of pseudo-sclerodermatous changes in the fingers.*

Cutaneous infections, especially folliculitis and candida, are more common in diabetics. Necrobiosis lipoidica and granuloma annulare are discussed in Chapter 6, as is scleroedema of Buschke (**Fig. 8.29**). Diabetic sclerosis or cheiroarthropathy is a term used to describe a stiffening and pseudo-sclerodermatous change of the hands and feet in patients with insulin-dependent diabetes (**Fig. 8.30**). As mentioned in Chapter 7, diabetics very occasionally develop bullae.

METABOLIC DISEASE

A number of 'metabolic diseases' present with skin manifestations.

Tophi are common in gout (**Fig. 8.31**). Fatty deposits in the skin — xanthomas (**Fig. 8.32a**) and xanthelasmas (**Fig. 8.32b**) — may reflect underlying hyperlipidaemia. Xanthelasmas in particular, however, frequently occur without any associated abnormality.

Several nutritional deficiencies of vitamins cause cutaneous changes. Notable among these are:

- Scurvy, in which gum bleeding accompanies purpuric skin changes (**Fig. 8.33**) and 'corkscrew' hairs. Scurvy is due to deficiency of vitamin C.
- Pellagra, in which a photosensitive dermatitis often accompanies diarrhoea and dementia. Pellagra is caused by nicotinic acid deficiency.

Skin signs associated with metabolic disease

Gout
Tophi
Hyperlipidaemia
Xanthomas
Xanthelasmas
Nutritional deficiency
Vitamin A
• follicular hyperkeratosis
Vitamin C
• scurvy
Nicotinic acid
• pellagra
Porphyrias
See Figure 8.34

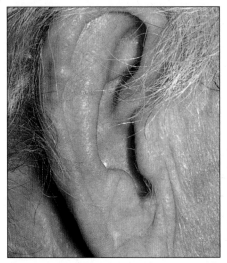

Fig. 8.31 *Tophi on the ears in a man with gout.*

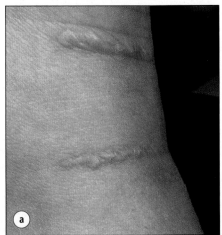

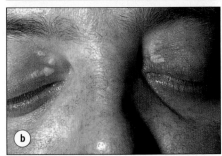

Fig. 8.32 *(a) Xanthomas in a child with familial hyperlipidaemia; (b) xanthelasmas.*

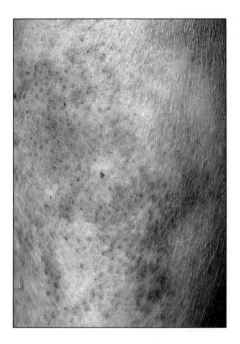

Fig. 8.33 *Purpura due to scurvy (vitamin C deficiency).*

The porphyrias

Skin changes are also seen in some of the porphyrias, a group of conditions caused by enzyme abnormalities in the metabolic pathways leading to the manufacture of haem (Fig. 8.34).

The porphyrias with cutaneous manifestations	
Disease	**Enzyme abnormality**
Erythropoietic porphyria	Uroporphyrinogen III Co-synthetase
Erythropoietic protoporphyria	Ferrochelatase
Porphyria cutanea tarda	Uroporphyrinogen decarboxylase
Variegate porphyria	Protoporphyrinogen oxidase
Hereditary coproporphyria	Coproporphyrinogen oxidase

Fig. 8.34 *The porphyrias with cutaneous manifestations.*

Erythropoietic porphyria is also known as Gunter's disease. It is very rare and is inherited as an autosomal recessive condition. Patients are severely photosensitive and develop marked scarring and hypertrichosis. They are also anaemic, due to haemolysis and hypersplenism, and generally ill. Their teeth fluoresce pink.

Erythropoietic protoporphyria (EPP) is encountered relatively frequently, at least in northern Europe and the United States. Both autosomal dominant and recessive patterns have been reported in families and there is undoubtedly a degree of heterogeneity in the clinical expression of the condition. Presentation is usually in childhood, with photosensitivity. As with other porphyrias, burning may occur indoors because window

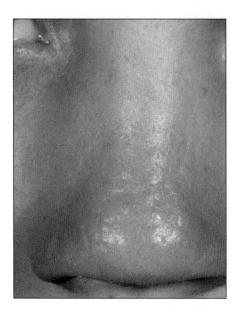

Fig. 8.35 *Waxy areas on the nose of a child with erythropoietic protoporphyria.*

glass is not protective against UVA, which is largely responsible. The skin becomes red and sore, but settles fairly quickly. Repeated episodes lead to subtle, waxy changes over exposed sites (**Fig. 8.35**). Most patients respond to some extent to β-carotene as a photoprotective agent. Liver damage has been reported, but is uncommon.

Porphyria cutanea tarda (PCT) generally presents in later life (hence, of course, 'tarda'), although families with a history of an early onset do exist. The enzyme that is deficient is manufactured in the liver and most patients have some evidence of liver disease, often alcoholic. Attacks can be precipitated by drugs — notably oestrogens, barbiturates, and ethanol. Patients present with blisters on exposed sites (**Fig. 8.36a**). Lesions heal to leave scars, milia, and hypertrichosis (**Fig. 8.36b**). Occasionally, severe sclerodermatous changes develop. Patients must avoid alcohol and other precipitating drugs. Chloroquine is effective in reducing photosensitivity and patients also respond to venesection.

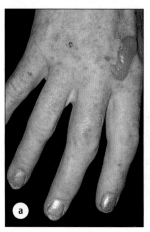
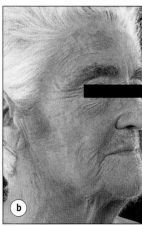

Fig. 8.36 *Porphyria cutanea tarda —*
(a) blisters and scarring on exposed sites;
(b) hypertrichosis on the face.

Variegate porphyria is very rare except in countries with a large population of Dutch extraction. The cutaneous features are similar to those of PCT, but there may also be abdominal and neurological problems similar to those seen in acute intermittent porphyria.

Hereditary coproporphyria is a rare cause of photosensitivity. The skin becomes waxy, like that in EPP. Patients also suffer bouts of jaundice and symptoms similar to those of acute intermittent porphyria.

Investigation of a patient with suspected porphyria

Blood, urine, and stools are vehicles for porphyrins, and abnormal quantities of various compounds may be found in any or all of them in the various types of porphyria. Most laboratories can screen for the presence of excess quantities — further analysis can then be undertaken as necessary. In some types of porphyria, genetic markers have also been identified.

- Skin changes in diabetes are common and include neuropathic ulceration and cutaneous infections, especially folliculitis and candida.
- Nutritional deficiencies of vitamins cause cutaneous changes, notable scurvy in vitamin C deficiency and pellagra with nicotinic acid deficiency.
- Skin changes are seen in some porphyrias with impaired manufacture of haem.

SKIN CHANGES CAUSED BY A PATHOPHYSIOLOGICAL PROCESS

This section is designed to deal with the skin signs of disorders that may involve more than one organ. We shall cover the important skin signs of internal malignancy, a group of disorders often called 'the connective tissue diseases', multisystem diseases, and pregnancy (acknowledging that pregnancy is entirely physiological).

SKIN SIGNS OF INTERNAL MALIGNANCY

The box on next page gives a list of some of the most important and best-documented skin markers of internal malignancy. The mechanisms for many of these changes are very poorly understood. Some of these signs are covered in other sections of this chapter or other chapters of the book.

Metastasis to the skin is not common, but it is important that such lesions — which are usually rather non-specific-looking nodules (**Fig. 8.37**) — are recognized for what they are. The term Sister Joseph's nodule is used to describe metastasis from an upper gastrointestinal cancer to the umbilicus. Direct extension of cancers from underlying tissues is more common, particularly on the breast (**Fig. 8.38**). Here, the change known as *peau d'orange* is due to lymphatic invasion of the dermis. An extreme form of this change resembles acute erysipelas and is known as carcinoma erysipelatoides.

Bizarre, serpiginous, and 'gyrate' erythemas — especially the classical but exceptionally rare erythema gyratum repens — are important markers of internal cancers. The patient illustrated in **Figure 8.39** had a carcinoma of the bronchus. The full-blown picture of erythema gyratum repens is said to resemble the rings or wood grains in a cut tree branch or trunk.

309

Skin signs of internal malignancy

Cutaneous metastasis

Cutaneous extension, infiltration, and spread

Paget's disease (*see* Chapter 4)

Pruritus

Any cancer, but lymphomas in particular — Hodgkin's disease

Dermatomyositis

Any cancer

Erythema gyratum repens and other 'gyrate' erythemas

Any cancer

Necrolytic migratory erythema

Glucagonoma — (*see* Fig. 8.23)

The sign of Leser–Trélat

Any cancer

Acanthosis nigricans

Adenocarcinoma of the foregut

Acquired ichthyosis

Lymphomas, especially Hodgkin's

Erythroderma

Lymphomas, especially T-cell — *see* Chapter 5

Hypertrichosis lanuginosa

Late-stage disease

Telangiectases

Carcinoid syndrome – (*see* also Fig. 8.22)

Thrombophlebitis migrans

Pancreatic cancer

Arsenical keratoses

Inherited syndromes in which skin changes accompany systemic cancers:

e.g. Bazex; Cowden's; Gardner's; Rothmund–Thomson; xeroderma pigmentosum; Bloom's; Howel–Evans — *see* Chapter 11.

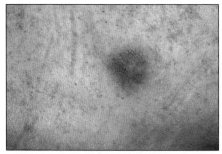

Fig. 8.37 *Cutaneous metastasis. A diagnosis of oat cell carcinoma was made on biopsying this nodule.*

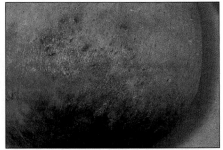

Fig. 8.38 *Cutaneous infiltration of the breast by an underlying carcinoma.*

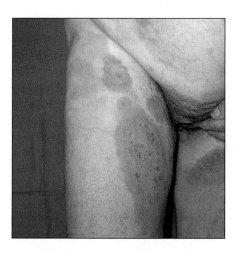

Fig. 8.39 *Gyrate erythema in a patient with squamous cell carcinoma of the bronchus.*

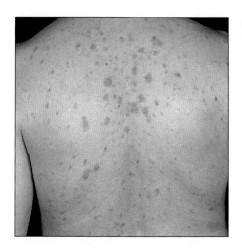

Fig. 8.40 *Multiple, eruptive, seborrhoeic warts (the sign of Leser–Trélat).*

The sign of Leser–Trélat is also very rare. **Figure 8.40** is of a man who described the sudden appearance of itchy seborrhoeic warts and was found to have an adenocarcinoma of the colon. Whether such associations are genuine or due to chance is open to debate. Acquired ichthyosis has been associated with lymphomas, particularly Hodgkin's disease (*see also* Chapter 11). Some very cachectic cancer patients develop a profuse growth of fine lanugo hair. The same occurs occasionally in anorexia nervosa. It is now very rare to meet a patient who has been given large quantities of arsenic, but punctate palmar keratoses occur in such patients. They also develop cutaneous and internal malignancies.

As indicated in the box above there are many congenital syndromes in which systemic cancers occur. These are covered briefly in Chapter 11.

311

SKIN SIGNS OF CONNECTIVE TISSUE DISEASE

The skin is prominently involved in the group of conditions frequently brought together under the general heading 'connective tissue disease'.

Skin signs associated with connective tissue disease

Systemic lupus erythematosus (SLE)
Facial erythema, photosensitivity, hair loss, oral and nasal ulceration, discoid lupus erythematosus, urticarial vasculitis (*see* Chapter 5), erythema-multiforme-like lesions, bullae, Raynaud's phenomenon

Systemic sclerosis
Acrosclerosis, Raynaud's phenomenon, 'mat-like' telangiectases, cutaneous calcinosis, beaked nose, small mouth with perioral furrows

Morphoea
Localized, generalized, or linear cutaneous sclerosis

Dermatomyositis
Periorbital oedema, periorbital rash (heliotrope), lichenoid rash often on extensor surfaces, rash on dorsum of phalanges, Gottron's papules, ragged cuticles poikilodermatous changes, cutaneous calcinosis

Mixed connective tissue disease
Various combinations of the features listed above

Polyarteritis nodosa
Livedo reticularis, ulceration

Rheumatoid arthritis
See box on page 317

Relapsing polychondritis
Red, inflamed ears

Lupus erythematosus

Lupus erythematosus (LE) derives its name from the ravaged appearance that both this condition and the common lupus ('vulgaris' — now known to be due to tuberculosis) creates on the skin of the head and neck. However, the label covers a large range of symptoms and signs associated with a multisystem disorder characterized by the development of cytotoxic antibodies and immune complexes. The cutaneous forms have been addressed in Chapter 5, but it should be noted that all the forms discussed in that section may be seen in patients with systemic LE (SLE). Occasionally, too, patients with chronic discoid LE, subacute cutaneous LE, and chilblain LE progress to full-blown SLE.

SLE classically — but not exclusively — affects young women. It has very significant effects on many internal organs. In addition to the skin conditions described in Chapter 5, patients often suffer from Raynaud's phenomenon, ulcers in the nose and mouth, diffuse, rather patchy, hair loss, marked photosensitivity, and vasculitis. The most often quoted cutaneous manifestation the so-called butterfly erythema, is not really well described by this term — any facial eruption affecting both cheeks and bridging the nose looks like a butterfly: notably, rosacea and various forms of eczema, especially seborrhoeic eczema. In fact, the blotchy, evanescent, erythematous rash of SLE is often much more widely

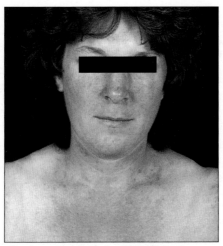

Fig. 8.41 *Systemic lupus erythematosus: this woman's widespread rash was light-provoked and light-exacerbated.*

distributed and is also often light-provoked (**Fig. 8.41**). The investigation and management of a patient with SLE is a matter for joint arrangements between appropriate specialists: nephrologists, rheumatologists, cardiologists, and dermatologists. Most patients have strongly positive antinuclear antibodies and there are various subtypes with different serological markers. Of particular relevance to dermatology, one notable type is characterized by the presence of a clotting promoter, paradoxically called the lupus anticoagulant. Patients with this form of SLE are prone to thrombotic episodes. Female patients may suffer recurrent abortions or give birth to children with heart block, other internal problems, and cutaneous livedo (congenital lupus). Patients usually need immunosuppressive treatment, often involving corticosteroids and azathioprine. Antimalarial drugs also have a role in some patients and are particularly useful in cutaneous SLE.

Systemic sclerosis and morphoea

Although essentially unrelated, systemic sclerosis and morphoea are usually considered together because they have one important clinical feature in common: primary cutaneous sclerosis. Systemic sclerosis is characterized by progressive changes in many organs (especially the lungs, heart, gut, and kidneys), as well as highly characteristic skin features:

- Raynaud's phenomenon.
- Tendency to cutaneous calcinosis.
- Sclerosis and, sometimes, thickening of the skin of the digits, hands, and feet (**Fig. 8.42a**).
- 'Mat-like' telangiectases (**Fig. 8.42b**).
- Progressive beaking of the nose and narrowing of the mouth with perioral furrows (**Fig. 8.42c**).

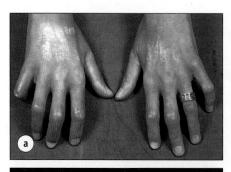

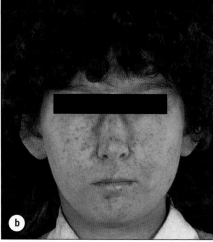

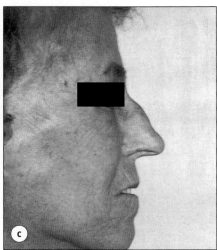

Fig. 8.42 Systemic sclerosis/CREST — *(a) sclerodactyly; (b) mat-like telangiectases; (c) beaking of the nose and perioral furrowing.*

A somewhat less aggressive variant is often encountered, in which anticentromere antibodies are often positive. This syndrome embraces the calcinosis, sclerodactyly, Raynaud's, oesophageal dysmotility, telangiectases of the more serious form and is known as the CREST syndrome. Internal organ involvement is less common and less severe.

Morphoea is the term used to describe cutaneous sclerosis without systemic features. There are four main forms encountered in clinical practice:

- Localized — here, an area or areas of skin become thickened, hard, and inflexible (**Fig. 8.43**). The areas usually slowly extend or remain static over many years, but may eventually disappear.

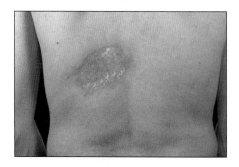

Fig. 8.43 An area of localized scleroderma (morphoea).

- Generalized — here, the changes spread to involve virtually the entire body surface, sometimes with serious consequences. Patients have restricted joint and chest movement and are very uncomfortable.
- Linear — plaques of cutaneous sclerosis follow a psuedo-dermatomal distribution along a limb or may affect the scalp and face. In a child, this may have significant implications, because growth may become markedly asymmetrical.
- A hyperpigmented, slightly atrophic form, called the atrophoderma of Pasini and Pierini, in which pale-brown areas appear, usually on the trunk

There is no treatment that has been shown conclusively to be effective in this group of disorders.

Dermatomyositis

As the name implies, dermatomyositis is a disorder in which inflammation of the skin and muscles predominates. Some patients have inflammation of only one of these tissues. The cutaneous changes are striking and unmistakeable:

- A purplish rash, which may be widespread but has a predilection for the face, periorbital skin (**Fig. 8.44a**), elbows and knees, and the dorsum of the phalanges (**Fig. 8.44b**) — because of its distinctive colour, this rash has been labelled 'heliotrope' for the horticulturally minded.
- Periorbital oedema, especially in adults.
- Ragged cuticles with nail-fold haemorrhages (**Fig. 8.44c**).
- Flat-topped papules on the fingers (Gottron's papules).

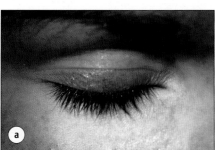

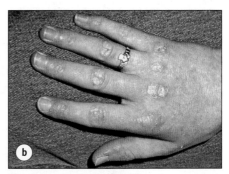

Fig. 8.44 *Dermatomyositis* — *(a) violatious rash on eyelid; (b) lesions tend to be linear over the knuckles; (c) typical nail-fold appearance.*

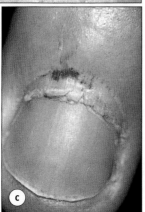

- Poikilodermatous (irregular pigmentary) changes, sometimes with atrophy and ulceration (especially in juvenile disease).
- Calcinosis (especially in juvenile disease).
- The myositis typically affects proximal muscle groups: shoulders, buttocks, and thighs. The muscles are tender and may be weak.

Investigations should include an assessment of the muscles: levels of muscle enzymes or urinary creatine, EMG, and muscle biopsy. There is debate as when to initiate a search for an internal cancer in older adults. There is no doubt that dermatomyositis occurs as a sequel to cancer, but it is not clear how often this is the case, nor at what age this association becomes significant enough to warrant invasive investigation. If no cancer is found, patients need to be treated with oral corticosteroids and immunosuppressive agents. High doses may be required until the rash improves and the muscle inflammation comes under control, and patients often need to continue therapy for many years.

Juvenile dermatomyositis

There is a distinct age-peak of dermatomyositis in childhood and the disease behaves somewhat differently in this form: internal cancer is not a feature, but the muscle disease is often more aggressive, resulting in permanent muscle-wasting and contractures; calcinosis is also more common. Such patients should be treated very aggressively to try and avoid permanent damage if at all possible. The condition usually burns itself out eventually.

Mixed connective tissue disease

Patients present to various specialists with 'overlap' features of the three major connective tissue diseases mentioned in this section. The clinical features are as described.

Polyarteritis nodosa

The skin may be involved in polyarteritis nodosa (PAN), usually with the onset of permanent livedo reticularis (**Fig. 8.45**), although more serious damage from the underlying vascular disease may result in ulceration and gangrene. Similar changes occasionally occur with Wegener's granulomatosis. Some patients with PAN seem only to have the arteritic changes in the skin and in subcutaneous fat.

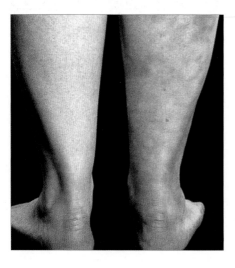

Fig. 8.45 *Asymmetrical livedo reticularis in a patient with cutaneous polyarteritis nodosa.*

Rheumatoid arthritis

The most important cutaneous manifestations of rheumatoid disease are listed below.

Skin signs associated with rheumatoid arthritis

- Vasculitis
- Nodules
- Leg ulcers
- Pyoderma gangrenosum
- Nail-fold infarcts (Bywater's lesions)
- Nocturnal urticarial rash (in Still's disease)

Most of these have been described previously in this section. One very remarkable phenomenon is the occurrence of a nocturnal (-only) urticarial eruption in juvenile rheumatoid arthritis (Still's disease — **Fig. 8.46**).

Relapsing polychondritis

Another disorder in which connective tissue (in this case, cartilage) is inflamed is relapsing polychondritis. Patients may present to the dermatologist with a red, sore ear, but only the cartilaginous part is involved (**Fig. 8.47**).

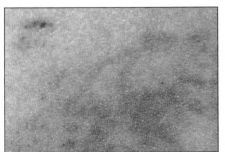

Fig. 8.46 *An urticarial eruption that appeared only in the late evenings in a child with juvenile rheumatoid arthritis.*

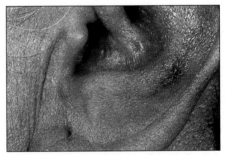

Fig. 8.47 *Relapsing polychondritis. The cartilagenous part of the ear is reddened; the lobe is normal.*

Behçet's disease

Behçet's disease is a complex of multi-organ problems, most prominently:
- Oral ulceration (**Fig. 8.48a**).
- Genital ulceration (**Fig. 8.48b**).
- Uveitis.
- Arthritis.
- Neurological signs.
- Thrombophlebitis.

The disease is rare, but is much more common in the Middle East and Japan. The main pathological process involved is thought to be a vasculitis. Treatment remains difficult and the condition may be a source of considerable disability.

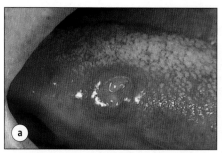

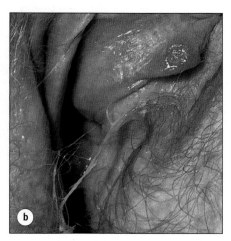

Fig. 8.48 *Behçet's disease* — *this young woman had recurrent* *(a)* *oral and* *(b)* *genital ulceration, anterior uveitis, and arthritis.*

SKIN SIGNS OF PREGNANCY

The skin signs of pregnancy are listed below.

Skin signs of pregnancy

- Pruritus
- Striae distense
- Vascular changes
  - palmar erythema
  - spider telangiectases
  - growth of vascular tumours
- Increased pigmentation, including chloasma/melasma
- Enhanced hair growth
- Polymorphic eruption of pregnancy [Pruritic papules and urticarial plaques of pregnancy — PUPPP (the US name for polymorphic eruption of pregnancy)]

Pregnant women often complain of itching (without visible primary skin lesions), thought to be due to cholestasis. This can be very severe and tends to resist all forms of treatment (except parturition).

Pregnant women often develop palmar erythema and vascular spiders (*see* Fig. 8.17) which may fade after childbirth. Women also notice a general increase in pigmentation, and moles may darken. Facial pigmentation (chloasma/melasma) is common (*see* Chapter 10). Hair growth is often luxuriant during pregnancy, but many women also record a marked hair loss (due to a telogen effluvium — *see* Chapter 9) a few weeks after birth. Another common phenomenon is an odd cutaneous disorder known in the United Kingdom as polymorphic eruption of pregnancy and in the United States as pruritic urticarial papules and plaques of pregnancy (or PUPPP). The condition produces irritable papules and plaques with a predilection for abdominal striae (**Fig. 8.49**). Herpes (pemphigoid) gestationis has already been discussed in Chapter 7.

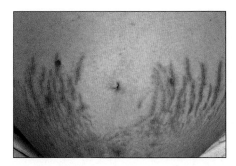

Fig. 8.49 *Polymorphic eruption of pregnancy, showing the typical predilection for abdominal striae.*

- Some skin changes can be important markers of internal malignancy.
- 'Butterfly' erythema in SLE can be widely distributed (not just bridging the nose) and is often light-provoked.
- Systemic sclerosis can be characterized by cutaneous changes including Raynaud's phenomenon, cutaneous calcinosis, sclerosis and skin thickening, telangiectases and beaking of the nose, and narrowing of the mouth with perioral furrows.
- Dermatomyositis is a disorder in which inflammation of the skin and muscles predominates.
- Polyarteritis nodosa can present with the onset of permanent livedo reticularis.
- Behçet's disease commonly presents with oral and genital ulceration uveitis and arthritis.
- Pregnant women often complain of itching and may develop palmar erythema and vascular spiders.

SKIN CHANGES CAUSED BY DRUGS GIVEN FOR SYSTEMIC OR CUTANEOUS DISEASE

Cutaneous reactions to drugs are very common. Most are relatively non-specific, morbilliform eruptions (**Fig. 8.50a**) that are due to type IV hypersensitivity, but some have very characteristic features.

Fixed drug eruptions are very curious. Lesions come up shortly after the offending agent has been taken and are always in the same place (hence 'fixed'). They are typically round or oval areas, with a dusky centre (**Fig. 8.50b**). Occasionally, they also have a bulla (*see* Chapter 7). They fade to leave quite pronounced hyperpigmentation. Lichenoid eruptions may resemble lichen planus clinically, but are often more eczematous or have a mixed morphology. However, lichenoid histological features are prominent.

Light may interact with drugs to cause reactions either by allergic or direct chemical pathways (**Fig. 8.50c**). A number of important and common agents are associated with such reactions (**Fig. 8.51**).

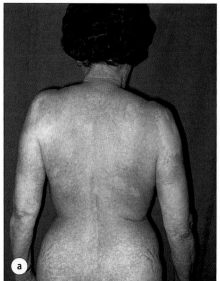

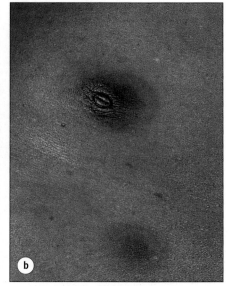

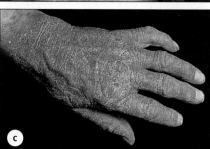

Fig. 8.50 *Drug eruptions —*
(a) morbilliform — a widespread, symmetrical eruption, in this case due to a semi-synthetic penicillin; (b) a good example of a fixed drug eruption, showing the typical oval, dusky appearance — there are two lesions, one of which involves the nipple; (c) photosensitivity due to quinine.

Additionally pre-existing skin disease can be exacerbated by a number of drugs:
- Acne — by androgens (testosterone and its derivatives, danazol, stanozolol), oral contraceptives, and corticosteroids.
- Psoriasis — by lithium and antimalarials.
- SLE — by penicillin and sulphonamides.
- Porphyrias — *see* page 307.

- Most cutaneous reactions to drugs are non-specific, morbilliform eruptions due to type IV hypersensitivity.
- Light may interact with drugs to cause reactions either by allergic or direct chemical pathways.

Important drug eruptions and their causes	
Type of reaction	**Common causes***
Morbilliform (*see* Fig. 8.50a)	Antibiotics, antihypertensives, non-steroidal anti-inflammatory drugs (NSAIDs), barbiturates, hydantoins
Urticaria and anaphylaxis (*see* Chapter 5)	Penicillin, vaccines, toxoids
Fixed (*see* Fig. 8.50b)	Phenolphthalein, tetracyclines, sulphonamides, quinine, paracetamol, chlordiazepoxide
Lichenoid	β-blockers, antimalarials, thiazides, gold, penicillamine, phenothiazines
Vasculitis	Thiazides, allopurinol, penicillin, captopril, sulphonamides, quinolones
Erythema multiforme	*see* Fig. 8.11
Autoimmune bullous disorders (*see* Chapter 7)	Penicillamine, captopril, rifampicin
Lupus-erythematosus-like syndrome	Hydantoins, hydralazine, griseofulvin, methyldopa, chlorpromazine, isoniazid
Photosensitivity (*see* Fig. 8.50c)	Amiodarone, chlorpromazine, nalidixic acid, sulphonamides, tetracyclines, thiazides, quinine, quinolones
Acneiform eruptions	Steroids, androgens, lithium, iodides
Pigmentation (*see* Chapter 10) Contact dermatitis (*see* Chapter 5)	
*NB This list is not comprehensive	

Fig. 8.51 *Important drug eruptions and their causes.*

THE CUTANEOUS EFFECTS OF PSYCHOLOGICAL DISTURBANCES

A full discussion of the possible interactions between the skin and the psyche is not feasible here because of the restraints of space. However, there are a number of important areas that need to be considered in a little detail.

STRESS AND THE SKIN

Firstly, there are many skin conditions that are commonly thought (at least by the general public) to be triggered or exacerbated by psychological stress. These include psoriasis, eczema, acne, urticaria, lichen planus, alopecia, and vitiligo. There is a limited volume of evidence to support this view in some of these conditions — psoriasis, for example.

There is, however, no doubt that having skin disease is a cause of unhappiness in its own right. Males with bad psoriasis are more likely to be heavy drinkers. There have been suicides attributed to acne in teenagers. Reducing other aspects of stress in a patient's life is, therefore, something that makes common sense, if it can be achieved.

DISORDERS IN WHICH PSYCHOLOGICAL FACTORS MAY BE IMPORTANT

'Neurodermatitis' and 'neurotic excoriations'

As the names imply, the terms neurodermatitis and neurotic excoriations are given to disorders that cause patients to itch and scratch and pick at lesions on their skin, the aetiology for which a simple, primary dermatological explanation is not always apparent. Affected patients are often tense, and admit to being 'under stress'. The same is true of some patients with pruritus ani and pruritus vulvae. The term neurodermatitis is also used alongside lichen simplex chronicus (*see* Chapter 5) and can be applied to heavily lichenified and excoriated atopic dermatitis.

Trichotillomania (see also Chapter 10)

Some patients repeatedly tug and pull at their hair, causing bald patches to form. This is quite common in the mentally subnormal and in the severely disturbed, but is also seen in apparently normal people, especially children. This is usually a compulsive habit, but it may mask some unhappiness at school or at work.

DISORDERS IN WHICH PSYCHOLOGICAL FACTORS ARE IMPORTANT

Skin conditions exist in which psychological disturbances are primarily involved in the cutaneous problem. There may be seen features of anxiety or depression, an abnormal (often obsessional or hysterical) personality trait, or a true psychosis.

Cutaneous Munchausen's syndrome and dermatitis artefacta

Some patients inflict skin lesions upon themselves. There are two main groups of such patients. In one group, this is a quite deliberate attempt at deception and the disorder can be considered to be a cutaneous form of Munchausen's syndrome. In the other, there are much more complex emotional and psychological factors at play and the patient may be seemingly unaware of the true nature of the lesions. Such a situation is best classified separately, as dermatitis artefacta.

The lesions in both types of disorder may be bizarre and unlike those of any normal, endogenous pathological process (**Fig. 8.52a**), or they may be much more difficult to diagnose as being due to external factors. This situation often occurs when a patient has been exposed to genuine skin disease themselves or in others and recognizes a way of simulating it. The repeated manifestation of skin lesions resembling genuine disease, such as cutaneous LE or severe eczema (**Fig. 8.52b**), but which are induced by the patient, is sometimes termed dermatological pathomimicry.

Many of these patients find the deliberate self-harm 'necessary' only for a limited period. This is especially true of adolescents who may be going through some sort of crisis (such as a family break-up). A few, however, develop a pattern of continual self-traumatization that can last indefinitely. Presumably, the presence of the skin lesions is in some way helpful to them psychologically. Even the most expert of psychiatrists often fail to deal with such patients adequately.

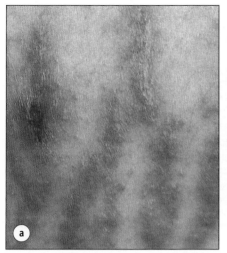 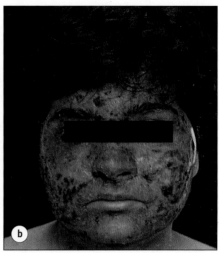

Fig. 8.52 *Skin disorders due to psychological factors — (a)* linear skin lesions, clearly due to external scratching, in a young girl whose parents were in the process of 'splitting up'; *(b)* this young man had observed a relative's treatment for eczema and induced these awful changes on his face with various caustic substances.

Dermatological 'non-disease'

Some patients complain bitterly about symptoms and describe physical changes in great detail, but never have any physical changes visible on examination. Severe burning or itching sensations in the scalp, mouth, nails, and perineum are common forms of this 'syndrome'. It is difficult to convince the patient that there is nothing physically wrong and they usually consult doctors of different disciplines in an almost endless search for someone who will agree to find something out of the ordinary.

Delusional parasitophobia

Perhaps the most bizarre psychocutaneous disease of all is delusional parasitophobia (sometime 'parasitosis'). Patients believe (and cannot be swayed from their conviction) that they, or their surroundings, or both, are infested with some creatures, usually insects or worms. They describe crawling sensations, offer explanations as to the type of creature involved (they have always seen it and are usually great experts on its anatomy and physiology), and may present the dermatologist with concrete 'evidence' to prove their point. This is sometimes in the form of debris that they have dug out of their skin, or, occasionally, supporting statements from witnesses who have seen the creatures or from laboratory personnel who have been asked to examine material by the patient.

Trying to change these beliefs is hopeless. It is said that some patients respond to pimozide, but this is often of little value — largely because the patients will not agree to take it. Risperidone is better tolerated and may be more effective.

- Evidence is lacking to support a definite link between psychological stress and skin disorders (e.g. psoriasis) but skin disease can in itself be an important cause of stress.
- Neurodermatitis occurs when patients itch and pick excessively at skin lesions.
- Trichotillomania occurs when patients repeatedly pull at hair causing bald patches.
- Some patients may inflict skin lesions upon themselves; others may complain of symptoms or physical changes not apparent on examination.
- Delusional parasitophobia is a term applied to patients with an obsessional belief that they and/or their surroundings are infested by parasites or other creatures.

chapter 9

Disorders of Hair and Nails

INTRODUCTION

As discussed in Chapter 1, hair and nails are formed from appendageal invaginations of the epidermis. Both may be affected by congenital abnormalities or by acquired diseases. In some instances, both hair and nails are affected by the same process, but either may, of course, be affected independently.

For convenience, we shall consider disorders of hair first, although, where these involve nail changes that are closely linked, the latter will be discussed at the same time. We shall then cover other important nail disorders.

Congenital syndromes associated with abnormal hair	
Monilethrix	Beaded hair; short, sparse scalp hair; follicular papules at the nape of neck; mild mental retardation; no biochemical abnormalities; autosomal dominant.
Netherton syndrome	Trichorrhexis invaginata; *see also* Chapter 11.
Trichothiodystrophy	Deficiency of sulphur-containing amino acids; brittle hair with a variety of microscopic changes, including trichorrhexis nodosa (*see* Fig. 9.2); variable mental retardation; infertility; short stature; autosomal recessive.
Marie–Unna alopecia	Sparse hair, gradually deteriorating with progressive scarring; hairs coarse, twisted, and fluted; autosomal dominant.
Ectodermal dysplasias	*see* Chapter 11.
Conradi–Hunerman syndrome	*see* Chapter 11.
Pili annulati	Dark and light bands along hair shafts; autosomal dominant.
Woolly hair and woolly-hair naevus	Hairs are oval in cross-section; scalp hair very curly.
Uncombable hair	Silvery-blonde, 'fly-away' hair; hair shafts triangular with longitudinal grooves; autosomal dominant.
Premature greying	Early-onset greying is often inherited.

Fig. 9.1 *Congenital syndromes associated with abnormal hair.*

DISORDERS OF HAIR

Broadly speaking, three basic problems with hair result in patients seeking attention:
- Disorders of texture and colour.
- Too much hair.
- Too little hair.

DISORDERS OF TEXTURE AND COLOUR

A number of congenital syndromes exist in which hair texture and colour are abnormal. **Figure 9.1** lists some of the more important (*see also* Chapter 11).

Microscopy of hair is helpful in distinguishing between these disorders, but is something that most general dermatologists undertake only infrequently. It may therefore be wise to seek the opinion of a specialist. A urinary screen for abnormalities in amino acid excretion is also advisable.

Textural and colour changes may also be acquired:
- Greying of hair — this is, of course, a perfectly natural process in most individuals. However, in some, greying occurs at a much earlier age than usual. When this is not an inherited tendency, it may be associated with pernicious anaemia (**Fig. 9.1**).
- Kinking — progressive, acquired kinking of the hair occurs in some males, usually as an early feature of male pattern, or androgenetic alopecia (*see* page 330).
- 'Dryness' — weathering and damage by chemicals, heat, and harsh hairdressing techniques (including bleaching and back-combing) may lead to permanent changes in the texture of the hair.

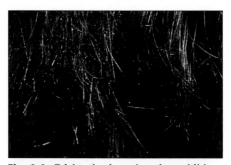

Fig. 9.2 *Trichorrhexis nodosa in a child with trichothiodystrophy.* The hairs in this disorder fracture and fray. The microscopic appearance has been likened to the ends of brushes pushed together. In this case, the child was otherwise entirely well.

TOO MUCH HAIR

Society dictates certain 'standards' regarding the normal amount of hair that is acceptable. In most Western cultures, for example, women are generally expected to have minimal facial hair, although some quite normally have relatively strong facial hair growth. It is conventional to consider excessive hair growth under two broad headings: hirsutism and hypertrichosis.

Box 9.1

Excessive hair growth

Hirsutism
Excess hair in a sexual distribution.
Hypertrichosis
Excess hair in a general distribution.

Hirsutism

Essentially a problem in women, too much hair on the upper lip, face (**Fig. 9.3**), chest, and abdominal wall may be genetically determined and, effectively, 'normal' for that individual and the women in her family. Sometimes, however, there are underlying factors involved. The most common of these is the polycystic ovary syndrome, in which ovarian cysts are associated with peripheral hyperandrogenism. In addition to excess hair in a 'male' secondary sexual distribution, there may be acne and a tendency to a male body shape.

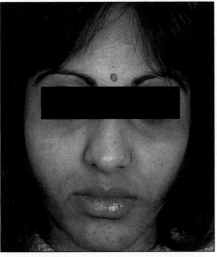

Fig. 9.3 *Hirsuties in an otherwise healthy girl. There was no family history, but ultrasound of the pelvis revealed polycystic ovary syndrome.*

Much less commonly, there may be a significant endocrinological problem. Hirsuties in a child, for example, may be associated with congenital adrenal hyperplasia. Androgen-secreting tumours may also result in hirsuties, as may Cushing's syndrome. Appropriate investigations should be considered if there is any doubt.

The hair can be destroyed physically in a variety of ways: shaving, plucking, depilatories, electrolysis, and laser treatment. Cyproterone acetate may also reduce the excessive hairiness gradually.

Hypertrichosis

Once again, this is frequently genetically determined (**Fig. 9.4**). However, hypertrichosis is a feature of some congenital disorders, such as the Cornelia de Lange syndrome (microcephaly; mental retardation; thick, bushy eyebrows and low hairline; generalized hypertrichosis). Some drugs — minoxidil (*see* page 330), ciclosporin (cyclosporin), hydantoins, steroids — induce hypertrichosis, sometimes quite marked. It is also a feature of porphyria cutanea tarda (*see* Chapter 8) and may occur in patients with cachexia and in those with anorexia nervosa, as a result of a marked increase in lanugo hair (*see* Chapter 1). Localized areas of hypertrichosis are seen in pretibial myxoedema (*see* Chapter 8) and in the 'faun tail' overlying spina bifida occulta (**Fig. 9.5**).

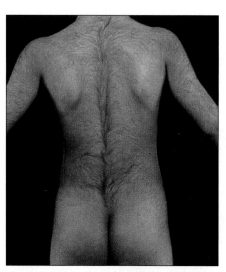

Fig. 9.4 *Generalized hypertrichosis in a teenage girl* — *this was normal for this family.*

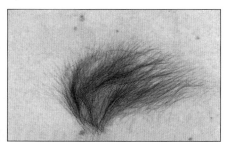

Fig. 9.5 *A localized area of hypertrichosis over the lower back ('faun tail') in a patient with occult spina bifida.*

TOO LITTLE HAIR

In addition to the disorders listed in Figure 9.1, scalp hair density may be abnormal from birth, due to localized failure of development of the hair-bearing skin (aplasia cutis), other scalp lesions (e.g. naevus sebaceous — *see* Chapter 4), or scarring from injury. The normal density of hair for any individual is maintained by the fact that normal hair-loss is matched by an equivalent rate of hair replacement.

Box 9.2

Alopecia
Any situation in which the quantity of hair becomes perceptibly reduced; multiple causes, some based primarily on an absolute increase in loss of hair or on destruction of follicles, and others on more subtle alterations in the homeostatic balance between loss and replacement.

Alopecia may affect any part of the body, but is most noticeable and most frequently symptomatic when it affects the scalp. **Figure 9.6** lists the main conditions to be considered in a patient presenting with scalp hair loss. Some of these have already been discussed in the appropriate chapters and will not be considered further here (e.g. basal cell carcinoma, cicatricial pemphigoid). Alopecia of other hair-bearing areas will be discussed briefly in the accounts of each condition that follow.

Causes of alopecia			
Diffuse Scalp normal	**Diffuse Scalp abnormal**	**Localized Scalp normal**	**Localized Scalp abnormal**
Front and crown	**Inflammatory**	**Scalp margins**	**No scarring**
Androgenetic alopecia	Dermatitis, Psoriasis, Pityriasis amiantacea	Traction, Alopecia areata	Tinea capitis, Pityriasis amiantacea, Psoriasis, Alopecia mucinosa
Generalized		**Anywhere**	**With scarring/ loss of tissue***
Telogen effluvium, Drug-induced, Thyroid disease, Syphilis, Systemic LE, Iron deficiency, Trichotillomania, Alopecia totalis/ Universalis		Alopecia areata, Trichotillomania	Discoid LE, Lichen planus, 'Pseudo-pelade', tumours e.g. basal cell carcinoma, Trigeminal trophic syndrome, Folliculitis decalvans, Morphoea, Tinea capitis, Cicatricial pemphigoid, Lupus vulgaris, Atypical necrobiosis

* **Cicatricial alopecia:**many of these conditions are discussed in other chapters,
LE = lupus erythematosus

Fig. 9.6 *Causes of alopecia.*

Androgenetic alopecia

The most common form of alopecia is that labelled androgenetic. This affects both men and women although, by and large, it is worse and more likely to begin at an early age in men.

In men, the appearances are well known and there is often a strong family history. It can, however, be a cause of extreme distress, particularly if the onset is at a very young age. Typically, the hair loss begins with temporal recession and is followed by a thinning and loss of hair over the crown. A rim of hair is retained around the parietal and occipital regions. In women, the condition seldom progresses to such an extreme degree, at least before the menopause. However, thinning of the crown may commence early in life (**Fig. 9.7a**) and may become quite marked (**Fig. 9.7b**), particularly if there is a strong family tendency.

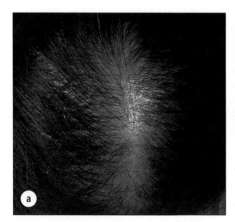

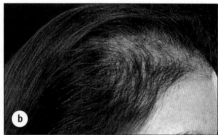

Fig. 9.7 *Androgenetic alopecia* — *(a) hair thinning over the crown in a 30-year-old woman; **(b)** more marked thinning in a young woman whose father was bald.*

Treatment is difficult. Various replacement techniques using artificial hair are available, including hair transplantation (which relies on the permanence of the occipitoparietal follicles), hair weaving, and toupées and wigs. More recently, minoxidil, if used daily over long periods, has been shown to restrain and even restore hair loss if started early enough. A topical lotion is commercially available.

Telogen effluvium

As discussed in Chapter 1, human hair grows in asynchronous cycles. However, some 'life events' are capable of altering hair growth and accelerating a rapid transition of many hairs into a resting phase together. This is followed some weeks later by a moult, as the old hairs are released from the follicles to allow their replacements to succeed them. This results in a sudden and alarming shedding of hair known as a telogen effluvium. Common triggers include parturition, coming off oral contraceptives, severe feverish illnesses, operations, and, perhaps, extreme stress. The condition will settle over time, but it can unmask an underlying androgenetic alopecia, and scalp hair density may never return completely to pre-effluvium levels.

Drug-induced alopecia

A number of drugs can induce hair loss (**Fig. 9.8**).

Some important drug causes of alopecia
Cytotoxic drugs
Antithyroid drugs
Anticoagulants
Retinoids

Fig. 9.8 *Some important drug causes of alopecia.*

Other causes of generalized hair loss with a normal scalp

A patient presenting with a generalized loss of hair should be screened for evidence of thyroid dysfunction and for iron deficiency. Both secondary syphilis and systemic lupus erythematosus are associated with a rather patchy, but diffuse, alopecia.

Trichotillomania

The term *trichotillomania* describes the deliberate traction of hair, leading to fracture of the hair shafts and a consequent alopecia (**Fig. 9.9**). It is most commonly seen in children, but can occur in adults. The scalp skin is usually normal, but can be mildly inflamed and scaly. The traction often results from a repeated twisting and tugging action that may simply be a habit tic. There may, however, be more serious psychopathology present.

Traction alopecia and other physical causes of hair loss

Constant tension on hair follicles also results in damage, breakage, and potentially permanent loss of follicles. This may result from particular hairdressing styles (**Fig. 9.10**). Some people with very curly hair, especially Afro-Caribbeans, may damage the hair follicles with hot waxes and combs designed to straighten the hair shaft. Some chemicals (such as perming solutions) can damage hair shafts, resulting in breakage, but permanent loss is very unusual. Repetitive trauma to the scalp may occur if sensation is abnormal. One cause of this is postherpetic neuralgia, and the resulting damage is known as the trigeminal trophic syndrome.

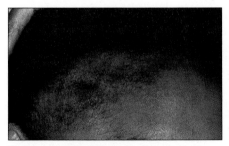

Fig. 9.9 *Trichotillomania. This girl had developed a habit of pulling and twisting the hair over her right temple.*

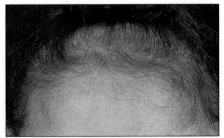

Fig. 9.10 *Traction alopecia — this Sikh boy has lost follicles around the front of his scalp. Similar changes occur with ponytails.*

331

Inflammatory causes of alopecia without scarring

Severe scalp psoriasis and dermatitis may result in temporary hair loss. Occasionally, psoriasis or seborrhoeic dermatitis may present with an extreme accumulation of scale, known as pityriasis amiantacea (**Fig. 9.11**). If the scale is removed, hair comes away as well. This hair loss is generally temporary, but is occasionally permanent.

Cicatricial alopecia

Scalp hair loss with loss of follicles or with scalp atrophy is known as cicatricial alopecia (**Fig. 9.12**). The term retains some value because the cause of such changes is not always apparent at first presentation. Indeed, there are some patients in whom an inflammatory process, affecting the scalp and causing scarring, is as near to a definitive diagnosis as it is possible to get, at least initially. However, the two most important primary skin disorders that give rise to this appearance are lichen planus (*see* Chapter 5) and chronic discoid lupus erythematosus (*see* Chapters 5 and 8), but Figure 9.6 lists several others. One clinical appearance or condition that gives rise to confusion is pseudo-pelade (of Brocq). This title is applied to a particular change in which small, oval or round patches of alopecia appear, with little or no preceding inflammation, but with loss of follicles. It is said to resemble 'footprints' (**Fig. 9.13**).

The investigation of a patient with cicatricial alopecia should include a careful clinical examination for evidence of skin disease elsewhere and for the nail changes of lichen planus, a biopsy for histology, immunofluorescence, and a screen for lupus erythematosus. Treatment is mostly symptomatic, but some patients respond well to topical, intralesional, or systemic steroids.

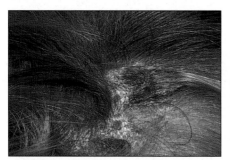

Fig. 9.11 *Pityriasis amiantacea — there is thick, adherent scale appearing to cling to a bunch of hair follicles. When this scale is lifted away, the hairs usually come away too.*

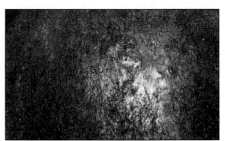

Fig. 9.12 *Cicatricial alopecia, showing widespread hair loss and loss of follicles.*

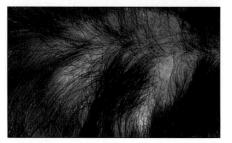

Fig. 9.13 *Pseudo-pelade — small, circumscribed areas of cicatricial alopecia with no other distinguishing features.*

Alopecia areata, totalis, and universalis

Alopecia areata is a very variable disorder and is thought to be an autoimmune process. Certainly, organ-specific autoantibodies are found in some patients and there is an association with vitiligo (*see* Chapter 10). Very rarely, alopecia areata is part of a multisystem autoimmune syndrome, including myasthenia gravis, thymomas, and other conditions. Alopecia areata is also seen in patients with Down syndrome (*see* Chapter 11).

The typical appearances are of circumscribed patches of hair loss with no cutaneous alteration at all (**Fig. 9.14a**), but there may occasionally be mild redness. The cardinal sign

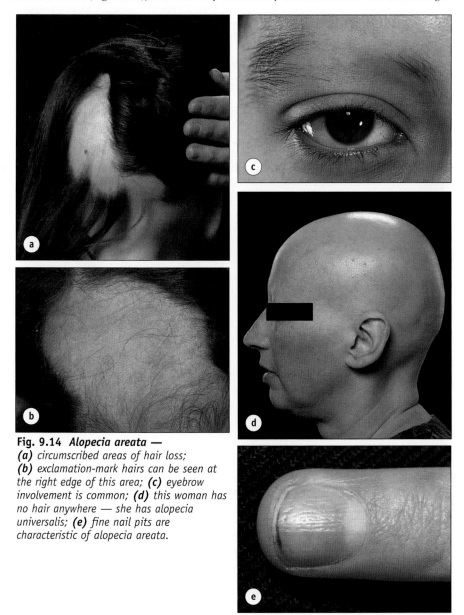

Fig. 9.14 *Alopecia areata —*
(a) circumscribed areas of hair loss; (b) exclamation-mark hairs can be seen at the right edge of this area; (c) eyebrow involvement is common; (d) this woman has no hair anywhere — she has alopecia universalis; (e) fine nail pits are characteristic of alopecia areata.

of this condition is the presence, usually at the edge of the area, of short, stubby hairs that taper towards the base — so-called exclamation-mark hairs (**Fig. 9.14b**). Areas other than the scalp are often involved, especially the eyebrows (**Fig. 9.14c**), eyelashes, and beard. If the condition affects the whole scalp, it is known as alopecia totalis; if the whole body is affected, it is called alopecia universalis (**Fig. 9.14d**). This nomenclature may seem somewhat artificial, since these clinical manifestations are one and the same pathologically; however, prognostically, the more extensive the process becomes, the less likely it is that it will resolve. Patients often have fine pits in the nails (**Fig. 9.14e**), especially in more extensive disease.

The natural history is generally good. Smaller areas will regrow in most instances. Exceptions, where the prognosis is generally poor, include very extensive alopecia and areas around the nape of the neck.

Treatment with intralesional steroids may help. There is no proof that topical steroids are of value, but they are frequently offered. Systemic steroids may bring about temporary hair growth. Topical sensitization therapy with diphencyprone may be of value. Here, a contact dermatitis is deliberately induced and the skin is repeatedly challenged with the antigen. Good results have been achieved with diphencyprone, but it is difficult to assess how much is due to the therapy and how much to spontaneous recovery.

Alopecia mucinosa (follicular mucinosis)

Alopecia mucinosa comprises a rare mucinous infiltration within hair follicles (*see* Chapter 6). Clinically, hairs are often lost and plugs develop in the follicular orifices. The condition may be associated with a cutaneous T-cell lymphoma.

- Hirsutism can be 'normal' in women but appropriate investigations should be considered if there is any doubt as to causes (endocrinological problem).
- Androgenetic alopecia affects both men and women. Temporal recession is characteristic in men while in women hair loss is more prominent on the crown.
- Cicatricial alopecia is scalp hair loss with loss of follicles and scarring.
- Alopecia areata is characterized by circular patches of hair loss and exclamation-mark hairs and is thought to be an autoimmune process.

DISORDERS OF THE NAILS

CHANGES OF TEXTURE AND SHAPE

Nails are subject to repeated trauma in normal daily life. It is hardly surprising, therefore, that they may be texturally abnormal or become physically damaged as a consequence. However, there are some changes that are worthy of specific mention because they are encountered frequently or because they represent significant pathology:

- Lamellar dystrophy — the nails split and flake horizontally (**Fig. 9.15**). This change is relatively common in the middle-aged. There are no significant systemic associations in the vast majority of patients.
- Onychogryphosis — the nails become grossly thickened and distorted (**Fig. 9.16**).
- Brittleness — some people complain that their nails are brittle. This is usually an ageing change.

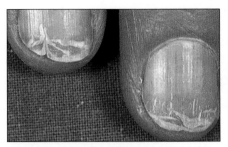

Fig. 9.15 *Lamellar nail dystrophy.*

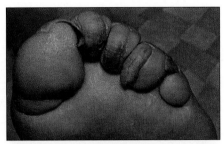

Fig. 9.16 *Onychogryphosis.*

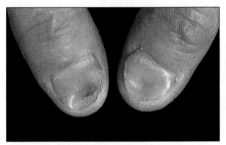

Fig. 9.17 *Koilonychia. This woman's mother and daughter had similar nails.*

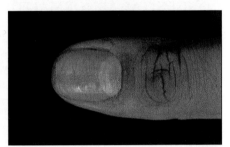

Fig. 9.18 *Median nail dystrophy. There are horizontal ridges down the centre of the nail — sometimes known as washboard nail. The appearance is due to habitual minor trauma to the paronychium.*

- Koilonychia — is a classical sign of iron deficiency (**Fig. 9.17**) and is more commonly seen as an inherited tendency.
- Median nail dystrophy — a habit-tic of 'fiddling' with the central paronychial area can lead to permanent nail-plate changes (**Fig. 9.18**). Very rarely, a primary defect results in similar, but more dramatic, changes.
- Pits — seen in psoriasis (*see* Chapter 4) and alopecia areata. Coarse dents and ridges may occur in the eczemas.
- Beau's lines — arrested nail growth, due to systemic illness or upset, may lead to a horizontal depression (**Fig. 9.19**). Occasionally, the nails may be lost temporarily.
- Clubbing — this is really an expansion of the finger-end, but is an important sign of malignancy, and of liver and cardiopulmonary disease.
- Onycholysis — lifting of the nail plate is common in psoriasis (*see* Chapter 5) and fungal infections (*see* Chapter 3). It may occur as an isolated phenomenon or, rarely, may be seen in thyrotoxicosis.
- Leuconychia — white marks in the nails are almost universal. Occasionally, longitudinal streaks are seen, which may be a feature of Darier's disease (*see* Chapter 11). Pale nails are a sign of hypoalbuminaemia (*see* Chapter 8).
- Yellow nails — fungal infections and onycholysis (*see* above) give rise to a yellow colour. The yellow-nail syndrome is discussed on page 337.
- Blue nails — some drugs (e.g. antimalarials) may cause blue colouration of the nails. Blue lunulae are seen in Wilson disease.
- Blue-green nails — pseudomonal infection of the nails.
- Black areas — an important sign of subungual melanoma (*see* Chapter 4).

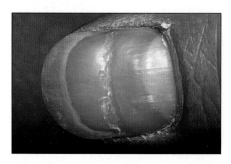

Fig. 9.19 *Beau's lines.*

CONGENITAL ABNORMALITIES OF THE NAILS

Almost any change may occur as a developmental defect, from relatively trivial abnormalities to complete absence of all nails. **Figure 9.20** lists some important congenital abnormalities — including paronychia congenita (**Fig. 9.21**) and dystrophy of the great toenail (**Fig. 9.22**) — and the syndromes in which some occur.

Congenital abnormalities of the nails	
Ectodermal dysplasias	*see* Chapter 11
Pachyonychia congenita	Wedge-shaped nails (*see* Fig. 9.21); associated palmoplantar keratoderma; oral leukoplakia; cysts (in type II); mental retardation (in type IV)
Palmoplantar keratodermas	*see* Chapter 11
Dystrophy of the great toenail	Isolated dystrophy and malalignment of great toenails (*see* Fig. 9.22)
Nail–patella syndrome	Hypoplastic nails (especially of thumbs); triangle lunalae, absent or rudimentary patellae, renal anomalies

Fig. 9.20 *Congenital abnormalities of the nails.*

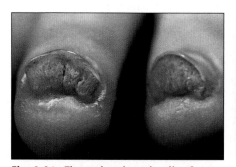

Fig. 9.21 *The wedge-shaped nails of pachyonychia congenita.*

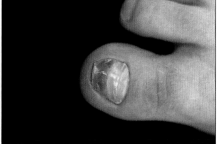

Fig. 9.22 *Great-toenail dystrophy.*

NAIL CHANGES ASSOCIATED WITH ACQUIRED DISEASE

The various nail changes and associated conditions are described at the beginning of this section. The nail changes of psoriasis and lichen planus are discussed in Chapter 5. Those seen in alopecia areata are illustrated in Figure 9.14e. There are a number of other conditions with relatively characteristic nail changes which deserve specific mention.

The yellow-nail syndrome

The yellow-nail syndrome is seen almost exclusively in adults. The nails in this disorder are overcurved, yellow, and hardly grow (**Fig. 9.23**). Patients notice a gradual change in their nails. However, once the changes are established, the nails remain unchanged for the rest of the patient's life. There are a number of important associations: lymphoedema, pleural effusions, and bronchiectasis. This syndrome has also been described in AIDS.

Trachyonychia and twenty-nail dystrophy

Children occasionally present with an onset of roughness (trachyonychia) that affects all twenty nails — although not always all at once (**Fig. 9.24**). The appearances are very similar to those seen when there is very extensive pitting, and some children have had, have, or will develop, alopecia areata. The histology in some instances is lichenoid.

Exostoses and other space-occupying lesions of the nail bed

Any tumour or mass beneath the nail may cause it to lift from its base. One very common lesion is an exostosis of the terminal phalanx (**Fig. 9.25**), which can easily be seen on X-ray. Surgical excision cures the problem. Other tumours may also develop under the nail. Melanoma has been discussed in Chapter 4. Naevi can arise in the nail bed and give rise to longitudinal brown streaks. Glomus tumours, although rare, are also classically found in the nails. They are usually exquisitely painful.

Paronychial disorders

Acute paronychia (or 'whitlow') is usually due to a staphylococcal infection. Herpetic infections may occur in the periungual area, as may warts. Large masses of viral wart in the paronychium can be a real nuisance and are very difficult to treat.

Ingrowing toenails are painful and unpleasant. They are due to lateral overcurvature of the nails, with the edges digging into the paronychial tissue, and cause chronic or acute-on-chronic sepsis. Wedge excisions may help, but complete nail-plate ablation may be required.

Chronic swelling and inflammation of the paronychium (**Fig. 9.26**) is often due to a combination of factors. Repeated damage and friction from occupational activities (packing, washing up, catering), especially if associated with damp conditions, predispose to the development of chronic paronychia. Candidal superinfection may also be important.

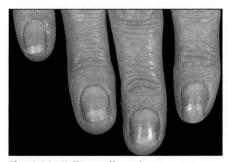

Fig. 9.23 *Yellow-nail syndrome.*

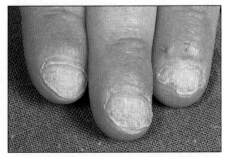

Fig. 9.24 *Twenty-nail dystrophy. This girl's nails cleared spontaneously after about 3 years.*

337

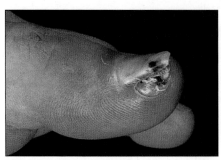

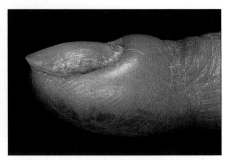

Fig. 9.25 *An exostosis was clearly visible on X-ray of this man's toe.*

Fig. 9.26 *Typical chronic paronychia.*

Treatment is very difficult. Gloves often make matters worse by causing the hands to sweat. Anti-candidal agents may help, but the condition frequently persists, despite the best endeavours of patient and physician alike.

Myxoid cysts

Another common presentation is of a small lump (or lumps) near the nail (or nails) of either hands or feet. If punctured, these exude a clear, gelatinous fluid. There is often a longitudinal depression in the nail (**Fig. 9.27**).

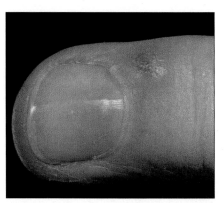

Fig. 9.27 *A slightly inflamed myxoid cyst with a depressed proximal nail and a longitudinal groove in the nail plate.*

- Nails are subject to repeated trauma in normal daily life and often become texturally abnormal or damaged, but some changes may represent significant pathology (e.g. clubbing or subungal pigmentation).
- Nail changes occur in a range of developmental defects from the 'trivial' to complete absence of all nails.
- Acute paronychia (or 'whitlow') is usually due to a staphylococcal infection; chronic paronychia can be associated with candidal infection.
- Any tumour or mass beneath the nail may cause it to lift from its base.

chapter 10

Disorders of Pigmentation

NORMAL PIGMENTATION

Normal melanization and pigmentary changes are also discussed briefly in Chapter 1.

Humans produce two main types of pigment: the dark granules known as eumelanin and the red pigment phaeomelanin. The main agent responsible for the colour of skin — hair, and eyes is eumelanin. The amount of eumelanin present in these structures is genetically determined, although, as mentioned in Chapter 1, exposure to ultraviolet radiation increases the amount of pigment concentrated in keratinocytes and causes a darkening of the skin — the much-glorified tan.

The result of the normal operation of the genetic processes controlling pigmentation is a range of complexions, conventionally, but somewhat arbitrarily, classified by Fitzpatrick into six 'skin types':

I   genetically 'white' but burns easily, never tans.

II genetically 'white' but burns easily, tans with difficulty.

III genetically 'white' but burns occasionally, tans well.

IV genetically 'white' but tans well, never burns.

V   genetically brown (Asian — Indo-Asian, Chinese, Japanese).

VI black (Afro-Caribbean).

Each of these 'skin types' will be accompanied, in the normal course of events, by appropriate hair and eye colour. Above and beyond this, the presence or absence of phaeomelanin modifies the phenotype by adding or removing a reddish hue to or from the hair. This is most commonly seen in fair-skinned individuals who often also have greenish eyes and many freckles (ephelides — see Chapter 4).

It is normal for the level of pigmentation to increase a little as the individual matures. Hair, of course, may cease to be pigmented quite early in life (*see* Chapter 9).

These mechanisms may be altered by genetic defects or acquired disease processes. In essence, there are two types of pigmentary disturbance: those with increased (hyper-) pigmentation and those with reduced (hypo-) or no pigmentation.

It is important to note, however, that skin colour may be altered by pigments other than melanin. Exogenously applied materials are often used deliberately, both on the surface of the skin (make-up and decorative paints) and within the skin (tattoos — *see* Chapter 1). The skin also takes on the colour of some ingested pigments (e.g. carotenes) and may be coloured by endogenously produced, non-melanin pigments such as bilirubin and haemosiderin, the breakdown product of haemoglobin.

Alteration to the 'normal' range of pigmentation has major social and psychological effects.

HYPERPIGMENTATION

CONGENITAL CAUSES

Figure 10.1 lists some important congenital disorders in which hyperpigmentation is a significant feature, and a brief account of these will be given here and in Chapter 11.

Congenital disorders associated with hyperpigmentation	
Freckles (ephelides) (Chapter 4)	
Syndromes featuring lentiginoses **(*see* Fig. 10.2)**	
Neurofibromatosis	Café-au-lait macules; Axillary freckling
Incontinentia pigmenti	Whorled pigmentary streaks
McCune–Albright syndrome	Brown patches with sharply demarcated margins
Xeroderma pigmentosum	
Xeroderma pigmentosum variant	Increasing freckles, lentigines, and pigmentation
Dowling–Degos disease∗	Reticulate pigmentation; Comedone-like lesions
Reticulate acral pigmentation∗	Similar changes to Dowling–Degos, but more acrally distributed
Becker's naevus (usually only ppears in adolescence)	Brown, hairy area over upper trunk/shoulder

∗There is considerable overlap between these two 'syndromes', and they may represent a spectrum of changes in one disorder.

Fig 10.1 *Congenital disorders associated with hyperpigmentation.*

Freckles are, as mentioned already, extremely common and represent a phenotypic variation on normal cutaneous pigmentation (*see* Chapter 4).

Lentigines are discrete, flat, permanent, pigmented areas that may occur in isolation as an acquired phenomenon (*see* Chapter 4), but are also seen as part of some rare multisystem congenital syndromes. The cardinal features of the most important of these are listed in **Figure 10.2**, and the clinical features of one, Peutz–Jeghers syndrome, are illustrated in **Figure 10.3**.

Incontinentia pigmenti (or Bloch–Sulzberger disease) is a rare X-linked disorder (*see also* Chapters 7 and 11). The pigmentary anomalies left by the inflammatory lesions follow Blaschko's lines.

Pigmented areas known as café-au-lait macules are one of the hallmarks of neurofibromatosis (**Fig. 10.4**). These are not unique to neurofibromatosis, however — it is not unusual for a child to have one or two such areas without any other abnormality, and similar lesions are sometimes seen in tuberous sclerosis (Chapter 11).

The McCune–Albright syndrome is another rare congenital disorder. Very striking brown patches with sharply demarcated borders (**Fig. 10.5**) are seen in association with polyostotic fibrous dysplasia and, in girls, with precocious puberty.

Xeroderma pigmentosum and its less drastic variant are discussed in Chapter 11. Dowling–Degos disease and reticulate acral pigmentation (of Kitamura) are probably variants of the same disorder. Both are extremely rare. As the second name implies, there is an increasing tendency to develop reticulate pigmented areas (**Fig. 10.6**). The distribution may be different in different family pedigrees.

Becker's naevus has been discussed in Chapter 4.

Syndromes in which multiple lentigines are seen	
LEOPARD syndrome	**L**entigines; **E**CG abnormalities; **O**cular hypertelorism; **P**ulmonary stenosis; **A**bnormal genitalia; **R**etardation of growth; **D**eafness
NAME syndrome	**N**aevi; **A**trial myxomas; **M**yxomas of skin; **E**phelides
LAMB syndrome	**L**entigines; **A**trial myxoma; **M**ucocutaneous myxoma; **B**lue naevi
Peutz–Jeghers syndrome	Orofacial lentigines; lentigines on hands and feet; intestinal polyposis (with an increased risk of malignancy) (*see* Fig. 10.3)

Fig. 10.2 *Syndromes in which multiple lentigines are seen.*

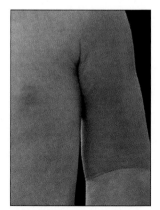

Fig. 10.3 *Peutz–Jeghers syndrome. This woman had multiple lentigines around the mouth and on the hands and feet.*

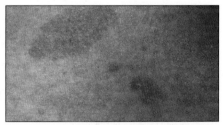

Fig. 10.4 *Café-au-lait macules on the trunk of a child with neurofibromatosis.*

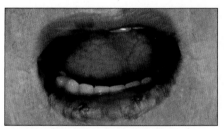

Fig. 10.5 *McCune–Albright syndrome. There is a clearly demarcated darker area on the inner aspect of this little boy's arm.*

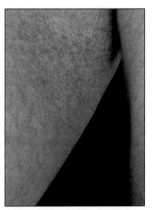

Fig. 10.6 *Dowling–Degos disease, showing reticulate pigmentation.*

ACQUIRED CAUSES

Some causes of acquired hyperpigmentation are listed in **Figure 10.7**.

By no means all hyperpigmentation is due to excess melanin (*see* Fig. 10.7).

Some causes of acquired hyperpigmentation	
Hypermelanosis	Postinflammatory hyperpigmentation, chloasma, poikiloderma of Civatte, Addison's disease, chronic renal disease, endogenous or exogenous excess of ACTH or ACTH-like agents, pregnancy, haemochromatosis, dermal melanocytosis (*see* Chapter 4), melanoma
Haemosiderosis	Ecchymoses and petechiae, stasis changes (*see* Chapter 8), pigmented purpuric eruptions (*see* Chapter 8), haemochromatosis
Hyperbilirubinaemia	Cholestasis, haemolysis
Carotenaemia	Idiopathic (enzyme deficiency), myxoedema, pernicious anaemia, exogenous consumption (e.g. 'fake tans'; photoprotective therapy in porphyrias)
Drugs and chemicals	Silver (argyria): slate grey chrysiasis (gold): blue–grey bismuthia (bismuth): blue–grey mepacrine: yellow minocycline: slate blue–black chloroquine: blue–black
Miscellaneous	Urticaria pigmentosa (*see* Chapter 4), confluent and reticulate papillomatosis (Gougerot–Carteaud), pityriasis versicolor (*see* Chapter 3)

Fig. 10.7 *Some causes of acquired hyperpigmentation*

One of the commonest causes of hypermelanosis is postinflammatory hyperpigmentation. This is extremely common following trauma to the skin and in those inflammatory skin disorders that disrupt the epidermis, especially the basal layer (e.g. lichen planus, discoid lupus erythematosus). The appearance is of a dusky, rather ill-defined pigmentation in the distribution of previous cutaneous inflammation (**Fig. 10.8**). Patients with darker skins are often more severely affected and may need much reassurance that lesions will fade in time.

Chloasma (melasma) is also extremely common. Increased pigmentation is typically seen across the forehead (**Fig. 10.9a**) and on the cheeks, upper lip, and chin (**Fig. 10.9b**). It is seen much more frequently in women than in men and may occur spontaneously or be associated with pregnancy or oestrogen consumption. Some patients benefit from the use of agents that hypopigment the skin, notably azaleic acid and hydroquinone (usually in a mixture as first described by Kligman or a modified version thereof: hydroquinone 2% + retinoic acid and dexamethasone). The effects are, however, unpredictable, and may make matters worse. The areas darken in the sun, therefore sun protection may help to reduce the cosmetic impact.

Poikiloderma of Civatte is a diagnostic label given to a change seen on the sides of the neck, especially in fair-skinned women. The skin becomes slightly mottled and rather reddened. The changes appear to be due largely to chronic sun damage, but perfumes may play a role. Similar changes may spread onto the face.

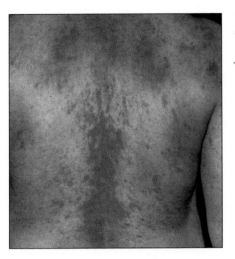

Fig. 10.8 *Post-inflammatory hyperpigmentation.* *This Asian man was left with widespread pigmentary changes following lichen planus.*

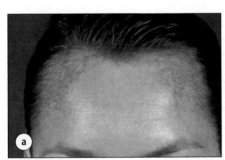 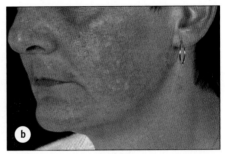

Fig. 10.9 *Chloasma —* (a) *hyperpigmentation around the hairline;* **(b)** *extensive changes on the face.*

The pigmentation associated with Addison's disease has been discussed (*see* page 300). Similar changes may occur with adrenocorticotrophic hormone (ACTH)-secreting tumours, or with exogenous ACTH or ACTH-like substances, because of their melanocyte-stimulating hormone (MSH)-like actions on melanocytes.

As mentioned in Chapter 8, pregnant women usually notice some increase in pigmentation, especially of the nipples and the linear alba (which becomes nigra), and chloasma is common.

The pigmentation of haemochromatosis is interesting because not only is there iron in the skin but there is also a marked increase in melanization, especially over light-exposed sites.

Very rarely, a patient with disseminated melanoma may develop widespread, deep pigmentation.

Haemosiderin is deposited in the skin in any situation in which red cells are extravasated and break down: bruises, petechiae, stasis changes, and capillaritis.

Carotenes are naturally occurring pigments. One of the commonest, b-carotene, is found in carrots, peppers, and many other orange or yellow fruits and vegetables. Some people have a relative deficiency of the hepatic enzyme responsible for metabolizing b-carotene and find that their skin becomes tinged with yellow or orange pigment, especially if they consume large quantities of carotene-containing foods. This is harmless, as is the similar colouration associated with myxoedema, pernicious anaemia, and deliberate treatment with high-dose b-carotene (which is, among other things, a useful photoprotective agent in erythropoietic protoporphyria). The distribution of the pigmentation is characteristic: palms and soles are typically noticeably high-coloured, as is the area around the nose and mouth. The sclerae, however, are spared, distinguishing carotenaemia from jaundice.

Several drugs and chemicals can pigment the skin: for example, **Figure 10.10** shows a woman who had been taking high-dose minocycline for 18 months (as a successful treatment for pyoderma gangrenosum). In some instances, the pigmentation with such chemicals is due solely to deposition of the material in the skin (e.g. argyria, chrysiasis); however, in others, there is a more complex chemical reaction, resulting in the formation of drug–melanin compounds (e.g. chloroquine, minocycline).

Urticaria pigmentosa, in which multiple pigmented lesions are due to accumulations of mast cells, is discussed in Chapter 6.

Confluent and reticulate papillomatosis of Gougerot–Carteaud is a rare disorder of unknown aetiology which is often difficult to distinguish from (and may indeed be related to) widespread hyperpigmenting pityriasis versicolor (*see* Chapter 3). Lesions are most common on the trunk and in the axillary regions (**Fig. 10.11**).

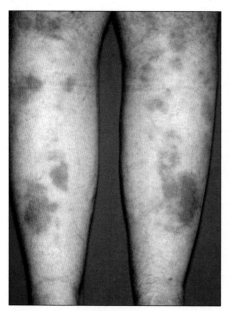

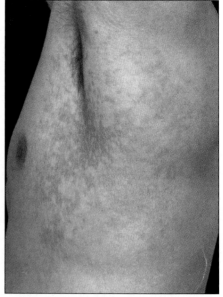

Fig. 10.10 *Pigmentation on the lower legs due to minocycline.* Minocycline deposition may also occur in areas of scarring.

Fig. 10.11 *Confluent and reticulate papillomatosis, showing scaly, reticulate, hyperpigmented patches on the trunk.*

REDUCED OR ABSENT PIGMENTATION

CONGENITAL CAUSES

Again, some of the more important congenital causes of reduced pigmentation are discussed in their own right in Chapter 11. However, **Figure 10.12** lists conditions that may need to be considered in the differential diagnosis of reduced or absent pigmentation in an infant or child.

Congenital causes of reduced or absent pigmentation	
Generalized loss of pigment	Oculocutaneous albinism tyrosinase-negative tyrosinase-positive Phenylketonuria
Patchy loss of pigment	Piebaldism, Waardenburg's syndrome, Tuberous sclerosis, Hypochromic naevi, Incontinentia pigmenti achromians (of Ito)

Fig. 10.12 *Congenital causes of reduced or absent pigmentation.*

The term albinism is applied to a group of genetic disorders in which the normal enzyme pathways involved in the production of melanin are defective. There are many variants but, broadly, patients may be grouped into those in whom tyrosine is absent and those in whom it is present but defective or in whom the defect occurs later in the chain of critical reactions. Many of the rarer types occur only in specific ethnic groups, many of which have traditionally been subject to isolation and in-breeding. Most are inherited as autosomal recessive traits. In some very rare syndromes, occultocutaneous albinism is associated with other defects (e.g. bleeding in the Hermansky–Pudlak syndrome, and recurrent infections in the Chediak–Higashi syndrome).

In tyrosinase-negative albinism (**Fig. 10.13a**), the skin is pink and remains pale throughout life. The eyes are severely affected, with complete absence of pigment and marked nystagmus. Skin cancers are very common in patients with this disorder living in sunny countries.

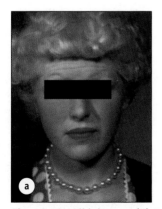 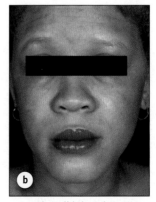

Fig. 10.13 *Albinism — (a) tyrosinase-negative albinism (courtesy of Dr D A Burns); (b) tyrosinase-positive albinism in a young Afro-Caribbean girl.*

Patients with tyrosinase-positive albinism are less pale. The skin in Afro-Caribbean patients is, in fact, quite frequently yellowish-brown (**Fig. 10.13b**). The hair is yellow and the eyes may show some pigmentation. Furthermore, the skin, hair, and eyes darken gradually as the patient ages. However, nystagmus and ocular problems are still common and skin cancers occur more frequently than among individuals of the same ethnic background but with normal pigmentary mechanisms.

Children with phenylketonuria also have pale skin, very fair hair, and pale eyes, because of defects in melanin production. Screening at birth enables early treatment, and, as such, has virtually eliminated the serious consequences of this disorder in Western societies.

The term piebaldism is used to describe the congenital occurrence of patchy depigmentation in an otherwise normal child. The white patches are indistinguishable from vitiligo (*see* page 347), but remain unchanged throughout life. One common form is the presence of a white forelock. Piebaldism associated with deafness and minor facial deformities is called Waardenberg's syndrome (gene locus 2q35, mutation in PAX3 gene which affects tyrosinase activation). Both this and isolated piebaldism (gene locus 4q12, mutations in the protooncongene which encodes a transmembrane tyrosine kinase) are inherited as autosomal dominant traits.

Pale macules are one of the key markers of tuberous sclerosis (**Fig. 10.14**), the main discussion of which appears in Chapter 11. These may be lanceolate (ash-leaf-shaped) or more irregular. Similar lesions may occur in isolation, when they are known as achromic naevi.

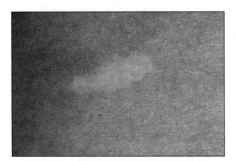

Fig. 10.14 *Tuberous sclerosis — a typical pale macule on the trunk of an infant.*

Incontinentia pigmenti achromians of Ito is a rare disorder in which areas of whorled hypopigmentation are present at birth. There are no preceding phases as in Bloch–Sulzberger disease (*see also* Chapter 11).

With the exception of phenylketonuria, there is no satisfactory treatment for any of these genetic disorders other than symptomatic control of associated problems and sun protection as appropriate.

ACQUIRED CAUSES

Acquired hypopigmentation (leucoderma) is a common problem in skin clinics. In some ethnic groups, leucoderma (usually due to vitiligo) is associated with severe stigmatization and has major cultural connotations. The most important causes are listed in **Figure 10.15**.

Acquired causes of hypopigmentation

Autoimmune
  Auto-immune vitiligo
  Sutton's halo naevus (*see* Chapter 4)
Post-inflammatory hypopigmentation
  Idiopathic guttate hypomelanosis
  Pityriasis alba
  Pityriasis lichenoides chronica
  Mycosis fungoides
  Sarcoidosis
Infections (*see* Chapter 3)
  Leprosy (indeterminate and tuberculoid)
  Pityriasis versicolor
  Pinta
  Postkala-azar dermal leishmaniasis
Drugs and chemicals
  Occupational leukoderma, self-inflicted

Fig. 10.15 *Acquired causes of hypopigmentation.*

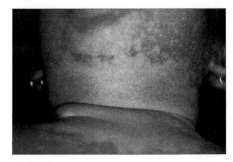

Fig. 10.16 *This Indo-Asian child has marked post-inflammatory hypopigmentation following infantile seborrhoeic dermatitis.*

Postinflammatory hypopigmentation is due to alteration of the normal pigment balance in the immediate aftermath of an inflammatory episode (**Fig. 10.16**). This will usually settle down and the skin colour will return to normal unless the damage is very severe. Many inflammatory disorders may result in temporary pigment loss. Psoriasis is particularly prone to do so, especially if the patient is treated with ultraviolet radiation. However, in more major trauma, including burns or freezing, the melanocytes may be permanently destroyed and the depigmentation may persist indefinitely.

Vitiligo is a very important condition and is the major acquired cause of widespread pigment loss. The condition is thought to be due to an autoimmune assault on the melanocytes, similar to that believed to occur in alopecia areata (*see* Chapter 9). Also, as in alopecia areata, organ-specific autoimmunity is more common in patients with vitiligo. Alopecia areata and vitiligo may occur together.

The characteristic appearance of vitiligo is of complete depigmentation of areas of the skin, without any other evidence of disease – in particular, scaling and inflammation are absent (**Fig. 10.17a**).

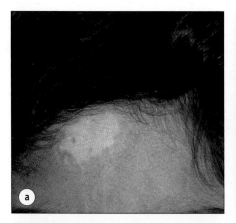

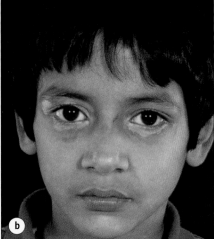

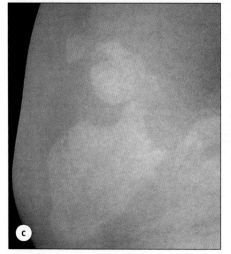

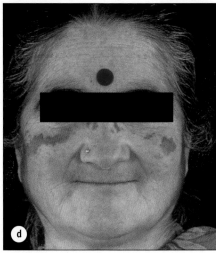

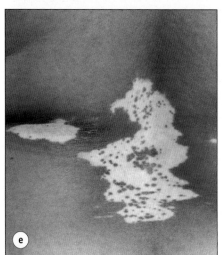

Fig. 10.17 Vitiligo — (a) *a patch of typical vitiligo on the forehead;* **(b)** *vitiligo is often symmetrical and the eyelids are frequently affected;* **(c)** *asymmetrical or segmental vitiligo;* **(d)** *this Indo-Asian woman's vitiligo is almost universal — only a few brown patches of normal-coloured skin remain;* **(e)** *repigmenting vitiligo — note the appearance of pigmentation in small spots and islands in the centre of the affected areas.*

The lesions are frequently remarkably symmetrical (**Fig. 10.17b**), affecting the skin around the right and left eyes, limbs, and hands and feet almost equally. In some cases, however, localized asymmetrical patches are present, often affecting one segment of the body and nowhere else (**Fig. 10.17c**). At its most extreme, vitiligo can lead to universal, or almost universal, depigmentation (**Fig. 10.17d**).

As can be imagined, such appearances give rise to a great deal of distress and misery. Vitiliginous skin burns easily while the surrounding skin tans normally, hence the problem is often perceptibly worse in summer months or on sunny holidays. Patients are often desperate to find something that will help. In children, repigmentation is comparatively common and a relatively positive prognosis is reasonable. When repigmenting, it is most common for areas of normal colour to return around hair follicles in the patches and for these spots to spread and coalesce (**Fig. 10.17e**), as well as for the edges to creep inwards. In adults, such repigmentation activity occurs much less commonly, but some patients respond to topical corticosteroids and these are worth a trial. PUVA can be effective, but it is very slow to act. In India, some dermatologists treat vitiligo as a systemic disease and claim success with high-dose steroids and other immunomodulators.

Many patients, sadly, have to settle for cosmetic camouflage and sun protection.

As mentioned in Chapter 4, changes identical to vitiligo may occur in the skin surrounding an apparently banal melanocytic naevus (and, rarely, a melanoma). Patients may also develop typical vitiligo on other areas.

Patients are occasionally encountered in whom multiple small 'guttate' areas of hypopigmentation appear to spread inexorably over the body surface. In the absence of another cause, the term idiopathic guttate hypomelanosis is applied here.

Pityriasis alba is another very common cause of hypopigmentation encountered in dermatological practice. The lesions are most typically seen on the cheeks (**Fig. 10.18**) and the upper outer arms, and become more noticeable in the summer months. The changes other than hypopigmentation can be very subtle, with only very fine scale (*see* **Fig. 10.18a**), or can be more obviously eczematous (*see* **Fig. 10.18b**). The histology is of a very mild dermatitis, and the condition usually responds to mild topical steroids, or moisturizers, or both. It also seems to improve at or around puberty and is quite uncommon in adults.

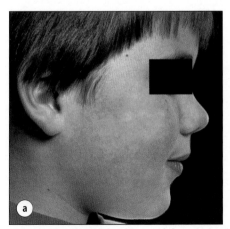
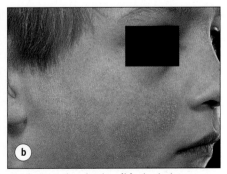

Fig. 10.18 *Pityriasis alba* — *(a) typical pale patches on the cheeks; (b) the lesions are sometimes very scaly.*

There have been reports of patients with pityriasis lichenoides chronica, mycosis fungoides, or sarcoidosis in whom the clinical presentation is of hypopigmented, macular or slightly scaly lesions.

The infective causes of hypopigmentation are discussed in Chapter 3. It is clearly important to differentiate leprosy from other causes of pale skin in a patient from an endemic area. Systemic leishmaniasis (kala-azar) may produce widespread, patchy hypopigmentation.

Certain drugs and chemicals can cause hypopigmentation, too. Outbreaks of whitening of the skin have occurred in workers exposed to the monobenzyl ether of hydroquinone and substituted phenols. Hydroquinone (which, as mentioned on page 342, is the active ingredient of a depigmenting lotion) is also available in various over-the-counter formulations of skin-lighteners. This chemical can have unpredictable effects, leading to bizarre, permanent hypopigmentation in some unfortunate patients.

- Two types of pigmentary disturbance: increased (hyper-) pigmentation and reduced (hypo-) pigmentation.
- Lentigines are discrete, flat, permanent, pigmented areas that may occur in isolation as an acquired phenomenon, but are also seen as part of some rare multisystem congenital syndromes.
- Pigmented areas known as café-au-lait macules are one of the hallmarks of neurofibromatosis.
- One of the commonest acquired causes of hypermelanosis is postinflammatory hyperpigmentation following trauma or disorders such as lichen planus.
- Several drugs and chemicals can pigment the skin (e.g. chloroquine, minocycline).
- Albinism occurs in genetic disorders in which the normal enzyme pathways involved in the production of melanin are defective.
- Leucoderma (usually due to vitiligo) is associated with severe stigmatization in some ethnic groups.
- Treatment of vitiligo is generally unsatisfactory and many patients have to settle for cosmetic camouflage and sun protection.

chapter 11

Genodermatoses

INTRODUCTION

In many ways it seems artificial to separate some dermatological conditions into a section which suggests that those covered in it, and only those, are genetically determined, because this is not the case. Genetic factors play a role in a huge number of dermatoses. There are also a great many genetically determined syndrome complexes in which cutaneous abnormalities are important features. Many of the skin disorders that have already been covered in the other chapters have genetic components (**Fig. 11.1**), but they have, in our judgement, been more appropriately dealt with alongside conditions with similar clinical, histological, or other features. In this chapter, we will cover some of the other dermatoses in which genetics play a major role — however, because of limitations of space, we have had to restrict ourselves to those that we judge to be the most important. Inevitably, the reader will want to turn to a fuller text for a more detailed account of those disorders we do address, and to search for many others that we have had to leave out.

INCONTINENTIA PIGMENTI (BLOCH–SULZBERGER DISEASE)

Incontinentia pigmenti (familial or IP2) and hypomelanosis of Ito (sporadic or IP1 — *see* page 346) — are examples of genetic mosaicism, where some clones of cells express genetic information on one chromosome of a pair, whereas other clones express it on the other. In the skin, disorders exhibiting genetic mosaicism often present with lesions that follow Blaschko's lines.

- Lesions are present in early infancy.
- Vesicular initially (**Fig. 11.2a**) and may be confused with a herpetic infection or other causes of blistering.
- Vesiculation settles leaving warty papules and plaques (**Fig. 11.2b**) which gradually flatten and disappear.
- All that is left in the end are streaks and whorls of hyperpigmentation (**Fig. 11.2c**).
- Some children with incontinentia pigmenti have other abnormalities:
  - anodontia, or peg-shaped teeth (**Fig. 11.2d**)
  - neurological delay and mental retardation
  - ocular anomalies (e.g. squint, cataract, optic atrophy).

Disorders with significant genetic factors covered elsewhere

Disorder	Gene	Chapter
Buschke–Ollendorff syndrome	Unknown	4
Atopic dermatitis	Multiple, including SPINK5, fc εRI-β, PHF11	5
Psoriasis	Multiple, including HLA-C, SLC9ARI, NAT9, PAPTOR, SLC12A8	5
Epidermolysis bullosa	Multiple, including keratin genes (EB simplex), laminin5, type xxvii collagen, α6β4 integrins (junctional), type vii collagen (dystrophic)	7
Hailey–Hailey disease	ATP2C1	7
LEOPARD and other syndromes with multiple lentiginoses	PTPN11	10
McCune–Albright syndrome*	GNAS1	10
Dowling–Degos disease and reticulate acral pigmentation	None as yet identified	10
Albinism	Tyrosinase gene	10
Phenylketonuria	Phenylalanine hydroxylase	10

*NB Not Albright's hereditary osteodystrophy, in which patients have pseudohypoparathyroidism or pseudopseudohypoparathyroidism and may develop cutaneous osteomas; remarkably, both of Albright's syndromes appear to be due to defects at the same gene locus.

Fig. 11.1 *Disorders with significant genetic factors covered in other chapters.*

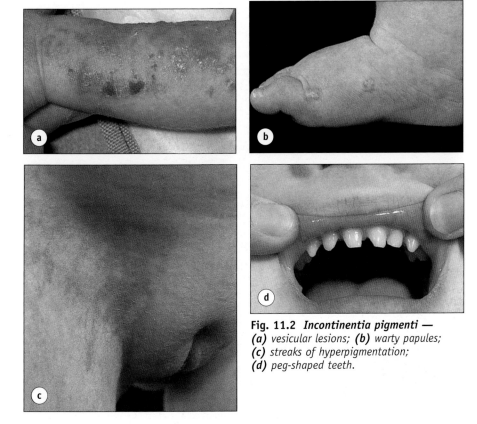

Fig. 11.2 *Incontinentia pigmenti —*
(a) vesicular lesions; (b) warty papules;
(c) streaks of hyperpigmentation;
(d) peg-shaped teeth.

The gene responsible for incontinentia pigmenti is the NEMO gene, located on the short arm of the X chromosome (Xq28) The disorder is usually lethal in normal XY males. Hypomelanosis of Ito is due to chromosomal aberration in the vicinity of the centromere and maps to Xp11.

These changes seem to be less common than was once thought. They may primarily be associated with the sporadic form of the disease, being less frequent in familial cases.

INCONTINENTIA PIGMENTI ACHROMIANS OR HYPOMELANOSIS OF ITO

Children (both boys and girls) present with whorls or streaks of hypopigmentation that follow Blaschko's lines, but with no preceding inflammatory component. There may be associated neurological, ocular, and skeletal defects.

ECTODERMAL DYSPLASIAS

There are a number of rare but important syndromes in which a variety of developmental anomalies of tissues derived from embryonic ectoderm are clustered together — over 120 have been described. The details of the clinical findings and inheritance of a few of the more important of these are listed in **Figure 11.3**. The conical incisor of a patient with hypohidrotic ectodermal dysplasia is shown in **Figure 11.4**.

Some of the ectodermal dysplasias	
Hidrotic ectodermal dysplasia*	Sparse, blonde hair, thickened nails, hyperkeratosis of palms and soles, mild mental retardation, normal sweating.
Hypohidrotic ectodermal dysplasia†‡	Partial or complete absence of sweat glands, few or no teeth, conical incisors (*see* Fig. 11.4), fine, sparse hair, thin nails, frontal bossing, saddle nose, maxillary hypoplasia, frequent infections.
Ectrodactyly–ectodermal dysplasia*	Lobster-claw deformity (syndactyly), sparse hair, abnormal teeth and nails, cleft lip and palate.
Orofaciodigital syndrome†§	Various oral, facial, and digital abnormalities.
Ankyloblepharon–ectodermal dysplasia*	Fusion of eyelids, sparse hair, hypohidrosis, cleft lip and palate, abnormal nails (may be absent).

*autosomal dominant
† autosomal recessive
‡ may also be X-linked recessive
§ may also be X-linked dominant (type I)

Fig. 11.3 *Some of the ectodermal dysplasias.*

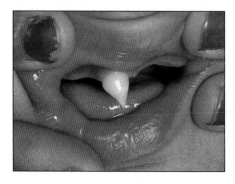

Fig. 11.4 *An isolated, conical incisor in a patient with hypohidrotic ectodermal dysplasia.*

GENETICS

In hidrotic ectodermal dysplasia the genetic defect is in GJB6, which codes for connexin-30, a gap protein important in communication between keratinocytes. The gene locus is 13q12. In hypohidrotic ectodermal dysplasia, the abnormality lies in the PKP1 gene, which codes for plakophilin 1, a desmosomal protein important in epidermal integrity. There is an X-linked form which is thought to be due to a mutation of the ectodysplasin A gene. Other genetic defects associated with forms of ectodermal dysplasia include: locus 7q11.2-q21.3 (ectrodactyly); CXORF5 gene at Xp22 (orofacialdigital syndrome type I); locus 3q27 — p63 (ankyloblepharon).

DISORDERS OF KERATINIZATION

A number of genetic diseases occur in which the process of keratinization is disordered in some way. Some are very rare, but some are common.

THE ICHTHYOSES

The ichthyoses are a group of genetically inherited conditions in which the epidermis is scaly and variably thickened. In some the changes are relatively mild, while in others they may be very troublesome.

Autosomal dominant ichthyosis vulgaris

Approximately 1 in 250 of the population have autosomal dominant ichthyosis vulgaris. The skin is generally rather 'dry' and flaky (**Fig. 11.5**). There is said to be an association with atopic dermatitis in about half of all patients, although this is difficult to quantify precisely since many patients with atopic dermatitis have similar skin changes. The changes are usually present at birth and persist throughout life. Emollients may help.

Gene: locus 1q21; reduced epidermal filaggrin and profilaggrin (responsible for intermediate filament assembly).

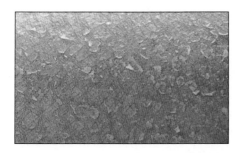

Fig. 11.5 *The typical fine scale of autosomal dominant ichthyosis vulgaris.*

X-Linked recessive ichthyosis vulgaris

An inherited deficiency of steroid sulphatase results in male children developing larger and darker scales than those found in the autosomal dominant form (**Fig. 11.6**), classically sparing the flexures. Some boys with this disorder also have corneal opacities. Steroid sulphatase, produced by the fetus, is required for the initiation of labour, and many pregnancies go beyond term and need induction.

Gene: ARSC1 gene, which encodes STS (arylsulphatase C).

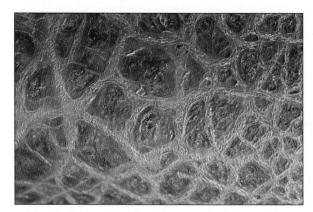

Fig. 11.6 *The scales in x-linked ichthyosis vulgaris are larger and much darker than they are in the autosomal dominant form.*

Bullous ichthyosiform erythroderma (or epidermolytic hyperkeratosis)

Bullous ichthyosiform is rare. Patients present with rather malodorous, red, scaly skin which blisters, particularly in infancy. In later life, there is, typically, a rippled hyperkeratosis over the knees and elbows, and a palmoplantar keratoderma. In some families, there is only a palmoplantar keratoderma. The disease is inherited as an autosomal dominant trait. Histologically, there is vacuolar degeneration of the mid-epidermis, a finding that is quite distinct from all the other ichthyoses and provides the basis for a simple way of confirming the diagnosis by skin biopsy.

Gene: Mutations in KRT1 and 10 (responsible for specific keratins).

Non-bullous ichthyosiform erythroderma and lamellar ichthyosis

There is some clinical overlap between non-bullous ichthyosiform erythroderma (NBIE) and lamellar ichthyosis — both are characterized by large, flat scales, but NBIE has comparatively more redness. Both are inherited as autosomal recessive conditions in most affected families. Both may also present in the collodion baby syndrome (*see* below).

Gene: TGM1 and lipoxygenase genes ALOX12B, ALOXE3.

Collodion baby and Harlequin fetus

Some infants are born with a tight membrane covering the whole body. This is known as the collodion baby syndrome. Although this membrane is shed in the weeks immediately after birth in most cases, the baby needs to be nursed with great care in the early days, with particular attention being paid to the eyes, because of ectropion, and to heat regulation and water loss. Most of the babies have an underlying ichthyotic disorder. The commonest is probably lamellar ichthyosis or NBIE, but some children have been described who have simple autosomal dominant ichthyosis vulgaris (**Fig. 11.7**).

Harlequin fetus is similar, but much more severe, and seems to be a separate entity, inherited in an autosomal recessive manner. Children only occasionally survive, and those that do require great efforts to be made on their behalf to avoid major complications, including life-threatening sepsis.

Rare ichthyoses and ichthyosis-associated syndromes

Figure 11.8 lists some of the rarer ichthyotic disorders, a few of which are associated with defects in other organ systems. Some children with severe immune deficiencies present with NBIE-like changes.

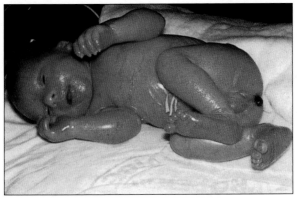

Fig. 11.7 Collodian baby. *The child is encased in a stiff membrane (courtesy of Dr D A Burns).*

Rare ichthyotic disorders	
Ichthyosis hystrix*	This term has been applied to a number of conditions, including linear or systematized epidermal naevi (these may represent mosaicism for non-bullous ichthyosiform erythroderma) and the 'porcupine men' — the Lambert family of Suffolk; there are no systemic features.
Netherton syndrome†	Various types of ichthyosis, most commonly ichthyosis linearis circumflexa (patches with a 'double-edged' scale), trichorrhexis invaginata ('bamboo hairs'), mental retardation, immune deficiency, aminoaciduria.
Refsum's disease†	Cerebellar ataxia, retinitis pigmentosa, peripheral neuropathy.
Sjögren–Larsson syndrome†	Mental retardation, spasticity.
Conradi–Hunerman syndrome (chondrodysplasia punctata)‡	Up to four types so far described — bony stippling of long bones (only seen in infancy), ichthyosiform erythroderma in early childhood, later follicular atrophoderma, alopecia — there may be severe dwarfism and mental retardation.

* autosomal dominant in the generalized conditions that bear this name
† autosomal recessive
‡ various inheritance patterns; the most severe form is autosomal recessive

Fig. 11.8 *Rare ichthyotic disorders*

Genes: Ichthyosis hystrix — keratin 1 mutation (locus 12q13); Netherton syndrome — 5q32, SPINK5; Refsum's — loci 8q31, 7q21-q22 (PEX1 or 2 genes); Sjogren Larsson — locus 17p11.2 (ALDh3 gene); Severe X-linked chondrodysplasia punctata — locus Xp22.3 (arylsulphatase).

PALMOPLANTAR KERATODERMA

Patients are commonly seen with congenital thickening of the palms and soles. The palmar and plantar surfaces are yellowish and may have a smooth or slightly roughened surface. This process may affect the whole surface or be more localized (**Fig. 11.9**). Such changes may be associated with other cutaneous manifestations or may occur as an isolated phenomenon. **Figure 11.10** lists some of the more important forms, their implications and the genes responsible where known.

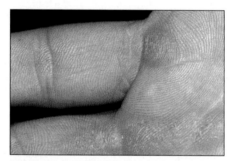

Fig. 11.9 *Localized form of palmoplantar keratoderma, showing yellowish, thickened plaques on the palm.*

DARIER'S DISEASE (KERATOSIS FOLLICULARIS)

Darier's disease is a relatively common genodermatosis in which crops of warty or greasy papules (**Fig. 11.11a**) usually begin to appear during childhood and gradually extend during adolescence. The underlying process is, histologically, one of dyskeratosis, with clefts and abnormal keratinocytes (known as grains and corps ronds) being present within the epidermis. The appearances resemble, to some extent, those seen in benign familial pemphigus (Hailey–Hailey disease — *see* Chapter 7).

Lesions can occur anywhere, but tend to be on the face — around the nose and mouth (**Fig. 11.11b**) and on the forehead, on the chest (**Fig. 11.11c**), and in the flexures, a distribution reminiscent of seborrhoeic dermatitis. The nails show characteristic white or red longitudinal streaks with 'V' notches (**Fig. 11.11d**). The dermatoglyphics are interrupted by small pits, and flat-topped warty papules are occasionally seen on the dorsa of the hands (clinically indistinguishable from acrokeratosis verruciformis of Hopf).

Patients with Darier's disease respond well to oral therapy with retinoid, but its use has to be balanced against the disadvantages, including hyperlipidaemia and teratogenicity. Darier's disease is an autosomal dominant condition.

Gene: locus 12q23-q24.1; ATP2A2 gene codes for sarcoplasmic endoplasmic reticulum calcium ATPase isoform 2 (SERCA2). This enzyme is critical for intracellular calcium transport and thus cell adhesion. Hailey–Hailey disease is caused by mutations in ATP2C1, which also codes for a calcium transporting ATPase (type 2c). This enzyme is magnesium dependent.

Palmoplantar keratodermas		
Form	Gene	Features
Diffuse (Unna-Thost)*	Locus 17q12-q21, keratin 9 and 16	Diffuse, sharp cut-off at wrists and heels, hyperkeratosis of knees/elbows, oral hyperkeratosis.
Localized/punctate*	Unknown	Usually no associated features, occasionally nail abnormalities.
Localized non-bullous icthyosiform erythroderma (NBIE)†	Unknown	Malodorous palmo-plantar thickening, no other features.
Howel-Evans†	Locus 17q25	Late onset diffuse, carcinoma of oesophagus.
Vohwinkel‡	Locus 1q21 (loricrin)	Diffuse with multiple pits, keratoses, constriction bands around digits.
Mal de Meleda§	8qter mutations in LSURO1 gene (SLURP1 protein)	Diffuse, hyperkeratotic patches on wrists and in flexures, abnormal nails.
Olmsted	Unknown	Painful, diffuse, hyperkeratotic plaques around mouth.
Papillon–Lefèvre§	Locus 11q14.1-q14.1 (cathepsin C gene)	Diffuse, red; periodontitis with loss of teeth.
Pachyonychia congenita	Keratins 6, 16, 17	see Chapter 9.

* autosomal dominant
† autosomal dominant or sporadic
‡ autosomal dominant or autosomal recessive
§ autosomal recessive

Fig. 11.10 *Palmoplantar keratodermas.*

KERATOSIS PILARIS AND KERATOSIS PILARIS ATROPHICANS

Keratosis pilaris is the term used to describe a very common inherited trait in which the hair follicles on the upper outer arms and on the thighs and cheeks have small, spiky projections (**Fig. 11.12a**). This is usually mild, but may be unsightly enough for patients to seek attention. Much less commonly, similar changes are associated with atrophy and loss of hair, a situation known as keratosis pilaris atrophicans. When this affects the scalp, the

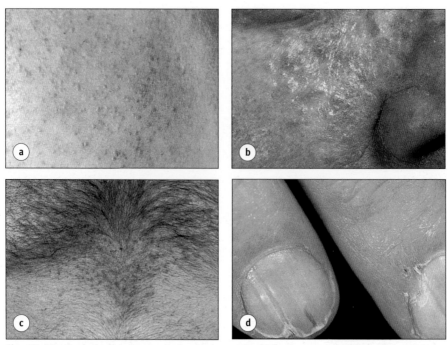

Fig. 11.11 *Darier's disease: typical greasy papules (a); the nasolabial area (b) and the chest (c) are sites of predilection; the typical nail changes (d).*

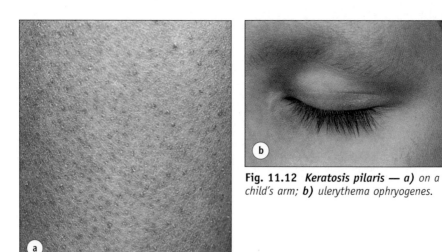

Fig. 11.12 *Keratosis pilaris — a) on a child's arm; b) ulerythema ophryogenes.*

term keratosis pilaris decalvans is used. Similar changes may affect the cheeks — leaving a reticulate, worm-like appearance (atrophoderma vermiculatum) — and the eyebrows (ulerythema ophryogenes — **Fig. 11.12b**).

Gene: ? locus18p.

FLEGEL DISEASE AND KYRLE DISEASE

Flegel disease (or hyperkeratosis lenticularis perstans) is a very rare, autosomal dominant condition in which hyperkeratotic papules appear on the limbs (**Fig. 11.13**). Similar lesions (but with a different histology) are seen in Kyrle disease (or hyperkeratosis follicularis et parafollicularis). Both conditions first present in adulthood.

Gene: unknown.

- Incontinentia pigmenti and hypomelanosis of Ito are examples of genetic mosaicism with lesions that present in early infancy, characteristically along Blaschko's lines.
- Ichthyoses are a group of genetically inherited conditions in which the epidermis is scaly and variably thickened.
- Palmoplantar keratoderma is characterized by congenital thickening of the palms and soles.
- Darier's disease is a relatively common genodermatosis in which crops of warty or greasy papules appear during childhood and extend during adolescence.
- Keratosis pilaris is a very common inherited trait in which hair follicles on the upper outer arms and on the thighs and cheeks have small, spiky projections.

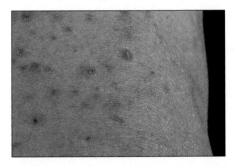

Fig. 11.13 *Flegel disease, showing reddish-brown, warty papules on the leg.*

BASAL CELL NAEVUS SYNDROME AND SYNDROMES ASSOCIATED WITH INCREASED SKIN CANCERS

Another autosomal dominant condition is Gorlin's, or the basal cell naevus, syndrome. In this disorder, multiple basal cell tumours (**Fig. 11.14a**) are associated with jaw cysts, hypertelorism, bifid ribs, palmar pits (**Fig. 11.14b**), and a variety of other changes.

Gene: locus9q31, 22.3; mutations in PATCHED, a tumour suppressor gene.

Bazex syndrome (follicular atrophoderma and basal cell carcinomas) is another rare, genetic disorder in which multiple basal cell carcinomas may occur. There is a characteristic pitted appearance of the dorsa of the hands, and of the elbows and face.

The dysplastic naevus syndrome is covered in Chapter 4.

Xeroderma pigmentosum (of which there are a number of subtypes, known as complementation groups) is due to a variety of defects of DNA repair, predominantly of excision enzymes. The less severe 'variant' is due to a defect of post-excision repair. Skin cancers occur at a very young age (*see also* Fig. 11.24).

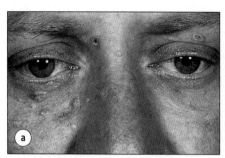

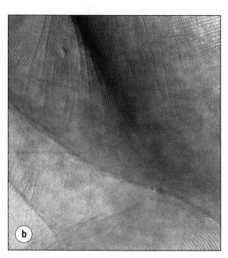

Fig. 11.14 *Gorlin's basal cell naevus syndrome — (a)* multiple basal cell carcinomas; *(b)* palmar pits.

NEUROFIBROMATOSIS

There are now known to be a number of genetic variants of neurofibromatosis (**Fig. 11.15** — *see also* Chapters 4 and 9).

Von Recklinghausen's disease (or NF-1) is the one that presents most frequently to the dermatologist.

Neurofibromatosis	
Von Recklinghausen's disease (NF-1)*†	see text
Acoustic neurofibromatosis (NF-2)*	VIIIth cranial nerve tumours, meningiomas, a few skin lesions.
Mixed central and peripheral (NF-3)	Multiple CNS tumours, skin lesions of NF-1.
Variant (NF-4)	Patients who are currently unclassifiable.
Segmental (NF-5)‡	Localized and segmental skin lesions; patients may have children with NF-1.

* autosomal dominant
† frequent new mutations
‡ mosaic?

Fig. 11.15 Neurofibromatosis

- Patients may have any or all of the following: café-au-lait patches (*see* Fig. 10.4), axillary freckles, cutaneous neurofibromas (**Fig. 11.16a**), and plexiform neuromas (**Fig. 11.16b**).
- Pigmented lesions in the iris (Lisch nodules) are also common, and other ocular lesions — notably retinoblastoma, glioma, and glaucoma — occur in some patients.
- Tumours may develop in the peripheral and central nervous system, and various skeletal anomalies have been described.
- Patients with NF-1 may also develop a variety of other tumours, including phaeochromocytoma, carcinoid tumours, and Wilms' tumour.
- Patients may or may not suffer from epilepsy and mental retardation.

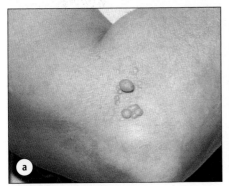

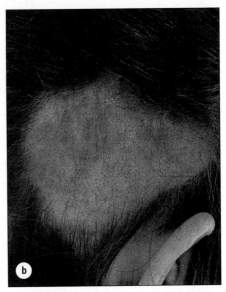

Fig. 11.16 *Neurofibromatosis —*
(a) typical neurofibromas; (b) a plexiform neuroma on the scalp.

The individual lesions can be removed, but this is usually not necessary except on cosmetic grounds. Rapidly growing lesions should be excised, as sarcomatous change can occur.

Tumours of the 8th cranial nerve, meningiomas, schwannomas, cataracts and small numbers of cutaneous lesions are seen in neurofibromatosis 2 (nf-2).

Occasionally, patients are encountered who have areas of skin in which lesions typical of neurofibromatosis are present but in whom the rest of the skin is normal. The term segmental neurofibromatosis is applied in such cases (*see* Fig. 11.15).

Patients with any form of neurofibromatosis need careful genetic counselling.

Gene: NF-1locus 17q11.2; NF-2 locus 22q12.2.

TUBEROUS SCLEROSIS

Another multisystem genetic disorder with cutaneous manifestations is tuberous sclerosis (epiloia).

- Hypopigmented macules (*see* Fig. 10.14) are often the first visible sign of the condition, although many patients present with fits in infancy and the pale patches are only then noticed (best seen under ultraviolet Wood's light).
- Patients later begin to develop angiofibromas (at one time erroneously labelled adenoma sebaceum) on the face (**Fig. 11.17a**), a connective tissue naevus (or Shagreen patch) on the trunk (**Fig. 11.17b**), and periungual fibromas (**Fig. 11.17c**).
- May be hamartomatous malformations in many organ systems, including the central nervous system, eyes, kidneys, heart, and lungs.

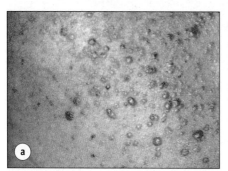
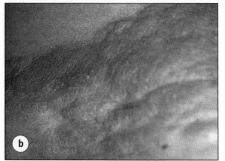
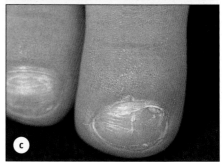

Fig. 11.17 *Tuberous sclerosis* —
(a) angiofibromas on the cheek (these were at one time called adenoma sebaceum); *(b)* Shagreen patch; *(c)* there is a small fibroma indenting the second toenail.

Tuberous sclerosis is an autosomal dominant trait, but the clinical features are very variable, even within families. As in neurofibromatosis, the disorder in many patients is said to represent new mutations.

Gene: 4 types currently known with genes at loci 16p13.3, 12q14 and 9q34.

DISORDERS OF CONNECTIVE TISSUE

There are several genetically determined diseases that are due to defects in the genes responsible for the production of collagens. They are often grouped together under the umbrella heading Ehlers–Danlos syndrome (**Fig. 11.18**). The clinical features are variable, but many of the disorders show a degree of skin laxity, or extensibility, or both, and joint hypermobility. Some are associated with serious complications.

Genes: a variety of genes are involved, but all are responsible for collagens, their precursors or coenzymes involved in the productionn of collagens.

Ehlers–Danlos syndrome		
Type	**Inheritance**	**Key clinical features**
IA/IB	AD	Skin fragility and hyperextensibility, easy bruising, atrophic scars, joint hypermobility.
II	AD	As above but less severe, mitral-valve prolapse.
III	AD	Marked joint hypermobility.
IV	AD or AR	Marked skin fragility with prematurely aged appearance (identical to acrogeria), easy bruising, arterial and internal-organ rupture, thin nose.
V	X-linked R	Virtually identical to type II.
VI	AR	Skin fragility, joint hypermobility, ocular abnormalities.
VII	AD or AR	Skin laxity, severe joint problems, including congenital dislocation of hip.
VIII	AD	Skin laxity, dental abnormalities.
IX	X-linked R	Skin laxity, hernias, bladder rupture, occipital horns, abnormal copper transport.
X	AR	Similar to type II, abnormal clotting.

Fig. 11.18a

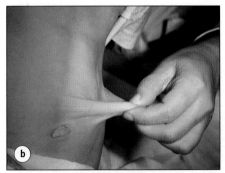
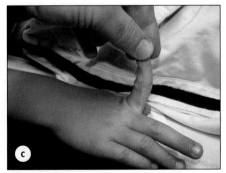

Fig. 11.18 *Ehlers–Danlos syndrome* — *(a)* box listing genetic defects and clinical features; *(b)* skin laxity and *(c)* joint laxity.

PSEUDOXANTHOMA ELASTICUM

In pseudoxanthoma elasticum, xanthoma-like papules appear on the sides of the neck (**Fig. 11.19**) and in flexural areas such as the antecubital fossae. There are several variants, some inherited in an autosomal dominant manner and some as recessive traits. In the most severe form (type IA), there are associated abnormalities of the eyes, leading to angioid

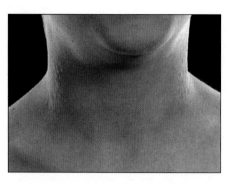

Fig. 11.19 *The typical yellowish papules of pseudoxanthoma elasticum.*

streaks in the retina, and abnormalities of major vessels, resulting in vascular rupture. Patients with type IB may develop mitral valve prolapse. Many of these patients only have skin manifestations.

Gene: locus 16p13.1; the ABCC6 gene responsible for elastic fibre assembly.

PREMATURE AGEING SYNDROMES

A very rare group of conditions is characterized by a greatly accelerated onset of ageing. This includes:

Progeria (Hutchinson–Gilford syndrome)	gene locus 1q21.2 (laminin A)
Pangeria (Werner syndrome)	gene locus 8p12-p11.2 (RECQL2 gene codes a DNA helicase)
Acrogeria (Gottron syndrome)	gene(s) unknown

SKIN MANIFESTATIONS OF CHROMOSOMAL DISORDERS

Figure 11.20 lists some of the commoner and more important chromosomal disorders that have significant cutaneous features, including Down syndrome (**Fig. 11.21**).

Chromosomal disorders with cutaneous manifestations	
Trisomy 21 (Down syndrome)	Cutis marmorata (see Fig. 11.21), elastosis perforans serpiginosa (may also occur in Ehlers Danlos syndrome and pseudoxanthoma elasticum)*, alopecia areata (*see* Chapter 9), fungal infections.
Turner syndrome (XO)	Webbed neck, lymphoedema, multiple moles.
Klinefelter's syndrome (XXY)	Leg ulcers. * small hyperkeratotic papules, arranged in irregular groups, histologically there is transepidermal elimination of altered collagen.

Fig. 11.20 *Chromosomal disorders with cutaneous manifestations.*

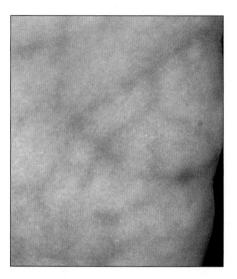

Fig. 11.21 *Cutis marmorata in a child with Down syndrome. Similar changes may occur sporadically without other features.*

VASCULAR DISORDERS

Hereditary haemorrhagic telangiectasia (or Osler–Weber–Rendou syndrome) is an autosomal dominant disorder characterized by the appearance of multiple telangiectases on the face, mouth, lips, and elsewhere (**Fig. 11.22**). Lesions are present in the oropharyngeal epithelium and in the gut, leading to recurrent epistaxes and gastrointestinal bleeds. Individual lesions can be treated with diathermy or laser.

Gene: locus 9q34.1.

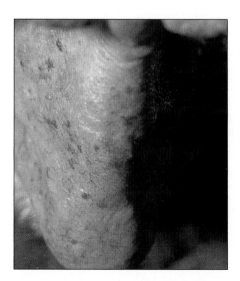

Fig. 11.22 *Telangiectases on the nose of a man with hereditary haemorrhagic telangiectasia.*

ANGIOKERATOMA CORPORIS DIFFUSUM (ANDERSON–FABRY DISEASE)

Multiple, small angiokeratomas appear in several inborn errors of metabolism, notably a-galactosidase deficiency, α-L-fucosidase deficiency (fucosidosis) and aspartylglycosaminuria. Lesions tend to cluster around the umbilicus and the groins, but may occur anywhere. A common finding is an abnormality of the cornea, known as cornea verticillata (corneal opacities and corneal dystrophy), and there are often dilated, tortuous conjunctival and retinal blood vessels present. Patients may also experience painful vascular spasms in the fingers and toes, and renal and cardiac defects may supervene. A full screening is therefore required in anyone presenting with angiokeratomas at a young age. Unfortunately, there is no specific treatment yet available for the enzyme defect(s) responsible.

SYNDROMES WITH IMMUNE DEFICIENCY

A number of conditions are characterized by recurrent infections resulting from congenital immune deficiency. The skin is often prominently involved and may provide important clues (Fig. 11.23).

Syndrome	Gene	Skin involvement
Agammaglobulinaemia	Xq21.3-q22 (regulation of B cell function)	Bacterial infections, eczema.
Severe combined immunodeficiency (SCID)	8q11 (protein kinase C)	Several forms, multiple, severe infections.
OMENN syndrome		Severe immunodeficiency and erythroderma.
Wiskott–Aldrich syndrome	Xp11.4p11.21 (WAS gene)	Atopic eczema.
Ataxia telangiectasia	11q23	Telangiectases of eyes and face, cerebellar ataxia, thymic dysfunction.
Epidermodysplasia verruciformis	17q25.3 (EVER1 gene)	*see* Chapter 3.
Chronic granulomatous disease	Xp21.1 (gene responsible for cytochrome b heavy chain)	Defective staphylococcal killing, recurrent infections.
Chronic mucocutaneous candidiasis	None as yet identified	Some types are inherited, *see* also Chapter 3.

Syndromes with immune deficiency and skin involvement

Fig. 11.23 *Syndromes with immune deficiency and skin involvement.*

There are a number of different inheritance patterns for several of these diseases. Some of these disorders, such as agammaglobulinaemia and chronic granulomatous disease, are X-linked and are predominantly disorders of males. Treatment is aimed at the underlying infection and, in appropriate cases, bone marrow transplantation is carried out.

Syndromes associated with cancers		
Syndrome	**Gene**	**Type of cancer**
Cowden syndrome	10q23.31, 10q22.3 (mutations of PTEN gene)	Multiple trichilemmomas (*see* Chapter 4), fibromas of the lips, acral keratoses, carcinoma of the breast, pancreas, and thyroid.
Gardner syndrome	5q21-q22 ('APC' gene)	Multiple epidermoid cysts, intestinal polyposis.
Rothmund–Thomson syndrome	8q24.3 (RECQL4, involved in DNA repair and ATP binding)	Poikiloderma (*see* Fig. 11.25), photosensitivity, short stature, skin and other cancers (e.g. osteosarcoma).
Xeroderma pigmentosum	Various DNA repair genes	Early onset of photosensitivity, excessive freckling, multiple skin cancers, some variants also develop internal cancers and CNS defects (Fig. 11.26a).
Xeroderma pigmentosum variant	Various DNA repair genes	Similar to xeroderma pigmentosum, but less severe changes and delayed onset (*see* Fig. 11.26b).
Bloom syndrome	15q26.1 (DNA function)	Growth retardation, pigmentary anomalies, leukaemia.
Howel–Evans syndrome	*see* Fig. 11.10	*see* Fig. 11.10 (palmoplantar keratodermas).
Muir–Torre syndrome	2p22-p21 (MSH2 gene)	Sebaceous gland carcinomas, colonic carcinomas.
Peutz–Jeghers syndrome	19p13.3 (STK11 — a tumour suppressor gene)	*see* Chapter 10, intestinal polyps occasionally undergo malignant transformation.

Fig. 11.24 *Syndromes associated with cancers*

INHERITED SYNDROMES IN WHICH SKIN CHANGES ACCOMPANY SYSTEMIC CANCERS

There are a number of genodermatoses in which cutaneous lesions are associated with a tendency to develop internal neoplasms, or cutaneous neoplasms, or both (**Figs 11.24–11.26**). In some of these, the defects are well understood and the genes have been mapped.

Patients with any of these syndromes need to be monitored carefully and referred to appropriate specialists when necessary.

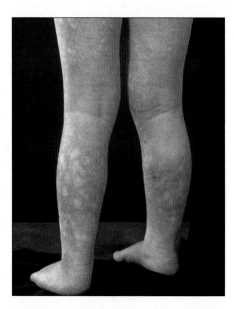

Fig. 11.25 *Poikilodermatous changes in a child with Rothmund–Thomson syndrome.* This little girl had an osteosarcoma.

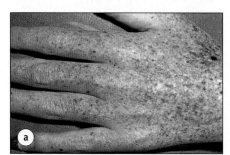

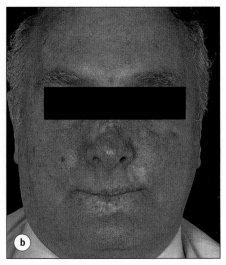

Fig. 11.26 *(a)* Multiple freckles (and a blue naevus) in a boy with xeroderma pigmentosum. *(b)* Xeroderma pigmentosum variant — this man has had multiple epithelial cancers and a melanoma removed over the years.

GENETIC COUNSELLING AND FURTHER MANAGEMENT

As more and more becomes known about these complex disorders it will become increasingly important for dermatologists to liaise with geneticists. Genetic counselling is important for families with any of the more severe of these conditions. Linkage studies have helped to map many of the responsible genes and tests will increasingly be available for the detection of carriers and homozygous states, including those in utero.

- Von Recklinghausen's disease is the most common genetic variant of neurofibromatosis and presents with café-au-lait patches, axillary freckles, cutaneous neurofibromas and plexiform neuromas.
- Tuberous sclerosis is a multisystem genetic order that presents initially with hypopigmented macules.
- Ehlers–Danlos syndrome is a group of disorders caused by defects in the genes responsible for the production of collagens and characterized by skin laxity and joint hypermobility.
- As more becomes known about the genodermatoses these complex disorders will become increasingly important for dermatologists to liaise with geneticists.

Index